Vasculitis

Editors

MAHMUD MOSSA-BASHA
CARLOS A. ZAMORA
MAURICIO CASTILLO

NEUROIMAGING CLINICS OF NORTH AMERICA

www.neuroimaging.theclinics.com

Consulting Editor
SURESH K. MUKHERJI

February 2024 • Volume 34 • Number 1

ELSEVIER

1600 John F. Kennedy Boulevard ● Suite 1800 ● Philadelphia, Pennsylvania, 19103-2899

http://www.neuroimaging.theclinics.com

NEUROIMAGING CLINICS OF NORTH AMERICA Volume 34, Number 1
February 2024 ISSN 1052-5149, ISBN 13: 978-0-443-18346-1

Editor: John Vassallo (j.vassallo@elsevier.com)
Developmental Editor: Saswoti Nath

Neuroimaging Clinics of North America (ISSN 1052-5149) is published quarterly by Elsevier Inc., 360 Park Avenue South, New York, NY 10010-1710. Months of issue are February, May, August, and November. Business and editorial offices: 1600 John F. Kennedy Blvd., Suite 1800, Philadelphia, PA 19103-2899. Business and editorial offices: 6277 Sea Harbor Drive, Orlando, FL 32887-4800. Periodicals postage paid at New York, NY, and additional mailing offices. Subscription prices are USD 430 per year for US individuals, USD 100 per year for US students and residents, USD 493 per year for Canadian individuals, USD 573 per year for international individuals, USD 100 per year for Canadian students and residents and USD 260 per year for foreign students and residents. For institutional access pricing please contact Customer Service via the contact information below. To receive student/resident rate, orders must be accompanied by name of affiliated institution, date of term, and the *signature* of program/residency coordinator on institution letterhead. Orders will be billed at individual rate until proof of status is received. Foreign air speed delivery is included in all *Clinics* subscription prices. All prices are subject to change without notice. POSTMASTER: Send address changes to *Neuroimaging Clinics of North America*, Elsevier Health Sciences Division, Subscription **Customer Service, 3251 Riverport Lane, Maryland Heights, MO 63043. Telephone: 1-800-654-2452 (U.S. and Canada); 314-447-8871 (outside U.S. and Canada). Fax: 314-447-8029. E-mail: journalscustomerservice-usa@elsevier.com (for print support); journalsonlinesupport-usa@elsevier.com (for online support).**

Reprints. For copies of 100 or more of articles in this publication, please contact the Commercial Reprints Department, Elsevier Inc., 360 Park Avenue South, New York, NY 10010-1710. Tel.: 212-633-3874; Fax: 212-633-3820; E-mail: reprints@elsevier.com.

Neuroimaging Clinics of North America is covered by *Excerpta Medical/EMBASE,* the RSNA Index of Imaging Literature, *MEDLINE/PubMed (Index Medicus),* MEDLINE/MEDLARS, SciSearch, Research Alert, and Neuroscience Citation Index.

PROGRAM OBJECTIVE

The goal of *Neuroimaging Clinics of North America* is to keep practicing radiologists and radiology residents up to date with current clinical practice in radiology by providing timely articles reviewing the state of the art in patient care.

TARGET AUDIENCE

Practicing radiologists, radiology residents, and other healthcare professionals who utilize neuroimaging findings to provide patient care.

LEARNING OBJECTIVES

Upon completion of this activity, participants will be able to:

1. Review crucial diagnostic criteria used to provide histologic proof of vasculitis.
2. Discuss the usefulness of different imaging methods in the diagnosis of vasculitides.
3. Recognize a stepwise approach and multidisciplinary team are vital in the evaluation of suspected cerebral vasculitis.

ACCREDITATION

The Elsevier Office of Continuing Medical Education (EOCME) is accredited by the Accreditation Council for Continuing Medical Education (ACCME) to provide continuing medical education for physicians.

The EOCME designates this journal-based CME activity for a maximum of 13 *AMA PRA Category 1 Credit*(s)™. Physicians should claim only the credit commensurate with the extent of their participation in the activity.

All other healthcare professionals requesting continuing education credit for this enduring material will be issued a certificate of participation.

DISCLOSURE OF CONFLICTS OF INTEREST

The EOCME assesses conflict of interest with its instructors, faculty, planners, and other individuals who are in a position to control the content of CME activities. All relevant conflicts of interest that are identified are thoroughly vetted by EOCME for fair balance, scientific objectivity, and patient care recommendations. EOCME is committed to providing its learners with CME activities that promote improvements or quality in healthcare and not a specific proprietary business or a commercial interest.

The planning committee, staff, authors, and editors listed below have identified no financial relationships or relationships to products or devices they or their spouse/life partner have with commercial interest related to the content of this CME activity:

Mehdi Abbasi, MD; Aaron Bangad; Bilal Battal, MD; Alison M. Bays, MD, MPH; Samuel C. Cartmell, MD; Mauricio Castillo, MD, FACR; Mauricio Castillo, MD; Benjamin Cho, MD; Diogo Goulart Corrêa, MD, PhD; Luiz Celso Hygino da Cruz, Jr, MD; Antônio José da Rocha, MD, PhD; Mona Dabiri, MD; Hubert de Boysson, MD, PhD; Ana Paula Alves Fonseca, MD; Carolina Guimaraes, MD; Omar Hamam, MB ChB; Sheng-Che Hung, MD, PhD; Kothainayaki Kulanthaivelu, BCA, MBA; Laurent Létourneau-Guillon, MD, MSc; Michelle Littlejohn; Christina M. Marra, MD; Kassie McCullagh, MD; Mahmud Mossa-Basha, MD; Ahmad Nehme, MD; Renato Hoffmann Nunes, MD; Felipe Torres Pacheco, MD, PhD; Igor Gomes Padilha, MD; Sam Payabvash, MD; Paulo Puac-Polanco, MD, MSc; Nabil Rahoui, MD; Francisco Rivas Rodriguez, MD; Javier M. Romero, MD; Griselda Romero-Sanchez, MD, MSc; Àlex Rovira, MD; Manish Kanti Saha, MD; Lubdha M. Shah, MD; Selima Siala, MD; Carlos Torres, MD, FRCPC, FCAR; Richard H. Wiggins, MD; Carlos Zamora, MD, PhD

The planning committee, staff, authors, and editors listed below have identified financial relationships or relationships to products or devices they or their spouse/life partner have with commercial interest related to the content of this CME activity:

Adam de Havenon, MD, MSCI: Consultant: Integra, Novo Nordisk; Ownership interest: Titin KM, Certus

UNAPPROVED/OFF-LABEL USE DISCLOSURE

The EOCME requires CME faculty to disclose to the participants:

1. When products or procedures being discussed are off-label, unlabelled, experimental, and/or investigational (not US Food and Drug Administration [FDA] approved); and
2. Any limitations on the information presented, such as data that are preliminary or that represent ongoing research, interim analyses, and/or unsupported opinions. Faculty may discuss information about pharmaceutical agents that is outside of FDA-approved labelling. This information is intended solely for CME and is not intended to promote off-label use of these medications. If you have any questions, contact the medical affairs department of the manufacturer for the most recent prescribing information.

TO ENROLL

To enroll in the *Neuroimaging Clinics of North America* Continuing Medical Education program, call customer service at 1-800-654-2452 or sign up online at http://www.theclinics.com/home/cme. The CME program is available to subscribers for an additional annual fee of USD 254.00.

METHOD OF PARTICIPATION

In order to claim credit, participants must complete the following:

1. Complete enrolment as indicated above.
2. Read the activity.
3. Complete the CME Test and Evaluation. Participants must achieve a score of 70% on the test. All CME Tests and Evaluations must be completed online.

CME INQUIRIES/SPECIAL NEEDS

For all CME inquiries or special needs, please contact elsevierCME@elsevier.com.

NEUROIMAGING CLINICS OF NORTH AMERICA

SERIES OF RELATED INTEREST

Advances in Clinical Radiology
Available at: https://www.advancesinclinicalradiology.com/
MRI Clinics of North America
Available at: https://www.mri.theclinics.com/
Neuroimaging Clinics
Available at: https://www.neuroimaging.theclinics.com/
PET Clinics
Available at: https://www.pet.theclinics.com/

Contributors

CONSULTING EDITOR

SURESH K. MUKHERJI, MD, MBA, FACR
Professor of Radiology and Radiation
Oncology, University of Louisville, Peoria,
Illinois, USA; Robert Wood Johnson Medical
School, Rutgers University, New Brunswick,
New Jersey, USA; Faculty, Otolaryngology
Head Neck Surgery, Michigan State University,
Farmington Hills, Michigan, USA; National
Director of Head and Neck Radiology, ProScan
Imaging, Carmel, Indiana, USA

EDITORS

MAHMUD MOSSA-BASHA, MD
Professor of Radiology, University of
Washington, Vice Chair of Clinical Research
and Clinical Transformation, Co-Director of the
Vascular Imaging Lab, Department of
Radiology, University of Washington School of
Medicine, Seattle, Washington, USA

CARLOS A. ZAMORA, MD, PhD
Associate Professor, Division of
Neuroradiology, Department of Radiology,
University of North Carolina School of
Medicine, Chapel Hill, North Carolina,
USA

MAURICIO CASTILLO, MD, FACR
Professor of Radiology, Division of
Neuroradiology, Department of Radiology,
University of North Carolina School of
Medicine, Chapel Hill, North Carolina,
USA

AUTHORS

MEHDI ABBASI, MD
Department of Neurology, Yale University, New
Haven, Connecticut, USA

AARON BANGAD, BA
Department of Neurology, Yale University, New
Haven, Connecticut, USA

BILAL BATTAL, MD
Division of Neuroradiology, Department of
Radiology, University of North Carolina School
of Medicine, Chapel Hill, North Carolina,
USA

ALISON M. BAYS, MD, MPH&TM
Assistant Professor of Rheumatology,
Department Medicine, University of
Washington, Seattle, Washington, USA

SAMUEL C. CARTMELL, MD
R.H Ackerman Neurovascular Laboratory,
Massachusetts General Hospital, Boston,
Massachusetts, USA

MAURICIO CASTILLO, MD, FACR
Professor of Radiology, Division of
Neuroradiology, Department of Radiology,
University of North Carolina School of
Medicine, Chapel Hill, North Carolina, USA

BENJAMIN CHO, MD
Department of Pathology and Laboratory
Medicine, University of North Carolina School
of Medicine, Chapel Hill, North Carolina,
USA

DIOGO GOULART CORRÊA, MD, PhD
Department of Radiology, Clínica de
Diagnóstico por Imagem (CDPI)/DASA, Rio de
Janeiro, Brazil; Department of Radiology,
Federal Fluminense University, Niterói, Rio de
Janeiro, Brazil

ANTÔNIO JOSÉ DA ROCHA, MD, PhD
Division of Neuroradiology, DASA -
Diagnósticos da América SA, São Paulo, São

Paulo, Brazil; Division of Neuroradiology, Santa Casa de São Paulo School of Medical Sciences, São Paulo, Brazil

MONA DABIRI, MD
Postdoctoral Research Fellow, Department of Radiology, Children's Medical Center, Tehran University of Medical Sciences, Tehran, Iran

HUBERT DE BOYSSON, MD, PhD
Departments of Neurology and Internal Medicine, Caen University Hospital, Caen, France

ADAM DE HAVENON, MD, MSCI
Department of Neurology, Center for Brain and Mind Health, Yale University, New Haven, Connecticut, USA

ANA PAULA ALVES FONSECA, MD
Division of Neuroradiology, DASA - Diagnósticos da América SA, São Paulo, São Paulo, Brazil

CAROLINA GUIMARAES, MD
Professor, Department of Radiology, University of North Carolina at Chapel Hill, Chapel Hill, North Carolina, USA

OMAR HAMAM, MD
R.H Ackerman Neurovascular Laboratory, Massachusetts General Hospital, Boston, Massachusetts, USA

SHENG-CHE HUNG, MD, PhD
Assistant Professor, Department of Radiology, University of North Carolina at Chapel Hill, Chapel Hill, North Carolina, USA

LUIZ CELSO HYGINO DA CRUZ JR, MD, PhD
Department of Radiology, Clínica de Diagnóstico por Imagem (CDPI)/DASA, Rio de Janeiro, Rio de Janeiro, Brazil

LAURENT LÉTOURNEAU-GUILLON, MD, MSc
Radiology Department, Centre Hospitalier de l'Université de Montréal (CHUM), Université de Montréal, Imaging and Engineering Axis, Centre de Recherche du Centre Hospitalier de l'Université de Montréal (CRCHUM), Montréal, Quebec, Canada

CHRISTINA M. MARRA, MD
Professor Emeritus, Department of Neurology, University of Washington, Seattle, Washington, USA

MAHMUD MOSSA-BASHA, MD
Professor of Radiology, University of Washington, Vice Chair of Clinical Research and Clinical Transformation, Co-Director of the Vascular Imaging Lab, Department of Radiology, University of Washington School of Medicine, Seattle, Washington, USA

AHMAD NEHME, MD, MSc
Department of Neurology, Caen University Hospital, Caen, France

RENATO HOFFMANN NUNES, MD
Division of Neuroradiology, DASA - Diagnósticos da América SA, São Paulo, São Paulo, Brazil

FELIPE TORRES PACHECO, MD, PhD
Division of Neuroradiology, Diagnó sticos da América SA - DASA, Division of Neuroradiology, Santa Casa de São Paulo School of Medical Sciences, São Paulo São Paulo, Brazil

IGOR GOMES PADILHA, MD
Division of Neuroradiology, Diagnósticos da América SA - DASA, Division of Neuroradiology, Santa Casa de São Paulo School of Medical Sciences, Division of Neuroradiology, United Health Group, São Paulo, São Paulo, Brazil; Radiology Department, Centre Hospitalier de l'Université de Montréal (CHUM), Université de Montréal, Montréal, Quebec, Canada

SAM PAYABVASH, MD
Center for Brain and Mind Health, Yale University, New Haven, Connecticut, USA

PAULO PUAC-POLANCO, MD, MSc
Assistant Professor, Department of Radiology, Radiation Oncology and Medical Physics, University of Ottawa, Ottawa, Ontario, Canada

NABIL RAHOUI, MD
Department of Pathology and Laboratory Medicine, University of North Carolina School of Medicine, Chapel Hill, North Carolina, USA

FRANCISCO RIVAS RODRIGUEZ, MD
Clinical Associate Professor, Division of
Neuroradiology, Department of Radiology,
University of Michigan, Michigan, USA

JAVIER M. ROMERO, MD
R.H Ackerman Neurovascular Laboratory,
Massachusetts General Hospital, Boston,
Massachusetts, USA

GRISELDA ROMERO-SANCHEZ, MD, MSc
Neuroradiology Faculty, Department of
Radiology, Instituto Nacional de Ciencias
Medicas y Nutricion Salvador Zubiran, Mexico
City, Mexico

ÀLEX ROVIRA, MD
Professor, Department of Radiology, Vall
D'Hebron University Hospital, Universitat
Autònoma de Barcelona, Barcelona,
Spain

MANISH KANTI SAHA, MD
Assistant Professor of Medicine, Internal
Medicine, University of North Carolina at
Chapel Hill, Chapel Hill, North Carolina,
USA

LUBDHA M. SHAH, MD
Associate Professor of Radiology, Division of
Neuroradiology, University of Utah, Salt Lake
City, USA

SELIMA SIALA, MD
Department of Radiology, University of North
Carolina School of Medicine, Chapel Hill, North
Carolina, USA

CARLOS TORRES, MD, FRCPC, FCAR
Professor, Department of Radiology, Radiation
Oncology and Medical Physics, University of
Ottawa, Ottawa, Ontario, Canada

RICHARD H. WIGGINS, MD
Professor, Department of Radiology and
Imaging Sciences, Associate Dean, University
of Utah School of Medicine, University of Utah
Health Sciences Center, Salt Lake City, Utah,
USA

CARLOS A. ZAMORA, MD, PhD
Associate Professor, Division of
Neuroradiology, Department of Radiology,
University of North Carolina School of
Medicine, Chapel Hill, North Carolina, USA

Contents

Vasculitis is characterized by the inflammation of blood vessels. Vasculitides refers to the different forms of vasculitis, often classified according to the size of the blood vessel that is involved. Vasculitis may occur as a primary process or secondary to many systemic diseases. This topic provides an overview of the clinical features, diagnosis, and classification of the different forms of vasculitides.

Stroke is a complication of many central nervous system (CNS) infections, but only a few present with stroke without other symptoms or signs of CNS infection. Chief among these are varicella zoster virus (VZV) and syphilis. Delayed cerebral vasculopathy after successful treatment of bacterial meningitis, most commonly pneumococcal, is an emerging entity with uncertain pathogenesis.

Primary central nervous system vasculitis (PCNSV) is a vasculitis limited to the brain and spinal cord. Induction therapy often consists of steroids and cyclophosphamide. Maintenance therapy includes a prednisone taper and may be combined with medications such as azathioprine or mycophenolate mofetil. Relapse is common in PCNSV and an increased dose of steroids is often given, sometimes with a change in therapy. Medications such as rituximab and mycophenolate mofetil may be good alternatives in those who do not respond to initial treatment or who have relapse of disease. Mortality rates of 8% to 9% are reported in the literature.

Primary angiitis of the central nervous system (PACNS) is a rare and potentially severe form of vasculitis that is limited to the brain, spinal cord, and meninges. Despite extensive research, the etiology and underlying immunologic mechanisms of PACNS remain largely unknown. PACNS presents with a variety of clinical, radiological, and pathologic features, but it is generally characterized by inflammation and destruction of the walls of blood vessels in the CNS, which can lead to tissue ischemia and/or hemorrhage. Three main histopathologic patterns have been identified, namely granulomatous, lymphocytic, and necrotizing vasculitis.

Assessment of cerebral vasculopathies is challenging and requires understanding the utility of different imaging methods. Various techniques are available to image the vessel lumen, each with unique advantages and disadvantages. Bolus-based CT and MR angiography requires careful timing of a contrast bolus to provide optimal luminal enhancement. Non-contrast MRA techniques do not require a contrast agent and can provide images with little venous contamination. Digital subtraction angiography remains the gold standard but is invasive, while VW-MRI provides a non-invasive way of assessing vessel wall pathology. Conventional brain MRI has high sensitivity in the diagnosis of vasculitis but findings are nonspecific.

Takayasu arteritis (TA) and Giant cell arteritis (GCA) are large vessel vasculitides, with TA targeting the aorta and its branches, and GCA targeting both large and medium-sized arteries. Early diagnosis of TA and GCA are of great importance, since delayed, inappropriate or no treatment can result in severe and permanent complications. Imaging plays a central role in establishing diagnosis, targeting lesions for confirmational diagnostic biopsy, specifically for GCA, and longitudinal disease evolution. In this article, we discuss imaging diagnosis of large artery vasculitis and the value of different imaging modalities.

Small artery vasculitis of the CNS is a rare and serious condition characterized by the inflammation of blood vessels within the brain and spinal cord. There are two groups of small artery vasculitis determined by the presence or absence of immunoglobulin complex deposition in the vessel wall. The former includes anti-glomerular basement membrane disease, cryoglobulinemic vasculitis, and IgA vasculitis. Absence of immune complex deposition is associated with anti-neutrophil cytoplasmic antibody (ANCA) and includes microscopic polyangiitis, granulomatosis with polyangiitis, eosinophilic granulomatosis with polyangiitis, and primary angiitis of the CNS. These conditions present a diagnostic challenge in which imaging plays a crucial role.

Vasculitides are characterized by inflammation of the vessel wall, with their categorization relying on clinical and paraclinical manifestations, vessel type, size, distribution, histological attributes, and associated conditions. This review delves into the salient neuroimaging hallmarks of central nervous system vasculitis associated with the most prevalent systemic diseases and highlightings potential pitfalls and diagnostic confounders.

Vasculitis is a complication of several infectious diseases affecting the central nervous system, which may result in ischemic and/or hemorrhagic stroke, transient ischemic attack, and aneurysm formation. Infectious agents may directly infect the

endothelium causing vasculitis or indirectly affect the vessel wall through an immunological cascade. Clinical manifestations usually overlap with those of noninfectious vascular diseases, making diagnosis challenging. Neuroimaging enables the
identification of inflammatory changes in intracranial vasculitis. In this article, we review the imaging features of infectious vasculitis of bacterial, viral, fungal and parasitic causes.

Illicit and recreational drugs, such as cocaine, heroin, amphetamines, and marijuana, can result in drug-related vasculitis or vasculopathy. Similarly, the use of certain antithyroid, oncologic, and immunosuppressive medications for therapeutic
purposes can lead to vasculopathy. This in turn may result in significant complications in the central nervous system, including intracranial hemorrhage and stroke.
Cocaine abuse can also lead to midline destructive lesions of the sinonasal complex.
MR imaging, Vessel Wall imaging, and CT/CTA are valuable imaging tools for the
evaluation of patients with suspected drug-induced vasculopathy or vasculitis.
This article reviews the pathomechanism, clinical presentation, and imaging findings
of vasculopathy related to drug abuse and prescribed medications.

PRES and RCVS are increasingly recognized due to the wider use of brain MRI and
increasing clinical awareness. Imaging plays a crucial role in confirming the diagnosis and guiding clinical management for PRES and RCVS. Imaging also has a pivotal
role in determining the temporal progression of these entities, detecting complications, and predicting prognosis. In this review, we aim to describe PRES and
RCVS, discuss their possible pathophysiological mechanisms, and discuss imaging
methods that are useful in the diagnosis, management, and follow-up of patients.

Childhood cerebral vasculitis is a condition that affects the blood vessels in the brain
of children and is rare but life-threatening. Imaging plays a crucial role in the diagnosis and monitoring of the disease. This article describes the classification, diagnostic
algorithm, and various imaging modalities used in the evaluation of childhood cerebral vasculitis and the imaging findings associated with primary and secondary vasculitis. Understanding the imaging features of this condition can assist in early
diagnosis, effective treatment, and improve outcomes.

Cerebral amyloid angiopathy (CAA) is a cerebrovascular disorder marked by the accumulation of amyloid-beta peptide (Aβ) within the leptomeninges and smaller blood
vessels of the brain. CAA can be both noninflammatory and inflammatory, and the
inflammatory version includes Aβ-related angiitis (ABRA). ABRA is a vasculitis of
the central nervous system related to an inflammatory response to Aβ in the vascular
walls, which necessitates differentiating ABRA from noninflammatory CAA, as ABRA
may require immunosuppressive treatment. MR imaging is typically the most effective imaging modality of choice to screen for these conditions, and they should be
obtained at varying time points to track disease progression.

Foreword

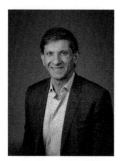

Suresh K. Mukherji, MD, MBA, FACR
Consulting Editor

I have always had challenges trying to determine when to suggest the possibility of vasculitis in patients with multiple white matter hyperintensities. I think we are familiar when to suggest white matter hyperintensities due to atherosclerotic disease ("small vessel disease") or demyelination. The challenge for myself (and I assume others as well) is, when should we appropriately initiate the complex and costly workup of a vasculitis due to an infectious or inflammatory cause when we encounter a patient with white matter hyperintensities?

This issue was developed to help better understand this perplexing topic and is a comprehensive issue devoted to all aspects of vasculitis and vasculopathies. There are numerous articles covering diagnostic guidelines, imaging techniques, and clinical review of various causes of vasculitis and vasculopathies along with treatment options.

I want to thank the guest editors and authors for their wonderful contributions. The articles provide practical clinical information and state-of-the-art reviews. The authors are world authorities on their subject matter, and the articles are beautifully illustrated. Finally, I would like to thank the Guest Editors, Drs Mahmud Mossa-Basha, Carlos Zamora, and Mauricio Castillo, for creating such a fantastic issue. My first faculty position was at the University of North Carolina, and I was delighted when these fellow "Tar Heels" and friends accepted our invitation to Guest Edit this challenging subject. Thanks so much to the Guest Editors and the article authors for creating such a valuable contribution that will improve our understanding of this challenging and important topic.

Suresh K. Mukherji, MD, MBA, FACR
Head and Neck Radiology
ProScan Imaging
1185 West Carmel Drive, Suite D, D1
Carmel, IN 46032, USA

E-mail address:
sureshmukherji@hotmail.com

Neuroimag Clin N Am 34 (2024) xv
https://doi.org/10.1016/j.nic.2023.09.002
1052-5149/24/© 2023 Published by Elsevier Inc.

Preface
Vasculitis: A Comprehensive Review

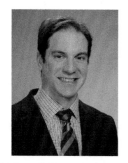

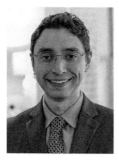

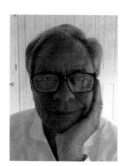

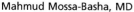

Mahmud Mossa-Basha, MD   Carlos A. Zamora, MD   Mauricio Castillo, MD

Editors

Inflammatory and infectious vasculopathies are an uncommon, although devastating cause of vascular injury, including arterial occlusion, rupture, and pseudoaneurysm formation, as well as end-organ damage resulting from ischemia or hemorrhage. While rare, these vasculopathies remain a constant concern for ordering providers and interpreting radiologists alike, due to their poor outcomes, as when detected late they overlap in imaging appearance and have nonspecific clinical presentations, and it is difficult to establish a final diagnosis. Conventional and advanced imaging plays a central role in the diagnosis of vasculitides. Conventional neuroimaging, specifically MR imaging, is very sensitive in the examination for CNS vasculitis; however, it lacks specificity. Similarly, for large-artery inflammatory vasculopathies, angiographic imaging is limited for the early detection of disease and may only detect disease once permanent inflammatory sequelae or complications have developed. Imaging, in addition to laboratory markers of inflammation, plays a central role in longitudinal evaluation of treatment response. Diagnostic imaging modalities for detection and follow-up evaluation of inflammatory vasculopathy include MR imaging, MR angiography, and CT angiography. Advanced imaging applications, including vessel wall MR imaging, perfusion, and PET/CT, can be used to detect nonstenotic disease, differentiate vasculopathies, confirm presence of inflammation, and/or assess end-organ damage or ischemic risk.

The current issue of *Neuroimaging Clinics* covers vasculopathies from multiple angles and includes discussions of classification and diagnostic guidelines for infectious and inflammatory vasculitis, pathologic considerations, treatment regimens, conventional imaging, and vessel wall MR imaging approaches for primary angiitis, imaging of large artery, small artery, drug-related, infectious, pediatric, amyloid-related and systemic vasculitides, and common vasculitis mimics.

This issue serves as a comprehensive discussion covering all important aspects of vasculitis diagnosis and treatment, providing a primer for readers to better understand expert radiologist and ordering provider perspectives on disease

Neuroimag Clin N Am 34 (2024) xvii–xviii
https://doi.org/10.1016/j.nic.2023.07.013
1052-5149/24/© 2023 Published by Elsevier Inc.

manifestation, diagnosis, evolution, and management strategies. This issue also introduces readers to cutting-edge imaging in vasculitis assessment that may serve as diagnostic and risk-stratification tools and may potentially stimulate future researchers on a career path investigating inflammatory arteritis. The authors and editors greatly enjoyed putting this issue together, and we hope our audience equally enjoys reading this work.

Mahmud Mossa-Basha, MD
Department of Radiology
University of Washington School of Medicine
1959 Northeast Pacific Street
Seattle, WA 98195, USA

Carlos A. Zamora, MD
Department of Radiology
University of North Carolina School of Medicine
Old Clinic Building CB# 7510
Chapel Hill, NC 27599-7510, USA

Mauricio Castillo, MD
Department of Radiology
University of North Carolina School of Medicine
Old Clinic Building CB# 7510
Chapel Hill, NC 27599-7510, USA

E-mail addresses:
mmossab@uw.edu (M. Mossa-Basha)
carlos_zamora@med.unc.edu (C.A. Zamora)
mauricio_castillo@med.unc.edu (M. Castillo)

Overview of Vasculitides in Adults

Manish K. Saha, MD*

KEYWORDS

• Vasculitis • Large-vessel • Medium-vessel • Small-vessel

KEY POINTS

- Vasculitis is defined as inflammation of blood vessel wall.
- Vasculitides could be primary or secondary to a systemic disease process.
- Vasulitides are differentiated based on size of involved vessel wall but the separation is not absolute.

OVERVIEW OF VASCULITIDES IN ADULTS

Vasculitis is defined as an inflammation of the blood vessel wall resulting in stenosis, occlusion, or aneurysms of involved vessels with consequential end-organ ischemia and tissue injury.[1,2] Large-vessel vasculitis (LVV) involves the aorta and its major branches, medium-vessel vasculitis affects visceral vessels and their initial branches, and small-vessel vasculitis involves arterioles, capillaries, intraparenchymal arteries, and venules.[3,4] Vasculitides are classified as primary or secondary to a systemic disease process, including connective tissue disorders, drugs, infections, and malignancies.[5,6] The various forms of vasculitides are distinguished based on definitions set by the Chapel Hill Consensus Conference (CHCC), 2012 – the purpose of which was to set up a nomenclature system rather than diagnostic criteria.[7] The various forms of vasculitis are distinguished by size of the blood vessel involved, but the separation is not absolute as there is a significant overlap–for example, in patients with biopsy-confirmed Giant Cell Arteritis (GCA, a form of LVV), there may be evidence of involvement of both medium (ciliary/retinal arteries) and small vessels (small branches of the ciliary artery).[7,8] Antineutrophil cytoplasmic antibody (ANCA)-associated vasculitis (AAV) usually affects the small blood vessels but may also present with aneurysms of medium-sized arteries, largely of the renal vasculature.[9]

An Overall Approach to a Patient with Vasculitis

Vasculitides are a heterogeneous group of disorders with clinical features that may overlap with many disease processes, including infections, malignancies, inflammatory conditions, and congenital disorders. A thorough history, detailed physical examination, and high degree of clinical suspicion is required in a multidisciplinary approach for timely diagnosis and treatment. There are no established diagnostic criteria for most forms of vasculitis. The criteria embedded in various classification systems should inform clinicians about typical clinical features but should not be used solely for diagnostic purposes. Upon diagnosis, disease activity and extent of injury should be assessed in all cases. Laboratory tests should be performed based on clinical suspicion–serum complement and cryoglobulin levels in patients with leukocytoclastic vasculitis with polyclonal staining on immunofluorescence (IF); ANCA serology in cases of recurrent non-infectious sinusitis or subglottic stenosis; the measurement of both CRP and ESR levels to evaluate a suspected case of large vessel vasculitis; infectious work-up should be considered in most cases of vasculitis. A tissue biopsy of the most accessible site with suspected active inflammation should be performed for histologic evaluation. A skin biopsy should be done in consultation with a dermatologist to ensure adequate sampling and

Division of Nephrology, University of North Carolina, Chapel Hill, NC, USA
* Division of Nephrology, University of North Carolina, Chapel Hill, NC 27519.
E-mail address: manish_saha@med.unc.edu

neuroimaging.theclinics.com

depth of tissue obtained , and perform appropriate immunohistochemistry analyses necessary to diagnose vasculitis or rule out secondary causes. Imaging studies should be tailored to the individual clinical scenario–in patients with end-stage kidney disease, CT angiogram may be preferred over MRA with gadolinium given risks of nephrogenic systemic fibrosis; conversely, in those requiring repeated imaging studies to evaluate for disease activity, MRA may be selected to reduce risks of radiation.

Mimics of Vasculitis

When evaluating a case of suspected vasculitis, it is critical to consider non-vasculitic etiologies that may have overlapping clinical features. Infection-related vasculopathy can mimic all forms of vasculitides, hypercoagulable conditions and calciphylaxis can have overlapping features of small vessel vasculitis, and lymphoma can mimic primary angiitis of the central nervous system (CNS).[4,10,11] Tuberculous aortitis is an important differential diagnosis for large vessel vasculitis, as it can cause aortitis and pseudoaneurysms, which can mimic classic symptoms of Takayasu's arteritis, or GCA with large vessel involvement.[12,13] Syphilitic aortitis can cause similar findings of aneurysms, aortic regurgitation, and coronary ostial lesions.[14] IgG4-related disease (IgG4-RD) may cause periarterial lesions mainly involving the thoracic and abdominal aorta and radiologically characterized by arterial wall thickening, precise circumscription, and dilated rather than stenotic luminal changes.[15] In surgically obtained tissue, there may be evidence of classical histologic changes of IgG4-RD including–lymphoplasmacytic infiltration, dominant IgG4+-plasma cells, and irregular/storiform fibrosis at the level of adventitia.[15] Non-Langerhans cell histiocytosis, such as Erdheim-Chester's disease, may also present with the periarterial thickening of the aorta and its major branches but histologically characterized by the presence of CD68+, CD1a(−) non-Langerhans histicoytes.[16] Genetic causes, including Marfan's syndrome and Ehler-Danlos, may present with aortic root dilatation and aneurysms but lack inflammatory features.[17]

Fibromuscular dysplasia (FMD) is an uncommon non-atherosclerotic arteriopathy seen predominantly in middle-aged women. Renal, external carotid, and vertebral arteries are most commonly involved. The cardinal clinical features are headache, pulsatile tinnitus, hypertension, and cervical or abdominal bruit. The classical CT or MR angiogram findings are a string of bead appearance of the renal arteries, concentric or tubular stenosis, and renal infarcts.[18,19]

Atherosclerosis may cause similar vascular imaging findings but is distinguished by the location, as atherosclerotic changes are mainly located at the ostium and proximal portion of vessels; in contrast, FMD changes are located at the middle-distal portion of the arteries.[20] The characteristics arterial wall edema/inflammationof LVV is absent in FMD as it is considered a non-inflammatory disorder.[20] Segmental arterial mediolysis may have features similar to FMD and is difficult to differentiate without tissue examination, which is characterized by vacuolization and lysis of outer arterial media.[21] Infectious etiologies should always be considered when appropriate, as infective endocarditis and mycotic aneurysms have been reported to mimic findings of vasculitis.[6,20,22,23]

Large Vessel Vasculitis

Takayasu's arteritis
Takayasu's arteritis (TA) is characterized by the inflammation of the of the aortic wall and its main branches.[4] Histologically, findings may vary from an active suppurative inflammation to chronic granulomatous changes along the media and adventitia layers of the involved vessel wall.[24] The entire length of aorta is predominantly involved, while the pulmonary arteries can be affected in 50% of cases.[25,26] TA predominantly affects women in their 2nd- 4th decade of life, particularly from Asian countries, but has a worldwide distribution.[27]

Immunopathogenesis
The underlying inciting mechanism is not very clear, but an unknown antigen/stimulus may cause – (1) expression of heat shock protein in the vessel wall which induces Major Histocompatibility Class I Chain-Related A on vascular cells resulting in acute vascular inflammation by release of perforin, (2) Th1-driven formation of giant cells through interferon-γ production, (3) potentially, the development of anti-endothelial antibodies resulting in complement-mediated cytotoxicity against endothelial cells.[28,29]

TA is a granulomatous arteritis with perivascular infiltrate around the vasa vasorum, while giant cells are predominantly found in the media of the large arteries.[30]

Clinical features
The presenting signs and symptoms may vary depending on the stage of presentation–the early phase, "pre-pulseless" is characterized by nonspecific symptoms of malaise, fever, night sweats, weight loss, and myalgia.[30] Serum inflammatory markers, ESR and CRP, are usually elevated. The early phase of the disease can go into spontaneous remission in a few months or progress to a chronic

inflammatory phase leading to arterial wall thickening, stenosis, and aneurysmal formation–a "pulseless" disease phase, clinically characterized by the presence of diminished pulse intensity, a discrepancy in blood pressure measurement between arms, limb claudication (due to occlusion of brachiocephalic and subclavian arteries); dizziness, vertigo, headache, stroke, decreased visual acuity (due to occlusion of carotid/vertebral arteries), renovascular hypertension, and mesenteric ischemia.[30–34] The most common ocular features are hypertensive retinopathy, Takayasu retinopathy, and ocular ischemic syndrome. In addition, treatment-related ocular complications may include cataracts and glaucoma secondary to corticosteroid therapy.[35] Cardiac involvement may present as myocarditis, coronary vasculitis, or dilated cardiomyopathy.[36]

A thorough clinical examination is essential in suspected cases of vasculitis. On physical examination, diminished pulse intensity may be more common in the upper than lower extremities; carotid-artery tenderness (carotidynia), and arterial bruit may be present.[37] There may be discrepancies in blood readings obtained from different extremities–those with significant stenosis will have lower readings. In some cases of severe patients with bilateral subclavian artery stenosis may have falsely normal blood pressure readings obtained from both arms with cuff monitors.[38]

Vascular Imaging Studies

One should investigate for presence of arterial wall inflammation, stenosis (long, smooth tapering of the involved vessel), occlusion, and aneurysmal changes on the different imaging modalities.[30] An intra-arterial angiogram is the gold standard method to evaluate the lumen of affected vessels; however, because of its invasive nature and inability to assess the arterial wall, noninvasive modalities such as MRI or CTA are used more frequently for diagnosis and follow-up studies.[26] 18F-fluorodeoxyglucose positron emission tomography (FDG-PET) is now being increasingly used. It has a sensitivity of 87% and specificity of 73% to 84% (depending on the type of disease activity criteria used) for diagnosis of TA; however, its utility in the follow-up of disease activity remains to be well defined.[39,40]

DIAGNOSIS

Although there are no established diagnostic criteria, typical signs and symptoms (diminished pulse, blood pressure difference between arms, arterial bruit) and imaging findings could be diagnostic. Tissue is rarely available for histologic

diagnosis other than that obtained during surgery or autopsy.[41] The 2022 American College of Rheumatology(ACR)/European Alliance of Associations for Rheumatology (EULAR) classification criteria was developed for research studies and clinical trials. The criteria and the associated weights are: female sex (+1), angina (+2), limb claudication (+2), arterial bruit (+2), reduced UE BP (+2), reduced pulse or tenderness of carotid artery (+2), blood pressure difference between arms ≥ 20 mm Hg, (+1), number of affected arterial territories (+1 to+3), paired artery involvement (+1), abdominal aorta plus renal or mesenteric involvement (+3). A patient could be classified as having TA if the cumulative score is ≥ 5 points.[42]

Giant Cell Arteritis

Giant cell arteritis, or temporal arteritis, is a transmural granulomatous inflammatory disorder of large- and medium-sized vessels.[43] GCA is the most common primary vasculitis in adults in the United States and Europe.[30] The incidence varies by geographic location and ranges from 1.6 to 32.8 per 100,000 persons ≥ 50 years of age.[44,45] GCA exclusively occurs in patients above 50 years of age and has a female predominance. The peak incidence is in the 7–8th decade of life and is common in patients with European ancestry, while it is uncommon in Asia and South America.[44,46] GCA primarily involves the extracranial branches of the carotid arteries (eg, temporal arteries) but may also affect the aorta and its major branches.[46]

Immunopathogenesis

Similar to TA, the underlying immunogenesis is not well-understood, but an unknown antigen/stimulus to dendritic cells results in the activation of Th1/Th17 cells, resulting in the production of cytokines and ensuing arterial wall inflammation.[47] Histologically, GCA is characterized by granulomatous arteritis.[48] Fibrinoid necrosis is rare and should raise suspicion for other diagnoses, that is, AAV and polyarteritis nodosa.[30]

Clinical Signs and Symptoms

Patients with GCA may present initially with constitutional symptoms followed by specific features resulting from the involvement of the cranial vasculature, large vessels, or both. Cranial GCA usually manifests as headache, scalp tenderness, jaw claudication, stroke, and vision changes. The involvement of the aorta and its major branches can cause limb claudication, decreased intensity of the pulse, and aortic aneurysms. Physical findings of asymmetric pulses, differences in blood pressure readings on both arms, vascular bruit, and aortic regurgitation murmur could be evident.[4,8,49,50]

Headache is the most common symptom in 70% to 85% of cases, usually located on the temporal side–described as a continuous and throbbing type that may be associated with scalp paresthesia. Headaches associated with jaw or tongue claudication and intermittent dysphagia are suggestive of GCA.[51,52]

A current or prior diagnosis of Polymyalgia Rheumatica (PMR), an inflammatory condtion affecting adults over the age of 50 causing stiffness and pain in the hips and shoulders, is important to recognize when considering a diagnosis of GCA as about 16-21% of patients with PMR may develop GCA.[53] Conversely, 40% to 60% of patients with GCA will have PMR symptoms, and clinicians should ask patients with suspected GCA about hip and shoulder stiffness and pain.[53,54]

Painless unilateral/bilateral vision loss is one of the most dreaded complications of GCA, commonly caused by anterior ischemic optic neuropathy and central retinal artery occlusion; therefore, early diagnosis with fundoscopic examination and prompt treatment is essential.[8,55] Acute ischemic stroke may occur in 10% to 16% of cases, more commonly in the vertebrobasilar than in the carotid artery territory.[8,50,52]

DIAGNOSIS

GCA is suspected in patients above > 50 years of age who present with cranial or LVV symptomatology. Serum inflammatory markers, ESR/CRP, are elevated in most cases of GCA, but about 4% of patients could have normal ESR/CRP. Although CRP is a more sensitive marker than ESR, measuring both tests at the initial evaluation increases the diagnostic sensitivity.[56] For patients with suspected GCA with cranial symptoms, unilateral long-segment (>1 cm) temporal artery biopsy (TAB) is recommended and is considered the gold standard methodology for diagnosis; a contralateral biopsy is only indicated in selective cases.[57]

The treatment for GCA should not be delayed to perform TAB– biopsy results can still be positive in 78% of cases treated with glucocorticoids for less than 2 weeks, 65% in those treated for 2 to 4 weeks, and 40% in those treated for more than 4 weeks.[58] In suspected cases of GCA with a negative TAB, MR/CT angiography of the neck, may be performed to investigate for the involvement of large vessels.[57]

Temporal artery ultrasound (TAS) is now being increasingly used to diagnose GCA–characterized by the presence of halo and compression signs– the halo signs reflects the presence of inflammatory infiltration of the vessel wall which appears as hypoechoic thickening of the vessel wall on ultrasound, while the compression sign denotes the inability to compress the involved vessel with an ultrasound probe compared to a healthy artery.[59–61] Although the current recommendation is to consider TAB over TAS for diagnosis, this modality can be complementary with increasing availability and operator experience.[57,62]

Classification System

There are no established diagnostic criteria for GCA. The ACR, 1990 classification included 5 criteria: age ≥ 50 years at disease onset, new onset of localized headache, temporal artery tenderness or decreased temporal artery pulse, elevated erythrocyte sedimentation rate ≥ 50 mm/hour, and biopsy sample showing necrotizing arteritis with predominant mononuclear cell infiltrates or granulomatous process with multinucleated giant cells. The presence of 3 of the 5 criteria was associated with a sensitivity of 93.5% and a specificity of 91.2% for classifying as GCA.[63] The ACR, 1990 classification criteria were developed by comparing those with GCA with other forms of vasculitis and not necessarily from non-vasculitis etiologies.[50,63] When applied as diagnostic criteria, the criteria performed poorly as the specificity decreased to 64.2% (95% CI, 52.8, 74.6).[64] Also, the ACR, 1990 criteria focuses on the cranial symptoms and not the large-vessel-related clinical features.[50]

The updated 2022 ACR/EULAR classification criteria validated for research purpose includes imaging modalities in addition to many of the previous ACR criteria–age ≥ 50 years is an absolute requirement, and positive TAB or temporal halo sign on ultrasound (+5 points), ESR ≥ 50 mm/hr or CRP ≥ 10 mg/L, sudden vision loss, morning stiffness in shoulder/neck, jaw or tongue claudication, new temporal headache, scalp tenderness, temporal artery abnormality on vascular examination, bilateral axillary involvement on imaging, and fluorodeoxyglucose-positron emission tomography activity throughout the aorta (+2 each). A patient can be classified as having GCA if the total score is ≥ 6 points with a specificity of 94.8% (95% CI 91.0–97.4).[50]

Medium Vessel Vasculitis

Polyarteritis nodosa

PAN is a rare systemic necrotizing vasculitis that mainly affects the medium size vessels and not associated with glomerulonephritis or involvement of small-sized vessels.[65] The prevalence of PAN is estimated between 2 and 33 per 100,000, with the difference primarily attributed to variable diagnostic criteria considered in different studies.[7,66] The disease process can manifest at any age but is more common in the 4–5th decade of life and has a male predominance.[67,68] Although most cases of PAN are considered primary, some may be secondary to viral infections, frequently hepatitis B (HBV).[69] The most typical presenting features are generalized non-specific symptoms (fever, weight loss, arthralgia, and myalgia) followed by neurologic symptoms (mononeuritis multiplex and peripheral neuropathy; CNS involvement is rare), skin involvement (nodules, purpura, and livedo reticularis), and gastrointestinal (post-prandial abdominal pain, bleeding). About one-third of patients may have hypertension. The most frequent renal manifestations are intrarenal aneurysms which can lead to the development of perirenal hematoma, renal infarct, and hypertension.[66,69–73]

There are no specific diagnostic serologic markers for PAN, although serum inflammatory markers such as ESR/CRP may be elevated at the time of active disease. ANCA serology by ELISA is usually negative, and a positive test should prompt an evaluation for AVV, as many signs/symptoms of AVV may overlap with PAN. Viral hepatitis serologies should be performed in all suspected cases of PAN.[3,70,74]

The diagnosis of PAN is made based on clinical signs/symptoms, histologic evidence, and imaging findings. Although histologic evidence of medium vessel arteritis/fibrinoid necrosis is considered diagnostic in a proper clinical scenario, a biopsy may not always be attainable or safe. In addition, the sensitivity could be variable as the vascular inflammatory lesions are segmental and predominate at branching points.[70]

Among the standard biopsy sites of skin, muscle, and the sensory nerve, the preferred location should match the clinical findings for a higher diagnostic yield. Those with visceral involvement require a prompt evaluation with a conventional or CT angiogram. Patients with PAN who presented with abdominal pain may have evidence of either microaneurysms or stenosis on celiomesentric angiogram–commonly involving renal, hepatic, and mesenteric vessels.[3,70,71,75] Fibromuscular dysplasia, AAV, and secondary vasculitis may have similar angiographic findings and are important differential diagnoses to consider.[3,70,75,76]

Deep skin biopsies should be performed to sample medium-sized vessels which is essential for higher sensitivity. In contrast, biopsies from an edge of an ulcer or livedo reticularis may have a lower yield for diagnosis.[71] In patients with peripheral neuropathy, a combined nerve and muscle biopsy can confirm the diagnosis in 80% of cases.[75,77] The

American College of Rheumatolgy,1990, classification criteria for poyarteritis nodosa are listed in **Box 1**.[78]

Kawasaki disease

Kawasaki disease is a form of febrile vasculitis that affects the small and medium sized vessels (typically coronary arteries), and predominantly occurs in children.[79] The topic has been recently reviewed by Shulman and colleagues[80]

Small Vessel Vasculitis

Antineutrophil cytoplasmic antibody-associated vasculitis

Antineutrophil cytoplasmic antibody (ANCA)-associated vasculitis (AAV) is a form of necrotizing small vessel vasculitis with scarce immune deposits, characterized by serologic evidence of ANCA–IgG autoantibodies directed against two cytoplasmic antigens present in a neutrophil, myeloperoxidase (MPO) and proteinase-3 (PR-3). In *vitro*, ANCA may create two distinct immunofluorescent staining patterns on ethanol-fixed neutrophils–cytoplasmic pattern (C-ANCA) is created when the autoantigen is PR-3, while perinuclear pattern (P- ANCA) is evident with MPO as the autoantigen.[81,82] At the CHCC, 2012, the various clinicopathologic variants were named as microscopic

---

Box 1
American College of Rheumatolgy, classification, 1990, Poyarteritis nodosa

- Weight loss $\geq$ 4 kg
- Livedo reticularis
- Testicular pain or tenderness
- Myalgia
- Mononeuropathy or polyneuropathy
- Diastolic blood pressure >90 mm Hg
- Elevated blood urea nitrogen or serum creatinine levels
- Presence of hepatitis B viral infection
- Arteriographic abnormalities –aneurysm or occlusion of visceral arteries not due to atherosclerosis, fibromuscular dysplasia, or other secondary causes
- Biopsy showing the infiltration of the vessel wall with granulocyte or mixed leukocyte infiltrate

The presence of 3 or more of these 10 criteria was associated with sensitivity and specificity of 82.2 and 86.6, respectively, for classifying patients with vasculitis as PAN.

polyangiitis (MPA), granulomatosis with polyangiitis (GPA) (formerly Wegener's granulomatosis) and eosinophilic granulomatosis with polyangiitis (EGPA) (formerly Churg-Strauss syndrome) and renal-limited vasculitis (RLV).[7]

Clinical Presentation

Patients usually present with constitutional symptoms of fatigue, low-degree fever, weight loss for months before developing organ-specific symptoms, commonly involving the kidney, and the upper and lower respiratory tract. Diffuse alveolar hemorrhage is a life-threatening manifestation; rapidly progressive glomerulonephritis can result in significant kidney injury while mononeuritis multiplex can result in peripheral neuropathy. Upper respiratory tract involvement can result in otitis media, sinusitis, nasal crusting, and subglottic stenosis.[83–85] Patients with EGPA present with asthma and peripheral eosinophilia. Although there is a significant overlap, patients with GPA usually present with upper/lower respiratory tract involvement and associated with positive ANCA-PR3 serology, and MPA presents skin and kidney disease and associated with a positive MPO-ANCA serology.[83,84,86–88]

Among all the different classification systems of the phenotypes including histology or GPA versus MPA subtypes, serotype associated disease processes–MPO-AAV vs. PR3-AAV has been most useful to estimate presenting clinical features and risks of relapse. While clinical features overlap, patients with PR3-AAV present with upper and lower respiratory tract diseases while those with MPO-AAV present with kidney, skin, and neural involvement. PR3-AAV is associated with a much higher risk of relapse of disease than MPO-AAV.[89,90]

Diagnosis

The diagnosis of AAV is usually based on typical clinical features in the presence of a positive ANCA serology, classic imaging findings, and/or histologic evidence. ANCA testing should include both immunofluorescence and ELISA assays. The common biopsy sites are skin and kidney– the classic renal lesion is pauci-immune cresentic glomerulonephritis with fibrinoid necrosis; skin lesions may show evidence of leukocytoclastic vasculitis.[85,91] Transbronchial biopsy usually has a low diagnostic yield and open lung biopsy is considered in selective cases.[92]

Pulmonary pathology may range from capillaritis, organizing pneumonia to granulomatous inflammation.[86,93] Secondary causes of a positive ANCA serology such as infections should always be considered; coversely, patients may present with classical clinical features of pauciimune small-vessel vasculitis in the absence of a positive ANCA serology (known as ANCA-negative vasculitis).

Cryoglobulinemic vasculitis

Cryoglobulinemic vasculitis (CGV) is characterized by the deposition of cryoglobulins/immune complexes in medium and small-sized vascular endothelium resulting in the development of an inflammatory cascade, with consequential generation of specific clinical signs and symptoms– purpuric rash, digital ulcers, arthralgia/arthritis, microscopic hematuria/kidney dysfunction, and peripheral neuropathy.[94,95] Cryoglobulins are immunoglobulins (Ig) that precipitate in vitro at low temperatures (below 37°C) and redissolve upon rewarming, primarily due to an alteration in their tertiary structures.[94,95] CGV is classified into three categories based on the type of Ig deposition– monoclonal Ig, usually IgM or IgG (Type 1), monoclonal IgM with rheumatoid factor (RF) activity and polyclonal IgG (type II), and only polyclonal IgM with RF activity and polyclonal IgG (type III). The underlying systemic processes that trigger cryoglobulin formation are listed in Table 1.[94,96,97]

Diagnosis

The diagnosis is based on clinical features and specific serological markers, including cryoglobulins in the serum. Histologic findings overlap with other forms of vasculitis but may be informative. Biopsy of a purpuric lesion may show evidence of leukocytoclastic vasculitis, while kidney biopsy may show hyaline thrombi in capillary lumen and organized substructures in a tubular or finger-like pattern on electron microscopy.[98,99] Serum levels of C4 may be low in mixed CGV while monoclonal Ig could activate the alternate complement pathway resulting in low C3 and C4.[100] Once a diagnosis of CGV is confirmed, additional serologic and imaging studies should be performed to investigate the underlying cause (see Box 1).[94,96,97,101] A stringent methodology for the collection and processing of blood sample is essential for the detection of cryoglobulins–upon the collection of a blood sample, it should be kept at 37°C to avoid the premature precipitation of cryoglobulins, and after warm centrifugation, the clear serum is observed at 4°C for the formation of cryoprecipitate.[96]

IgA vasculitis (formerly, henoch-schönlein purpura vasculitis)

IgAV mainly involves small-sized vessels and is caused by the deposition of immune complexes predominantly containing IgA and C3. IgAV is more common in children than adults – 3.5 to

Table 1
Systemic diseases associated with Cryoglobulinemic vasculitis

	Type I	Type II	Type III
Associated disorders	MGUS, CLL, Waldenstorm macroglobulinemia, Multiple myeloma	HCV, HBV Connective tissue diseases Lymphoproliferative disorder	HCV Infections CTD Autoimmune disorders

Abbreviations: CLL, chronic lymphocytic leukemia; CTD, connective tissue disorder; HBV, Hepatitis B virus; HCV, Hepatitis C virus; MGUS, monoclonal gammopathy of unclear significance.

26.7 cases per 100,000 children and 5 cases per 100,000 adults.[102,103] The mean age at onset of disease for adults is 50 years, with a male predominance. The typical symptoms are rash (virtually present in all patients), arthralgia/arthritis, and abdominal pain, while urine examination may show the presence of microscopic hematuria and proteinuria.[104] The rash is typically purpuric or petechial and commonly present in the lower than upper extremities; arthritis involves the large joints and is migratory; abdominal pain and intestinal bleeding may occur and usually manifest after the appearance of the rash.[105–107]

There are two classification criteria–ACR criteria of 1990, and European Alliance of Associations for Rheumatology/Pediatric Rheumatology International Trials Organisation/Pediatric Rheumatology European Society (EULAR/PRINTO/PRES) criteria of 2010, mainly designed for research studies and clinical trials and not for diagnostic purposes. The criteria included in the ACR, 1990 are: age ≤ 20 years at disease onset, palpable purpura, acute abdominal pain, and tissue biopsy evident for the presence of granulocytes in the walls of small arterioles or venules–the presence of 2 or more of these criteria distinguish IgAV from other forms of vasculitis.[108] The CHCC, 2012 defines IgAV as vasculitis with IgA1-dominant immune deposits affecting small blood vessels.[7]

The EULAR/PRINTO/PRES Classification criteria for pediatric IgAV includes: Purpura or petechiae (mandatory) with lower limb predominance and at least one of the four following criteria: (1) abdominal pain (diffuse colicky pain, may include intussusception or gastrointestinal bleeding), (2) histopathology (leukocytoclastic vasculitis with predominant IgA deposits, or proliferative glomerulonephritis with predominant IgA deposits), (3) arthritis or arthralgia, (4) kidney Involvement (proteinuria > 0.3 g/24h, > 5 red blood cells/hpf or red blood cell cast in urine sediment, or ≥ 2+ on dipstick).[109] When the same criteria was evaluated in a single-center retrospective study cohort of adult patients with IgAV, defined by CHCC, 2012 criteria, the diagnostic sensitivity and specificity

of the pediatric IgAV EULAR/PRINTO/PRES criteria were higher than the ACR criteria.[102]

Diagnosis of IgA Vasculitis (IgAV)

There are no established diagnostic criteria for IgAV in adults. Criteria from pediatric literature are often extrapolated to adults, namely, the finding of palpable purpura in the presence of at least one of the following: diffuse abdominal pain, arthritis/arthralgia, kidney involvement (hematuria/proteinuria), and a tissue biopsy showing predominant IgA deposition.[104,110]

Palpable purpura or a maculopapular rash of the lower extremities are the most common cutaneous lesions of vasculitis.[104] Histologic evidence of a fresh lesions could be diagnostic–leukocytoclastic vasculitis, characaterized by neutrophilic infiltration in and around the vessel wall, fibrinoid necrosis, and presence of nuclear dust.[111] Immunofluorescnce microscopy could be informative to differentiate IgAV from other causes of LCV including IgAV, CGV, AAV, and infection-associated vasculitis.

Variable vessel vasculitis

Behcet's disease (BD) is a rare form of vasculitis that may affect arteries and veins of any size and is characterized by recurrent oral and/or genital ulcers.[112,113] In a study from Olmsted County in Minnesota, the annual incidence of BD was 0.38 per 100,000 population, with a higher prevalence in women.[113] The most common dermatologic lesions are oral ulcers, genital ulcers, erythema nodosum-like lesion, and papulopustular lesions.[112] In addition, ocular lesions (uveitis, retinal vasculitis), vascular complications (superficial and deep vein thrombosis), and CNS system (migraine, stroke, aseptic meningitis) involvement may be present in some patients.[112,114]

Diagnosis: There are no diagnostic biomarkers or histologic findings for BD. The histologic findings may range from leucocytoclastic vasculitis of postcapillary venules to lymphocytic perivasculitis.[114] Inflammatory markers, ESR and CRP, may be elevated in active disease.[115] The diagnosis is usually informed by the International Criteria for

Bechet's disease, which includes recurrent oral ulceration (3 times in 12 months) and any 2 of the following: recurrent genital lesions, cutaneous lesions, eye lesions, and a positive pathergy test.[116]

Primary central nervous system vasculitis
CNS vasculitis is divided into two categories–primary or secondary to an identified secondary systemic disease process.[117] Primary central nervous system angiitis is a rare severe form of vasculitis that preferentially affects the CNS and spinal cord. The annual incidence in the USA is 2.4 per 1,000,000 person-years.[118] Headache is the most common symptom, followed by cognitive impairment, stroke, or hemiparesis. Visual field defect, diplopia, and decreased visual acuity are other symptoms. CSF analysis usually reveals increased total leukocyte count and/or protein concentration.[118–120] The typical findings on cerebral angiography are smooth-wall segmental narrowing or dilatation and occlusions in small- and large-sized arteries.[121] The diagnosis of PACNS requires a multidisciplinary approach–to evaluate for mimics of PACNS, appropriate imaging modalities, and consideration for leptomeningeal/brain biopsy in selective cases.[119] Histologically, three spectra of changes have been noted – (1) acute necrotizing vasculitis, (2) lymphocytic infiltration, and (3) granulomatous changes.[122] The diagnosed criteria proposed by Calabrese and Mallek could be informative and includes the following clinical features: a history of an unexplained neurologic deficit that remains after a vigorous diagnostic workup, including lumbar puncture and neuroimaging studies; either classic angiographic evidence of vasculitis or histopathologic evidence of vasculitis within the CNS; and no evidence of systemic vasculitis or any other condition to which the angiographic or pathologic evidence can be attributed.[120]

Other forms of vasculitis
About 10% of patients with connective tissue disorders may have features of vasculitis.[123] Patients with rheumatoid arthritis may present with vasculitic features involving the small- and medium-sized vessels, commonly of the peripheral nerve and skin. Sjogren's syndrome may be associated with vasculitis of medium-sized vessels and may mimic PAN.[124] About 11% to 36% of patients with SLE may present with lupus vasculitis which mainly involves the skin but may also affect the CNS, renal and retinal vessels.[125,126] Hypocomplementic urticarial vasculitis is an immune complex mediated vasculitis characterized by angioedema, leucocytoclastic vasculitis, glomerulonephritis, and uveitis, in the presence of hypocomplementemia and anti-C1q antibodies.[127,128] Cogan syndrome is another rare form of vasculitis characterized by ocular and audiovestibular symptoms.[129]

CLINICS CARE POINTS

- Multidisciplinary team approach is essential in evaluating and treating patients with vasculitis.
- Non-vasculitic etiologies may have overlapping features of vasculitis.
- Classification criteria could be informative but shouldnt be used soley for diagnosis.

DISCLOSURE

Honoraria from Travere, Calliditas, ChemoCentryx, and Elsevier.

REFERENCES

1. Langford CA. 15. Vasculitis. J Allergy Clin Immunol 2003;111:S602–12.
2. Kermani TA, Warrington KJ, Dua AB. Treatment Guidelines in Vasculitis. Rheumatic diseases clinics of North America 2022;48:705–24.
3. Saadoun D, Vautier M, Cacoub P. Medium- and Large-Vessel Vasculitis. Circulation 2021;143: 267–82.
4. Pugh D, et al. Large-vessel vasculitis. Nat Rev Dis Prim 2022;7:93.
5. Zarka F, Veillette C, Makhzoum JP. A Review of Primary Vasculitis Mimickers Based on the Chapel Hill Consensus Classification. Int J Rheumatol 2020; 2020:8392542.
6. Keser G, Aksu K. Diagnosis and differential diagnosis of large-vessel vasculitides. Rheumatol Int 2019;39:169–85.
7. Jennette JC, et al. 2012 revised International Chapel Hill Consensus Conference Nomenclature of Vasculitides. Arthritis Rheum 2013;65:1–11.
8. Hayreh SS. Giant cell arteritis: Its ophthalmic manifestations. Indian J Ophthalmol 2021;69:227–35.
9. Hankard A, et al. Characteristics of ANCA-associated vasculitis with aneurysms: Case series and review of the literature. Autoimmun Rev 2023; 22:103293.
10. Maningding E, Kermani TA. Mimics of vasculitis. Rheumatology 2021;60:34–47.
11. Molloy ES, Langford CA. Vasculitis mimics. Curr Opin Rheumatol 2008;20:29–34.
12. Adefuye MA, et al. Tuberculosis and Cardiovascular Complications: An Overview. Cureus 2022;14: e28268.

13. López-López JP, et al. Tuberculosis and the Heart. J Am Heart Assoc 2021;10:e019435.
14. Roberts WC, Barbin CM, Weissenborn MR, et al. Syphilis as a Cause of Thoracic Aortic Aneurysm. Am J Cardiol 2015;116:1298–303.
15. Zen Y, Kasashima S, Inoue D. Retroperitoneal and aortic manifestations of immunoglobulin G4-related disease. Semin Diagn Pathol 2012;29: 212–8.
16. Mazor RD, Manevich-Mazor M, Shoenfeld Y. Erdheim-Chester Disease: a comprehensive review of the literature. Orphanet J Rare Dis 2013;8:137.
17. Villatoro-Villar M, et al. Arterial involvement in Erdheim-Chester disease: A retrospective cohort study. Medicine (Baltim) 2018;97:e13452.
18. Shivapour DM, Erwin P, Kim E. Epidemiology of fibromuscular dysplasia: A review of the literature. Vasc Med 2016;21:376–81.
19. Gornik HL, et al. First International Consensus on the diagnosis and management of fibromuscular dysplasia. Vasc Med 2019;24:164–89.
20. Olin JW, et al. Fibromuscular dysplasia: state of the science and critical unanswered questions: a scientific statement from the American Heart Association. Circulation 2014;129:1048–78.
21. Pillai AK, Iqbal SI, Liu RW, et al. Segmental arterial mediolysis. Cardiovasc Intervent Radiol 2014;37: 604–12.
22. Heritz DM, Butany J, Johnston KW, et al. Intraabdominal hemorrhage as a result of segmental mediolytic arteritis of an omental artery: case report. J Vasc Surg 1990;12:561–5.
23. Mahr A, et al. Brief report: prevalence of antineutrophil cytoplasmic antibodies in infective endocarditis. Arthritis Rheumatol 2014;66:1672–7.
24. Hotchi M. Pathological studies on Takayasu arteritis. Heart Vessels Suppl 1992;7:11–7.
25. Mwipatayi BP, et al. Takayasu arteritis: clinical features and management: report of 272 cases. ANZ J Surg 2005;75:110–7.
26. Mason JC. Takayasu arteritis–advances in diagnosis and management. Nat Rev Rheumatol 2010; 6:406–15.
27. Espinoza JL, Ai S, Matsumura I. New Insights on the Pathogenesis of Takayasu Arteritis: Revisiting the Microbial Theory. Pathogens 2018;7. https://doi.org/10.3390/pathogens7030073.
28. Arnaud L, Haroche J, Mathian A, et al. Pathogenesis of Takayasu's arteritis: a 2011 update. Autoimmun Rev 2011;11:61–7.
29. Seko Y. Takayasu arteritis: insights into immunopathology. Jpn Heart J 2000;41:15–26.
30. Weyand CM, Vasculitides JJG. Primer on the Rheumatic Diseases 2008;398–450. https://doi.org/10.1007/978-0-387-68566-3_21.
31. Kerr GS, et al. Takayasu arteritis. Ann Intern Med 1994;120:919–29.
32. Joseph G, Goel R, Thomson VS, et al. Takayasu Arteritis: JACC Focus Seminar 3/4. J Am Coll Cardiol 2022. https://doi.org/10.1016/j.jacc.2022.09.051.
33. Schmidt WA, Nerenheim A, Seipelt E, et al. Diagnosis of early Takayasu arteritis with sonography. Rheumatology 2002;41:496–502.
34. Strachan RW. The natural history of takayasu's arteriopathy. Q J Med 1964;33:57–69.
35. Dammacco R, Cimino L, De Simone L, et al. Ocular Manifestations in an Italian Cohort of Patients with Takayasu Arteritis. Ocul Immunol Inflamm 2023; 31:945–54.
36. Kreidstein SH, Lytwyn A, Keystone EC. Takayasu arteritis with acute interstitial pneumonia and coronary vasculitis: expanding the spectrum. Report of a case. Arthritis Rheum 1993;36:1175–8.
37. Mayfield JJ, Hidano D, Torres JA, et al. The Young and the Breathless. N Engl J Med 2022;387: 67–73.
38. Sohn IS, et al. A case of concentric left ventricular hypertrophy with falsely normal blood pressure in patient with Takayasu's arteritis. Heart Ves 2008; 23:209–13.
39. Tombetti E, Mason JC. Application of imaging techniques for Takayasu arteritis. Presse Med 2017;46: e215–23.
40. Soussan M, et al. Management of large-vessel vasculitis with FDG-PET: a systematic literature review and meta-analysis. Medicine (Baltim) 2015;94:e622.
41. Vaideeswar P, Deshpande JR. Pathology of Takayasu arteritis: A brief review. Ann Pediatr Cardiol 2013;6(1):52–8.
42. Grayson PC, et al. 2022 American College of Rheumatology/EULAR classification criteria for Takayasu arteritis. Annals of the rheumatic diseases 2022;81: 1654–60.
43. Weyand CM, Liao YJ, Goronzy JJ. The immunopathology of giant cell arteritis: diagnostic and therapeutic implications. J Neuro Ophthalmol 2012;32: 259–65.
44. Alba MA, Mena-Madrazo JA, Reyes E, et al. Giant cell arteritis in Mexican patients. J Clin Rheumatol 2012;18:1–7.
45. Samec MJ, et al. Relapse Risk and Safety of Long-Term Tocilizumab Use Among Patients With Giant Cell Arteritis: A Single-Enterprise Cohort Study. J Rheumatol 2023. https://doi.org/10.3899/jrheum.2022-1214.
46. Gravanis MB. Giant cell arteritis and Takayasu aortitis: morphologic, pathogenetic and etiologic factors. Int J Cardiol 2000;75(Suppl 1):S21–33.
47. Ly KH, Régent A, Tamby MC, et al. Pathogenesis of giant cell arteritis: More than just an inflammatory condition? Autoimmun Rev 2010;9:635–45.
48. Robinette ML, Rao DA, Monach PA. The Immunopathology of Giant Cell Arteritis Across Disease Spectra. Front Immunol 2021;12:623716.

49. Koster MJ, Matteson EL, Warrington KJ. Large-vessel giant cell arteritis: diagnosis, monitoring and management. Rheumatology 2018;57:ii32–42.

50. Ponte C, Martins-Martinho J, Luqmani RA. Diagnosis of giant cell arteritis. Rheumatology 2020;59: iii5–16.

51. Smetana GW, Shmerling RH. Does this patient have temporal arteritis? JAMA 2002;287:92–101.

52. Soulages A, et al. Neurologic manifestations of giant cell arteritis. J Neurol 2022;269:3430–42.

53. Dejaco C, Duftner C, Buttgereit F, et al. The spectrum of giant cell arteritis and polymyalgia rheumatica: revisiting the concept of the disease. Rheumatology (Oxford) 2017;56(4):506–15.

54. Narváez J, et al. Prevalence of ischemic complications in patients with giant cell arteritis presenting with apparently isolated polymyalgia rheumatica. Semin Arthritis Rheum 2015;45:328–33.

55. Hayreh SS, Podhajsky PA, Zimmerman B. Ocular manifestations of giant cell arteritis. American journal of ophthalmology 1998;125:509–20.

56. Parikh M, et al. Prevalence of a normal C-reactive protein with an elevated erythrocyte sedimentation rate in biopsy-proven giant cell arteritis. Ophthalmology 2006;113:1842–5.

57. Maz M, et al. 2021 American College of Rheumatology/Vasculitis Foundation Guideline for the Management of Giant Cell Arteritis and Takayasu Arteritis. Arthritis Rheumatol 2021;73:1349–65.

58. Narváez J, et al. Influence of previous corticosteroid therapy on temporal artery biopsy yield in giant cell arteritis. Semin Arthritis Rheum 2007;37:13–9.

59. Berger CT, et al. The clinical benefit of imaging in the diagnosis and treatment of giant cell arteritis. Swiss Med Wkly 2018;148:w14661.

60. Dejaco C, et al. The provisional OMERACT ultrasonography score for giant cell arteritis. Ann Rheum Dis 2022. https://doi.org/10.1136/ard-2022-223367.

61. Schmidt WA, Kraft HE, Völker L, et al. Colour Doppler sonography to diagnose temporal arteritis. Lancet 1995;345:866.

62. Monti S, Schäfer VS, Muratore F, et al. Updates on the diagnosis and monitoring of giant cell arteritis. Front Med (Lausanne) 2023;10:1125141.

63. Hunder GG, et al. The American College of Rheumatology 1990 criteria for the classification of giant cell arteritis. Arthritis Rheum 1990;33:1122–8.

64. Seeliger B, et al. Are the 1990 American College of Rheumatology vasculitis classification criteria still valid? Rheumatology 2017;56:1154–61.

65. Jennette JC, Falk RJ, Hu P, et al. Pathogenesis of anti-neutrophil cytoplasmic autoantibody-associated small-vessel vasculitis. Annu Rev Pathol 2013;8: 139–60.

66. Mahr A, Guillevin L, Poissonnet M, et al. Prevalences of polyarteritis nodosa, microscopic polyangiitis, Wegener's granulomatosis, and Churg-Strauss syndrome in a French urban multiethnic population in 2000: a capture-recapture estimate. Arthritis Rheum 2004;51:92–9.

67. Huang Z, Li T, Nigrovic PA, Lee PY. Polyarteritis nodosa and deficiency of adenosine deaminase 2 - Shared genealogy, generations apart. Clin Immunol 2020;215:108411.

68. Erden A, Batu ED, Sönmez HE, et al. Comparing polyarteritis nodosa in children and adults: a single center study. Int J Rheum Dis 2017;20(8):1016–22.

69. Johnson RJ, Couser WG. Hepatitis B infection and renal disease: clinical, immunopathogenetic and therapeutic considerations. Kidney Int 1990;37: 663–76.

70. Hernández-Rodríguez J, Alba MA, Prieto-González S, et al. Diagnosis and classification of polyarteritis nodosa. J Autoimmun 2014;48-49:84–9.

71. Levine SM, Hellmann DB, Stone JH. Gastrointestinal involvement in polyarteritis nodosa (1986-2000): presentation and outcomes in 24 patients. Am J Med 2002;112:386–91.

72. Frohnert PP, Sheps SG. Long-term follow-up study of periarteritis nodosa. Am J Med 1967;43:8–14.

73. Symmers WS, Gillett R. Polyarteritis nodosa associated with malignant hypertension, disseminated platelet thrombosis, "wire loop" glomeruli, pulmonary silicotuberculosis, and sarcoidosis-like lymphadenopathy. A.M.A. Archives of Pathology 1951; 52:489–504.

74. Trepo C, Guillevin L. Polyarteritis nodosa and extrahepatic manifestations of HBV infection: the case against autoimmune intervention in pathogenesis. J Autoimmun 2001;16:269–74.

75. Pagnoux C, et al. Clinical features and outcomes in 348 patients with polyarteritis nodosa: a systematic retrospective study of patients diagnosed between 1963 and 2005 and entered into the French Vasculitis Study Group Database. Arthritis Rheum 2010; 62:616–26.

76. Henegar C, et al. A paradigm of diagnostic criteria for polyarteritis nodosa: analysis of a series of 949 patients with vasculitides. Arthritis Rheum 2008;58: 1528–38.

77. Lin YC, et al. Polyarteritis Nodosa: A Systematic Review of Test Accuracy and Benefits and Harms of Common Treatments. ACR Open Rheumatol 2021;3:91–100.

78. Lightfoot RW Jr, et al. The American College of Rheumatology 1990 criteria for the classification of polyarteritis nodosa. Arthritis Rheum 1990;33: 1088–93.

79. Agarwal S, Agrawal DK. Kawasaki disease: etiopathogenesis and novel treatment strategies. Expet Rev Clin Immunol 2017;13:247–58.

80. Shulman ST, Rowley AH. Kawasaki disease: insights into pathogenesis and approaches to treatment. Nat Rev Rheumatol 2015;11:475–82.

81. Weiner M, Segelmark M. The clinical presentation and therapy of diseases related to anti-neutrophil cytoplasmic antibodies (ANCA). Autoimmun Rev 2016;15:978–82.

82. Savige J, et al. International Consensus Statement on Testing and Reporting of Antineutrophil Cytoplasmic Antibodies (ANCA). Am J Clin Pathol 1999;111:507–13.

83. Quinn KA, et al. Subglottic stenosis and endobronchial disease in granulomatosis with polyangiitis. Rheumatology 2019;58:2203–11.

84. Comarmond C, Cacoub P. Granulomatosis with polyangiitis (Wegener): clinical aspects and treatment. Autoimmun Rev 2014;13:1121–5.

85. Jennette JC, Nachman PH. ANCA Glomerulonephritis and Vasculitis. Clin J Am Soc Nephrol 2017;12:1680–91.

86. Sacoto G, Boukhlal S, Specks U, et al. Lung involvement in ANCA-associated vasculitis. Presse Med 2020;49:104039.

87. Cornec D, Cornec-Le Gall E, Fervenza FC, et al. ANCA-associated vasculitis - clinical utility of using ANCA specificity to classify patients. Nat Rev Rheumatol 2016;12:570–9.

88. Comarmond C, et al. Eosinophilic granulomatosis with polyangiitis (Churg-Strauss): clinical characteristics and long-term followup of the 383 patients enrolled in the French Vasculitis Study Group cohort. Arthritis Rheum 2013;65:270–81.

89. Kitching AR, et al. ANCA-associated vasculitis. Nat Rev Dis Prim 2020;6:71.

90. Nachman PH, et al. Recurrent ANCA-associated small vessel vasculitis after transplantation: A pooled analysis. Kidney Int 1999;56:1544–50.

91. Yap BJM, et al. Unraveling the Immunopathogenesis and Genetic Variants in Vasculitis Toward Development of Personalized Medicine. Front Cardiovasc Med 2021;8:732369.

92. Schnabel A, Holl-Ulrich K, Dalhoff K, et al. Efficacy of transbronchial biopsy in pulmonary vaculitides. Eur Respir J 1997;10:2738–43.

93. Alba MA, et al. Interstital lung disease in ANCA vasculitis. Autoimmun Rev 2017;16:722–9.

94. Muchtar E, Magen H, Gertz MA. How I treat cryoglobulinemia. Blood 2017;129:289–98.

95. Dammacco F, Lauletta G, Vacca A. The wide spectrum of cryoglobulinemic vasculitis and an overview of therapeutic advancements. Clin Exp Med 2023;23:255–72.

96. Motyckova G, Murali M. Laboratory testing for cryoglobulins. Am J Hematol 2011;86:500–2.

97. Duvoux C, et al. Hepatitis C virus (HCV)-related cryoglobulinemia after liver transplantation for HCV cirrhosis. Transpl Int 2002;15:3–9.

98. Ogihara T, et al. Finger print deposits of the kidney in pure monoclonal IgG kappa cryoglobulinemia. Clin Nephrol 1979;12:186–90.

99. Menter T, Hopfer H. Renal disease in cryoglobulinemia. Glomerular Dis 2021;1:92–104.

100. Ravindran A, Fervenza FC, Smith RJH, et al. C3 glomerulopathy associated with monoclonal Ig is a distinct subtype. Kidney Int 2018;94:178–86.

101. Roccatello D, et al. Cryoglobulinaemia. nature reviews. Disease primers 2018;4:11.

102. Hočevar A, et al. IgA vasculitis in adults: the performance of the EULAR/PRINTO/PRES classification criteria in adults. Arthritis Res Ther 2016;18:58.

103. Hočevar A, et al. Incidence of IgA vasculitis in the adult Slovenian population. Br J Dermatol 2014;171:524–7.

104. Nachman P, Lerma E, Rheault M. Handbook of Glomerulonephritis. 1st edition. Philadelphia, PA: Lippincott Williams & Wilkins; 2023.

105. Audemard-Verger A, et al. Characteristics and management of iga vasculitis (henoch-schönlein) in adults: data from 260 patients included in a french multicenter retrospective survey. Arthritis Rheumatol 2017;69:1862–70.

106. Audemard-Verger A, Pillebout E, Guillevin L, et al. IgA vasculitis (Henoch-Shönlein purpura) in adults: diagnostic and therapeutic aspects. Autoimmun Rev 2015;14:579–85.

107. Linskey KR, Kroshinsky D, Mihm MC Jr, et al. Immunoglobulin-A–associated small-vessel vasculitis: a 10-year experience at the Massachusetts General Hospital. J Am Acad Dermatol 2012;66:813–22.

108. Mills JA, et al. The american college of rheumatology 1990 criteria for the classification of henoch-schönlein purpura. Arthritis Rheum 1990;33:1114–21.

109. Ozen S, et al. EULAR/PRINTO/PRES criteria for Henoch-Schönlein purpura, childhood polyarteritis nodosa, childhood Wegener granulomatosis and childhood Takayasu arteritis: Ankara 2008. Part II: Final classification criteria. Annals of the rheumatic diseases 2010;69:798–806.

110. Leung AKC, Barankin B, Leong KF. Henoch-Schönlein Purpura in Children: An Updated Review. Curr Pediatr Rev 2020;16:265–76.

111. Caproni M, Verdelli A. An update on the nomenclature for cutaneous vasculitis. Curr Opin Rheumatol 2019;31:46–52.

112. Alpsoy E, Bozca BC, Bilgic A. Behçet Disease: An Update for Dermatologists. Am J Clin Dermatol 2021;22:477–502.

113. Calamia KT, et al. Epidemiology and clinical characteristics of Behçet's disease in the US: a population-based study. Arthritis Rheum 2009;61:600–4.

114. Leccese P, Alpsoy E. Behçet's Disease: An Overview of Etiopathogenesis. Front Immunol 2019;10:1067.

115. Parsaei A, et al. Predictive value of erythrocyte sedimentation rate and C-reactive protein in Behcet's disease activity and manifestations: a cross-sectional study. BMC Rheumatol 2022;6:9.
116. Criteria for diagnosis of Behçet's disease. International Study Group for Behçet's Disease. Lancet 1990;335:1078–80.
117. Molloy ES, Hajj-Ali RA. Primary angiitis of the central nervous system. Curr Treat Options Neurol 2007;9:169–75.
118. Salvarani C, Brown RD Jr, Hunder GG. Adult primary central nervous system vasculitis. Lancet 2012;380:767–77.
119. Birnbaum J, Hellmann DB. Primary angiitis of the central nervous system. Arch Neurol 2009;66:704–9.
120. Calabrese LH, Mallek JA. Primary angiitis of the central nervous system. Report of 8 new cases, review of the literature, and proposal for diagnostic criteria. Medicine (Baltim) 1988;67:20–39.
121. Giannini C, Salvarani C, Hunder G, et al. Primary central nervous system vasculitis: pathology and mechanisms. Acta Neuropathol 2012;123:759–72.
122. Miller DV, et al. Biopsy findings in primary angiitis of the central nervous system. Am J Surg Pathol 2009;33:35–43.
123. Cozzani E, et al. Vasculitis associated with connective tissue diseases. G Ital Dermatol Venereol 2015;150:221–32.
124. Scofield RH. Vasculitis in Sjögren's Syndrome. Curr Rheumatol Rep 2011;13(6):482–8.
125. Barile-Fabris L, Hernández-Cabrera MF, Barragan-Garfias JA. Vasculitis in systemic lupus erythematosus. Curr Rheumatol Rep 2014;16:440.
126. Calle-Botero E, Abril A. Lupus vasculitis. Curr Rheumatol Rep 2020;22:71. https://doi.org/10.1007/s11926-020-00937-0.
127. Jara LJ, Navarro C, Medina G, et al. Hypocomplementemic urticarial vasculitis syndrome. Curr Rheumatol Rep 2009;11:410–5.
128. Wisnieski JJ, et al. Hypocomplementemic urticarial vasculitis syndrome. Clinical and serologic findings in 18 patients. Medicine (Baltim) 1995;74:24–41.
129. Greco A, et al. Cogan's syndrome: an autoimmune inner ear disease. Autoimmun Rev 2013;12:396–400.

Infectious and Postinfectious Vasculopathies

Christina M. Marra, MD*

KEYWORDS

- Central nervous system infection • Vasculitis • Varicella zoster virus • *Treponema pallidum*
- Syphilis • Delayed cerebral vasculopathy

KEY POINTS

- Only a few CNS infections present with stroke without other symptoms or signs of CNS infection, chiefly varicella zoster virus (VZV), and *Treponema pallidum*, the bacterium that causes syphilis.
- In about half of adults with VZV vasculopathy, there is no history of a shingles rash.
- Fifty to seventy percent of patients with meningovascular syphilis present solely with stroke, most often acutely, and the underlying syphilitic etiology is often initially missed.
- Delayed cerebral vasculopathy occurs most commonly in individuals with acute pneumococcal meningitis who have been treated with adjunctive dexamethasone.

INTRODUCTION

Stroke is a complication of many central nervous system (CNS) infections (reviewed in refs[1–3]). For example, in a meta-analysis of 1692 individuals with bacterial meningitis, stroke occurred in 332 (16%).[4] Tuberculous,[5] cryptococcal,[6] and coccidioidal[7] meningitis are commonly complicated by stroke. In these instances, infarction is likely a consequence of inflammation of cerebral vessels as they course through a purulent basilar infiltrate or due to stretching from concomitant hydrocephalus.[1] CNS infection with aspergillus[8] and the agents responsible for mucormycosis[9] may be angioinvasive, leading to destruction or occlusion of cerebral arteries, thereby causing hemorrhage or ischemic stroke. However, only a few CNS infections present with stroke without other symptoms or signs of CNS infection. Chief among these are varicella zoster virus (VZV) and syphilis. Early in the epidemic, HIV was believed to cause a cerebral vasculitis but subsequent work suggests that VZV may be the more likely culprit.[10] Delayed cerebral vasculopathy (DCV) after successful treatment of bacterial meningitis, most commonly pneumococcal, is an emerging entity with uncertain pathogenesis. In this article, the background, clinical manifestations, pathophysiology, and treatment, as well as a clinical vignette, for VZV vasculopathy, meningovascular syphilis, and DCV, are provided.

VARICELLA ZOSTER VIRUS
Background

VZV is the cause of chickenpox. After resolution of infection, the virus remains latent in cranial nerve, dorsal root, and autonomic ganglia. Reactivation occurs in the setting of waning immunity, usually related to age or to immunomodulatory medications, to cause the rash of shingles. After primary infection or reactivation in children, or reactivation in adults, CNS involvement in the form of encephalitis or vasculitis or both, may occur and may not be accompanied by rash.[11,12] Clinical findings include headache, change in mental status, and focal neurologic deficits.[11] VZV vasculopathy occurs in immunocompetent and immunocompromised individuals, and it affects CNS small and large cerebral arteries, or both, leading to

Department of Neurology, University of Washington, Seattle, WA, USA
* Harborview Medical Center Box 359775, 325 9th Avenue, Seattle, WA 98104-2499.
E-mail address: cmarra@uw.edu

Neuroimag Clin N Am 34 (2024) 13–21
https://doi.org/10.1016/j.nic.2023.06.001
1052-5149/24/© 2023 Elsevier Inc. All rights reserved.

transient ischemic attacks or focal or multifocal infarcts. Less commonly, the vasculopathy may cause aneurysms, subarachnoid hemorrhage, or intracranial hemorrhage.[13,14] Moyamoya collaterals have been described in children with VZV vasculopathy.[15]

Clinical Findings

Stroke days to weeks after an episode of shingles in the ophthalmic division of the trigeminal nerve, termed herpes zoster ophthalmicus with contralateral hemiplegia, has long been described as a rare cause of stroke. Studies in the 1970s showed angiographic evidence of vascular stenosis ipsilateral to the zoster rash,[16,17] and subsequent pathological studies confirmed VZV as the cause.[11,18] VZV vasculopathy, as it is now known, can be acute or chronic, and in adults it can cause recurrent stroke over several months to even years.[12]

A case report and review of 62 adults with serological or molecular confirmation of VZV vasculopathy documented a history of shingles in a little over half with an average of 57 days between rash and onset of neurologic symptoms; one individual and the authors' additional case had onset of shingles after the development of neurologic symptoms.[14] Small cerebral vessels alone were involved in 24 (38.7%), large cerebral vessels alone in 11 (17.7%), and both in 27 (43.5%).[14] In comparison to adults, a series of 22 children with VZV vasculopathy, in whom the course is generally monophasic, suggests that large cerebral arteries are more often involved than small arteries.[12]

Pathophysiology

VZV travels from trigeminal and autonomic ganglia of the head and neck transaxonally to cerebral arteries where they terminate in the adventitia, followed by transmural spread. Adventitial fibroblasts are one of the first vascular cells that are infected. The accompanying inflammation consists of neutrophils early in the course and T cells and macrophages throughout the course of infection. The elastic lamina is disrupted, the intima is thickened and there is loss of medial smooth muscle cells (reviewed in ref[19]). Vasculitis is patchy with identification of VZV DNA and antigen in arteries, but not in brain itself.[11]

In an in vitro study,[20] VZV infection of human brain vascular adventitial fibroblasts induced their transformation into myofibroblasts and increased their proliferation and ability to migrate. Incubation of human umbilical vein endothelial cells with conditioned media from VZV-infected human brain vascular adventitial fibroblasts led to endothelial activation. Centrifuged VZV-infected cells contained microparticles that included VZV and that were able to infect human brain vascular adventitial fibroblasts and to activate human umbilical vein endothelial cells. A transcriptional study of VZV-infected human brain vascular adventitial fibroblasts confirmed an increase in migratory phenotype.[21] These findings support a model of VZV vasculopathy pathogenesis in which VZV infection of adventitia is propagated, leading to arterial remodeling and endothelial activation. Additional studies suggest that the accumulation of amyloid may contribute to VZV vasculopathy.[21,22]

Diagnosis

VZV vasculopathy should be suspected in children with stroke and in adults with stroke with a history of zoster or current zoster or in those without traditional stroke risk factors. Angiography shows multifocal stenosis with post-stenotic dilation when large cerebral arteries are involved, and cerebrospinal fluid (CSF) pleocytosis is seen in 75% of affected individuals.[14] Black blood MR imaging may be able to distinguish between VZV vasculopathy and arteriosclerosis in the correct clinical setting by demonstrating circumferential vessel wall enhancement.[23] The best diagnostic test is detection of intrathecal synthesis of VZV immunoglobulin G (IgG) antibody. The detection of VZV DNA in CSF is diagnostic in the correct clinical setting but is less likely than detection of CSF IgG antibody synthesis. When both tests are negative, VZV vasculopathy is unlikely. Vaccination with the live zoster vaccine likely decreases the risk of VZV vasculopathy,[24] but whether there is a difference in risk after the preferred recombinant zoster vaccine is unknown.

Treatment

There have been no controlled studies of treatment of VZV vasculopathy. The recommendation based on expert opinion is intravenous acyclovir 10-15 mg/kg three times a day (dose may need to be adjusted based on renal function) for 14 days, with prednisone 1 mg/kg/day orally for the first 5 days of treatment. Symptoms may persist or recur after therapy, particularly in individuals who are immunocompromised. In this situation, the IV treatment course may be repeated, followed by valacyclovir 1 g orally three times a day for 1 to 2 months.[19,25]

In the 2013 review of 62 patients, 32 (51.6%) patients were treated with acyclovir alone, 21 (33.8%) received acyclovir with corticosteroids, and 9 (14.5%) received other therapy; overall 47 patients (75.8%) improved or stabilized. There was no difference in outcomes between the treatment groups.[14] A subsequent review of 30 immunosuppressed individuals with VZV vasculopathy suggested that 75% to 80% improved or stabilized on antivirals alone or in combination with corticosteroids.[23]

Clinical Vignette

A 32-year-old woman living with well controlled, but advanced, HIV developed acute onset of bilateral leg weakness, right arm weakness and tingling, and difficulty with speech that resolved after 15 minutes, recurred 5 minutes later and again resolved after 5 minutes. She had an episode of shingles 3 months before. CSF showed 64 white blood cells (WBCs)/μL (97% lymphocytes), normal glucose concentration, protein concentration 122 mg/dL, and 12,000 copies/mL of VZV DNA; no VZV DNA was detected in blood. MR imaging showed multifocal vascular stenoses with circumferential vessel wall enhancement with contrast (**Fig. 1**). Based on history, CSF findings, and neuroimaging, she was diagnosed with VZV vasculitis.

MENINGOVASCULAR SYPHILIS
Background

Syphilis is caused by the bacterium *Treponema pallidum* subspecies *pallidum* (hereafter *T pallidum*). Uncomplicated syphilis is traditionally categorized into stages. Primary syphilis is characterized by a chancre, a usually painless ulcer at the site of inoculation. Secondary syphilis is characterized by rash, mucosal, and intertriginous lesions; involvement of major organ systems can also occur. Primary and secondary syphilis are the most contagious forms of syphilis. In the United States, early latent syphilis refers to asymptomatic individuals with the evidence of *T pallidum* infection in the last year, whereas late latent syphilis refers to asymptomatic individuals with initial infection more than a year before; for the purposes of determining duration of therapy, individuals with syphilis of unknown duration are included in the category of late latent syphilis, which requires more prolonged therapy than primary, secondary, or early latent syphilis. In the United States, the rate of primary and secondary syphilis has progressively increased since 2000 when rates were historically low; between 2020 and 2021, this rate increased 29%.[26] Although syphilis disproportionately affects men who have sex with men, the United States is experiencing an ongoing epidemic in heterosexuals as well.[26] Other countries are similarly experiencing increasing incidence of syphilis.[27]

Neurosyphilis can occur at any time during infection. Inconsistent reporting underestimates the number of individuals with syphilis who develop neurosyphilis.[28] However, a study from King County, WA, in which patients were systematically interviewed about neurologic symptoms and medical charts were reviewed for confirmatory data, estimated that 3.5% of individuals with syphilis develop neurosyphilis. Neurosyphilis, like uncomplicated syphilis, is divided into stages. Early neurosyphilis includes asymptomatic and symptomatic meningitis and meningovascular disease, which often presents as stroke. Early neurosyphilis occurs within the first months to years after infection. Late neurosyphilis includes syphilitic dementia and tabes dorsalis, which presents as a spinal cord disorder with sensory ataxia and bowel and bladder incontinence. Late neurosyphilis occurs years to decades after initial infection. Persons living with HIV (PLWH) who are not receiving antiretroviral therapy or who have low peripheral blood CD4+ T-cell concentrations are at an increased risk of neurosyphilis.[29,30]

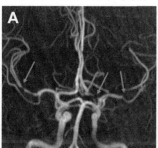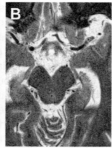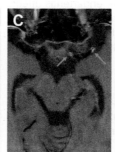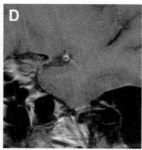

Fig. 1. Coronal maximum intensity projection (MIP) reformatted time-of-flight (TOF) magnetic resonance angiography (MRA) (*A*) shows multifocal stenoses involving the right and left M2 MCA branches, the left A2/A3 ACA branches (blue *arrows*). Axial T2-weighted vessel wall MR imaging (*B*) shows circumferential T2 hyperintense wall lesion involving the left M2 MCA (blue *arrow*). On Axial T1-weighted post-contrast vessel wall MR imaging (*C*), there are lesions involving the left M1 and M2 MCA (blue *arrows*), with the left M2 MCA lesion also seen on sagittal T1 post-contrast vessel wall MR imaging (*D*) (blue *arrow*). (*Courtesy* © 2023 Christina M. Mara.)

Clinical Findings

Much of what we know about neurosyphilis comes from studies conducted in the first half of the twentieth century. The largest series of meningovascular syphilis in this era was reported by Merritt and coworkers, and it included 42 individuals selected from a possible 250 cases.[31] Most patients were 30 to 50 years old, and presented within months to years after infection, with an average of seven years. Prodromal symptoms, such as headache, dizziness, and personality changes, for days or weeks, preceded the onset of ischemia or stroke in about half of individuals, and these symptoms were attributed to concomitant syphilitic meningitis. Onset of vascular symptoms was abrupt in three-fourths of patients, and hemiplegia or hemiparesis was the most common focal finding, followed by aphasia, reflecting preferential involvement of the middle cerebral artery (MCA) and its branches. The posterior circulation and even the spinal cord could also be involved.[32]

Modern studies document that patients with meningovascular neurosyphilis may have prodromal symptoms, including headaches, seizures, and personality changes, sometimes lasting for years before stroke onset.[33–35] However, 50% to 70% of patients present solely with stroke, most often acutely, and the underlying syphilitic etiology is often initially missed.[35]

Pathogenesis

Two forms of vasculitis occur in neurosyphilis.[31] Heubner arteritis affects large- or medium-sized cerebral arteries with infiltration primarily of the adventitia by lymphocytes and plasma cells, but sometimes also the media and intima, and there may be occlusion of the vasa vasorum. Fibroblast proliferation thickens the intima. With progression, there is medial necrosis and replacement by connective tissue. Nissl-Alzheimer endarteritis affects small cerebral vessels with endothelial and adventitial proliferation that leads to obliteration of the vessel lumen. This is not accompanied by inflammation.

Diagnosis

The diagnosis of uncomplicated syphilis relies on reactivity of serological tests, including nontreponemal or lipoidal, such as the rapid plasma reagin (RPR) or Venereal Disease Research Laboratory (VDRL) tests, with confirmation by treponemal tests, such as enzyme immunoassays using recombinant T pallidum antigens, or the T pallidum particle agglutination test or the fluorescent treponemal antibody absorption (FTA-ABS) test (reviewed in ref[36]).

There is no perfect test for diagnosis of neurosyphilis. A reactive CSF-VDRL rules in neurosyphilis with a high degree of certainty, but a nonreactive test does not exclude the diagnosis, particularly in early neurosyphilis. In such instances, reliance is made on identification of CSF pleocytosis.[37] In PLWH, CSF pleocytosis due to HIV itself may be seen, especially in those with peripheral blood CD4+ T-cell concentrations greater than 200/μL or in those with detectable plasma HIV RNA,[38] which can complicate neurosyphilis diagnosis. Although some algorithms rely on a nonreactive CSF treponemal test, such as the FTA-ABS test, in such situations to exclude a diagnosis of neurosyphilis, this is likely not appropriate for diagnosis of symptomatic forms of the disease.[39]

In the series by Merritt,[31] the CSF white blood cell count was greater than 10/μL in 63% and the CSF Wassermann (the predecessor of the CSF-VDRL) was reactive in 81%. Because there is no single diagnostic test for neurosyphilis, case reports and series vary in their definitions of neurosyphilis. As such, it is hard to determine with certainty how often patients with meningovascular syphilis have a reactive CSF-VDRL.

Neuroradiographic findings in neurosyphilis are recently reviewed.[40] In meningovascular neurosyphilis, brain computed tomographic and magnetic resonance scans show multiple areas of infarction, consistent with diffuse intracranial vasculitis. Angiographic findings include segmental arterial narrowing, focal narrowing, and dilatation and occlusion. The angiographic appearance may resemble spasm associated with subarachnoid hemorrhage or other infectious or noninfectious vasculitis.

Treatment

Penicillin is the recommended treatment for neurosyphilis, either aqueous crystalline penicillin G, 18 to 24 million units per day administered intravenously as 3 to 4 million units every four hours or 24 million units daily as a continuous infusion for 10 to 14 days; or procaine penicillin G, 2.4 million units intramuscularly per day, plus probenecid 500 mg orally four times a day, both for 10 to 14 days.[37] These recommendations are not based on large, controlled, randomized, trials, but their efficacy is supported by long-term clinical experience. Although also not supported by large, controlled, randomized trials, a potential alternative regimen is ceftriaxone 2 g intramuscularly or intravenously daily for 10 to 14 days based on a small randomized trial in PLWH[41] and a larger retrospective study in PLWH and individuals without HIV.[42]

Clinical Vignette

A 46-year-old man living with HIV complained of headache and photophobia of 2 months duration. Serum RPR was reactive with a titer of 1:1024. Neurologic examination was unremarkable. CSF showed 187 WBCs (95% lymphocytes) and protein 125 mg/dL. CSF-VDRL was reactive with a titer of 1:32. He began treatment with intramuscular or intramuscularly (IM) procaine penicillin G and oral probenecid for syphilitic meningitis, and he restarted his HIV medications. His symptoms improved. However, on day 5 of treatment, he was reevaluated because of recurrent headache, dizziness, diplopia, and memory loss. Neurologic examination was notable for impaired recall and ataxia. Neuroimaging showed punctate infarcts in the right MCA distribution and in the anterior-middle cerebral arteries border zone and stenoses in bilateral terminal carotid artery and MCAs (Fig. 2). Based on history, CSF abnormalities and neuroimaging findings, he was diagnosed with meningovascular syphilis. The relationship of meningovascular disease with initiation of treatment for meningeal neurosyphilis and HIV is the topic of a case report.[43]

DELAYED CEREBRAL VASCULOPATHY AFTER SUCCESSFUL TREATMENT OF ACUTE BACTERIAL MENINGITIS
Background

Stroke may occur in individuals with acute bacterial meningitis. It is most common with pneumococcal meningitis, but it may occur with other etiologies.[4] Stroke usually occurs within the first 7 days of infection.[4] In contrast, DCV, also called delayed cerebral thrombosis, occurs in individuals who initially recover from bacterial meningitis only to suddenly develop multiple infarcts, on average 14 days after initial presentation.[4] Death or severe disability is common. Of note, DCV has been observed only in the era of routine use of adjunctive dexamethasone for acute bacterial meningitis, and most affected individuals received adjunctive dexamethasone, although a few did not.[44] This complication may occur in 2% to 4% of individuals with pneumococcal meningitis.[45]

Clinical Findings

After initial recovery from acute bacterial meningitis, patients with DCV develop sudden clinical worsening, with fever, headache, change in mental status, focal neurologic findings, and seizures.[44,46] Onset usually occurs at about 14 days after admission, with a range of 5 to 42 days.[44,46] Repeat CSF may show persisting or recurrent inflammation, but cultures are negative. Neuroimaging shows multiple infarcts in anterior and posterior circulations. Rarely, a chronic, recurrent course is described,[47] sometimes with development of Moyamoya syndrome.[48,49] Angiographic evidence of vasculitis is often absent.

Pathophysiology

As noted above, DCV is a phenomenon seen since the routine use of adjunctive dexamethasone for acute bacterial meningitis. A review of 120 individuals with bacterial meningitis, 5 of whom developed DCV, showed that all 5 with DCV received dexamethasone compared with 35% of those who did not develop DCV, a difference that was statistically significant.[50]

Many theories have been advanced to explain the relationship between DCV and dexamethasone use. Chief among these are that high-dose glucocorticoids could "tip the balance" toward

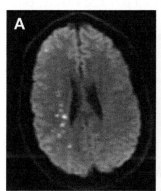
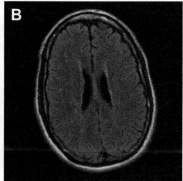
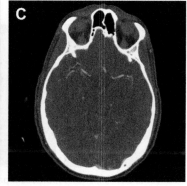

Fig. 2. Axial diffusion-weighted image (DWI) (*A*) shows multiple foci of diffusion restriction within the right MCA territory and right MCA–anterior cerebral artery (ACA) borderzone distribution, with corresponding hyperintensity on axial T2-fluid-attenuated inversion recovery (FLAIR) (*B*). Axial CTA source image (*C*) shows stenosis of the right greater than left carotid terminus and proximal M1 MCA. (*Courtesy* © 2023 Christina M. Mara.)

coagulation and platelet aggregation[44] that the abrupt discontinuation of dexamethasone after the recommended short course leads to rebound inflammation,[44] or that there is an immune response to vessels themselves.[49]

An autopsy study[45] showed no difference in meningeal artery inflammation and arterial thrombosis between individuals with pneumococcal meningitis who did ($n = 4$) and did not ($n = 8$) have DCV, but two of the individuals with DCV had infectious basilar artery aneurysms. Pneumococcal capsule was identified in meninges of both groups, even in an individual who underwent autopsy 35 days after presentation. The investigators concluded that there was a persistent pro-inflammatory response in pneumococcal meningitis. The same research group previously showed that variation in the complement factor 5 gene affects disease course in pneumococcal meningitis.[51] One way to tie the data and hypotheses together is to postulate that ongoing CNS inflammation leads to DCV in individuals with a genetic predisposition, such as those with a particular single nucleotide polymorphism in the C5 gene.

Diagnosis

For this discussion, I have referred to studies that define DCV as onset of multiple strokes in individuals who initially recovered from acute bacterial meningitis because it is the most common and the most rigorous definition. In all instances, repeat CSF cultures at the time of DCV diagnosis were negative. Other diagnostic criteria have been used. In a retrospective series from Spain,[52] DCV in individuals with pneumococcal meningitis was defined as (1) clinical worsening after 72 hours post-admission with new onset of fever, or neurologic symptoms, or both, without an alternative diagnosis; or (2) lack of improvement after 72 hours of adequate antimicrobial and corticosteroid treatment without

an alternative diagnosis. The certainty of diagnosis was based on pathology or brain imaging or vessel imaging. One hundred sixty-two episodes of pneumococcal meningitis were identified, and 17 (10.5%) individuals had DCV, with onset a median of 7 days after admission.[52] This finding suggests that the development of cerebral ischemia after diagnosis and initiation of treatment of pneumococcal meningitis is relatively common, although a biphasic course with improvement followed by abrupt worsening may not be seen.

Treatment

There is no consensus treatment for DCV. Most patients are treated with antibiotics until repeat CSF cultures are proven negative and high-dose steroids.[44,46] A longer initial course of dexamethasone for acute bacterial meningitis or a tapering course have been suggested as methods to avoid DCV, but the benefit of these approaches is unproven. Given that DCV is uncommon, and the benefit of dexamethasone in acute pneumococcal meningitis, dexamethasone should not be withheld because of concern for DCV.[46]

Clinical Vignette

A 70-year-old man was air lifted to our hospital because of concern for stroke. Brain MR imaging and computed tomography angiography (CTA) of the brain did not show abnormalities consistent with stroke. Shortly after admission the patient became obtunded with respiratory failure. CSF showed 875 WBCs/μL (77% neutrophils), glucose concentration less than 10 mg/dL, and protein concentration 1480 mg/dL. Gram stain showed gram positive cocci and culture grew pan-sensitive *Streptococcus pneumoniae*. Because he did not improve clinically, on hospital day 3 (brain MR imaging) and 4 (CTA brain), he underwent neuroimaging that showed punctate infarcts, diffuse

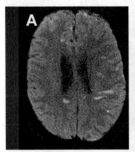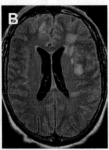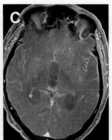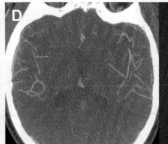

Fig. 3. Axial DWI (*A*) shows multifocal parenchymal diffusion restriction representing acute ischemic lesions, and multifocal sulcal DWI abnormality, representing leptomeningitis. Similar pattern of corresponding signal abnormality is seen on T2-FLAIR (*B*). Axial T1-weighted post-contrast imaging (*C*) shows extensive leptomeningitis. Axial CTA image (*D*) shows multifocal narrowing, most pronounced involving the left MCA M2 and M3 branches (blue *arrows*). (*Courtesy* © 2023 Christina M. Mara.)

leptomeningitis, and multifocal vascular narrowing (Fig. 3). Despite clearance of infection and treatment with high-dose corticosteroids, his course over the ensuing month was complicated by repeated infarcts. Although this patient does not meet the strict criteria for DCV, he does meet the criteria for that entity described in the Spanish series, and his course may be more characteristic of what an average clinician may see.

SUMMARY

Stroke can accompany many CNS infections, but only a few etiologies present with stroke without other evidence of CNS infection. Chief among these are VZV and *T pallidum*, the cause of syphilis; a high index of suspicion is required to not miss these diagnoses. Treatment with adjunctive dexamethasone is recommended for individuals with acute pneumococcal meningitis. However, in the era of this treatment a new syndrome, DCV (also termed delayed cerebral thrombosis) has emerged as a complication of adjunctive dexamethasone treatment.

CLINICS CARE POINTS

- Stroke is a complication of many central nervous system (CNS) infections, including acute bacterial meningitis and tuberculous, cryptococcal, and coccidioidal meningitis. *Aspergillus* species and the agents responsible for mucormycosis are angioinvasive.

- Only a few CNS infections present with stroke without other symptoms or signs of CNS infection, chiefly varicella zoster virus (VZV) and *T pallidum*.

- VZV vasculopathy occurs in immunocompetent and immunocompromised individuals, leading to transient ischemic attacks, or focal or multifocal infarcts.

- In about half of adults with VZV vasculopathy, there is no history of a shingles rash.

- In VZV vasculopathy in adults, small cerebral vessels or a combination of small and large cerebral vessels are involved, whereas in children with VZV vasculopathy, large cerebral vessels are more involved.

- Fifty to seventy percent of patients with meningovascular syphilis present solely with stroke, most often acutely, and the underlying syphilitic etiology is often initially missed.

- Delayed cerebral vasculopathy (DCV) occurs most commonly in individuals with acute pneumococcal meningitis.

- DCV is more common in individuals, who are treated with adjunctive dexamethasone, but this remains an uncommon complication, and the early benefits of dexamethasone continue to justify its use.

DISCLOSURE

The author reports no disclosures relevant to this work.

REFERENCES

1. Shulman JG, Cervantes-Arslanian AM. Infectious etiologies of stroke. Semin Neurol 2019;39(4):482–94.
2. Chow FC, Marra CM, Cho TA. Cerebrovascular disease in central nervous system infections. Semin Neurol 2011;31(3):286–306.
3. Pagliano P, Spera AM, Ascione T, et al. Infections causing stroke or stroke-like syndromes. Infection 2020;48(3):323–32.
4. Beuker C, Werring N, Bonberg N, et al. Stroke in patients with bacterial meningitis: a cohort study and meta-analysis. Ann Neurol 2023;93(6):1094–105.
5. Sy MCC, Espiritu AI, Pascual JLRt. Global frequency and clinical features of stroke in patients with tuberculous meningitis: a systematic review. JAMA Netw Open 2022;5(9):e2229282.
6. Vela-Duarte D, Nyberg E, Sillau S, et al. Lacunar stroke in cryptococcal meningitis: clinical and radiographic features. J Stroke Cerebrovasc Dis 2019; 28(6):1767–72.
7. Thompson GR 3rd, Blair JE, Wang S, et al. Adjunctive corticosteroid therapy in the treatment of coccidioidal meningitis. Clin Infect Dis 2017;65(2): 338–41.
8. Kleinschmidt-DeMasters BK. Central nervous system aspergillosis: a 20-year retrospective series. Hum Pathol 2002;33(1):116–24.
9. Ramachandran D, Aravind R, Panicker P, et al. The mucormycosis and stroke: the learning curve during the second COVID-19 pandemic. J Stroke Cerebrovasc Dis 2023;32(2):106819.
10. Gilden DH, Nagel M. Stroke caused by human immunodeficiency virus-associated vasculopathy? Arch Neurol 2007;64(5):763 [author reply: 763].
11. Gilden DH, Kleinschmidt-DeMasters BK, Wellish M, et al. Varicella zoster virus, a cause of waxing and waning vasculitis: the New England Journal of Medicine case 5-1995 revisited. Neurology 1996;47(6): 1441–6.
12. Amlie-Lefond C, Gilden D. Varicella zoster virus: a common cause of stroke in children and adults. J Stroke Cerebrovasc Dis 2016;25(7):1561–9.
13. Liberman AL, Nagel MA, Hurley MC, et al. Rapid development of 9 cerebral aneurysms in varicella-

zoster virus vasculopathy. Neurology 2014;82(23): 2139–41.

14. Gonzalez-Suarez I, Fuentes-Gimeno B, Ruiz-Ares G, et al. Varicella-zoster virus vasculopathy. A review description of a new case with multifocal brain hemorrhage. J Neurol Sci 2014;338(1–2):34–8.

15. Kumar S, Pillai SV. Moyamoya syndrome as a manifestation of varicella-associated cerebral vasculopathy-case report and review of literature. Childs Nerv Syst 2019;35(4):601–6.

16. Gilbert GJ. Herpes zoster ophthalmicus and delayed contralateral hemiparesis. Relationship of the syndrome to central nervous system granulomatous angiitis. JAMA 1974;229(3):302–4.

17. Walker RJ 3rd, el-Gammal T, Allen MB Jr. Cranial arteritis associated with herpes zoster. Case report with angiographic findings. Radiology 1973;107(1): 109–10.

18. Eidelberg D, Sotrel A, Horoupian DS, et al. Thrombotic cerebral vasculopathy associated with herpes zoster. Ann Neurol 1986;19(1):7–14.

19. Nagel MA, Bubak AN. Varicella zoster virus vasculopathy. J Infect Dis 2018;218(suppl_2):S107–12.

20. Eleftheriou D, Moraitis E, Hong Y, et al. Microparticle-mediated VZV propagation and endothelial activation: Mechanism of VZV vasculopathy. Neurology 2020;94(5):e474–80.

21. Bubak AN, Como CN, Hassell JE Jr. et al. Targeted RNA sequencing of VZV-infected brain vascular adventitial fibroblasts indicates that amyloid may be involved in VZV vasculopathy, Neurol Neuroimmunol Neuroinflamm, 9 (1), 2021:e1103.

22. Bubak AN, Beseler C, Como CN, et al. Amylin, Abeta42, and amyloid in varicella zoster virus vasculopathy cerebrospinal fluid and infected vascular cells. J Infect Dis 2021;223(7):1284–94.

23. Shah J, Poonawala H, Keay SK, et al. Varicella-zoster virus vasculopathy: a case report demonstrating vasculitis using black-blood MRI. J Neurol Neurophysiol 2015;6(6):1000342.

24. Yawn BP, Lindsay AC, Yousefi M, et al. Risk of, and risk factors for, vasculopathy associated with acute herpes zoster. J Stroke Cerebrovasc Dis 2023; 32(2):106891.

25. Gilden D, Cohrs RJ, Mahalingam R, et al. Varicella zoster virus vasculopathies: diverse clinical manifestations, laboratory features, pathogenesis, and treatment. Lancet Neurol 2009;8(8):731–40.

26. Centers for Disease Control and Prevention. Sexually Transmitted Disease Surveillance, 2021. Available at: https://www.cdc.gov/std/statistics/2021/default.htm. Published 2023. Accessed April 23, 2023.

27. Du M, Yan W, Jing W, et al. Increasing incidence rates of sexually transmitted infections from 2010 to 2019: an analysis of temporal trends by geographical regions and age groups from the 2019 Global Burden of Disease Study. BMC Infect Dis 2022;22(1):574.

28. Burghardt NO, Nelson LN, Tang EC, et al. Neurosyphilis surveillance: exploring the use of multiple data sources to better understand morbidity in california. Sex Transm Dis 2021;48(8S):S11–3.

29. Ghanem KG, Moore RD, Rompalo AM, et al. Neurosyphilis in a clinical cohort of HIV-1-infected patients. Aids 2008;22(10):1145–51.

30. Marra CM, Sahi SK, Tantalo LC, et al. Toll-like receptor polymorphisms are associated with increased neurosyphilis risk. Sex Transm Dis 2014;41(7):440–6.

31. Merritt HH, Adams RD, Solomon HC. Neurosyphilis. New York: Oxford; 1946.

32. Adams RD, Merritt HH. Meningeal and vascular syphilis of the spinal cord. Medicine (Baltim) 1944; 23:181–214.

33. Ahbeddou N, El Alaoui Taoussi K, Ibrahimi A, et al. Stroke and syphilis: a retrospective study of 53 patients. Paris): Rev Neurol; 2018.

34. Aziouaz F, Mabrouki FZ, Chraa M, et al. Analysis of fourteen new cases of meningovascular syphilis: renewed interest in an old problem. Cureus 2021; 13(8):e16951.

35. Liu LL, Zheng WH, Tong ML, et al. Ischemic stroke as a primary symptom of neurosyphilis among HIV-negative emergency patients. J Neurol Sci 2012; 317(1–2):35–9.

36. Ramchandani MS, Cannon CA, Marra CM. Syphilis: a modern resurgence. Infect Dis Clin 2023;37(2): 195–222.

37. Workowski KA, Bachmann LH, Chan PA, et al. Sexually transmitted infections treatment guidelines, 2021. MMWR Recomm Rep (Morb Mortal Wkly Rep) 2021;70(4):1–187.

38. Marra CM, Maxwell CL, Collier AC, et al. Interpreting cerebrospinal fluid pleocytosis in HIV in the era of potent antiretroviral therapy. BMC Infect Dis 2007; 7:37.

39. Harding AS, Ghanem KG. The performance of cerebrospinal fluid treponemal-specific antibody tests in neurosyphilis: a systematic review. Sex Transm Dis 2012;39(4):291–7.

40. Correa DG, de Souza SR, Freddi TAL, et al. Imaging features of neurosyphilis. J Neuroradiol 2023;50(2): 241–52.

41. Marra CM, Boutin P, McArthur JC, et al. A pilot study evaluating ceftriaxone and penicillin G as treatment agents for neurosyphilis in human immunodeficiency virus-infected individuals. Clin Infect Dis 2000;30(3):540–4.

42. Bettuzzi T, Jourdes A, Robineau O, et al. Ceftriaxone compared with benzylpenicillin in the treatment of neurosyphilis in France: a retrospective multicentre study. Lancet Infect Dis 2021;21(10):1441–7.

43. Bucher JB, Golden MR, Heald AE, et al. Stroke in a patient with human immunodeficiency virus and syphilis treated with penicillin and antiretroviral therapy. Sex Transm Dis 2011;38(5):442–4.

44. Schut ES, Brouwer MC, de Gans J, et al. Delayed cerebral thrombosis after initial good recovery from pneumococcal meningitis. Neurology 2009;73(23):1988–95.

45. Engelen-Lee JY, Brouwer MC, Aronica E, et al. Delayed cerebral thrombosis complicating pneumococcal meningitis: an autopsy study. Ann Intensive Care 2018;8(1):20.

46. Lucas MJ, Brouwer MC, van de Beek D. Delayed cerebral thrombosis in bacterial meningitis: a prospective cohort study. Intensive Care Med 2013;39(5):866–71.

47. Kim HK, Jang Y, Seo T, et al. Chronic recurrent delayed cerebral vasculopathy after pneumococcal meningitis, *Acta Neurol Belg*, 2022, Online ahead of print.

48. Dou Z, Chen H, Cheng H, et al. Moyamoya syndrome after bacterial meningitis. Pediatr Investig 2018;2(2):134–6.

49. Czartoski T, Hallam D, Lacy JM, et al. Postinfectious vasculopathy with evolution to Moyamoya syndrome. J Neurol Neurosurg Psychiatr 2005;76(2):256–9.

50. Gallegos C, Tobolowsky F, Nigo M, et al. Delayed cerebral injury in adults with bacterial meningitis: a novel complication of adjunctive steroids? Crit Care Med 2018;46(8):e811–4.

51. Woehrl B, Brouwer MC, Murr C, et al. Complement component 5 contributes to poor disease outcome in humans and mice with pneumococcal meningitis. J Clin Investig 2011;121(10):3943–53.

52. Boix-Palop L, Fernandez T, Pelegrin I, et al. Delayed cerebral vasculopathy in pneumococcal meningitis: epidemiology and clinical outcome. a cohort study. Int J Infect Dis 2020;97:283–9.

Treatment of Primary Angiitis of the Central Nervous System

Alison M. Bays, MD, MPH&TM

KEYWORDS

- CNS vasculitis • Cyclophosphamide • Primary angiitis

KEY POINTS

- Diagnosis for PCNSV should include angiography and brain biopsy
- Induction therapy for PCNSV often includes steroids and cyclophosphamide.
- Maintenance therapy should be considered in all patients; azathioprine is the most often used for maintenance.
- Rituximab and mycophenolate mofetil may be good alternatives in patients who do not respond to initial therapy or those with relapse.

INTRODUCTION

Primary central nervous system vasculitis (PCNSV) is an autoimmune disease resulting in the inflammation of the blood vessels, limited to the brain and spinal cord. It was first described in the 1950s, with some case reports dating back to 1922.[1,2] Calabrese and Mallek first proposed criteria for PCNSV in 1988 that included all three of the following: an otherwise unexplained neurologic deficit, angiographic or histopathological features consistent with PCNSV and lack of systemic vasculitis or other explanation for the findings.[3] PCNSV does not include central nervous system (CNS) involvement of other systemic vasculitides, such as Behçet's Disease. These proposed criteria were not validated due to disease rarity.

The average age of onset of PCNSV is 50 years old and it affects men and women equally.[4,5] The most common symptoms are headache and cognitive dysfunction, while some have hemiparesis and persistent neurologic deficit or stroke.[4] Diagnosis is made primarily on the basis of brain biopsy and angiography and may be supported by lumbar puncture and MRI. Brain biopsy is important not only to confirm the diagnosis, but to rule out other entities such as intravascular lymphoma.

A lumbar puncture is frequently done to aid in the diagnosis. More than 90% of patients have an abnormal spinal fluid analysis, with increased leukocytes over 5/mm^3, and elevated total protein over 0.5 g/dl.[4,6] Acute phase reactants such as erythrocyte sedimentation rate and C-reactive protein as well as anti-nuclear antibodies and anti-cytoplasmic nuclear antibodies (ANCA) are most often normal or negative.

There are two major subsets of PCNSV by vessel size (Table 1). The "small vessel" disease subset tends to be positive by biopsy but angiography is often negative. Biopsy can be characterized as granulomatous, lymphocytic, or necrotizing. This group includes patients diagnosed with Aß-related angiitis (ABRA). Patients may have leptomeningeal enhancement on MRI and typically there are no cerebral infarcts. These patients often respond well to initial therapy, but may be at higher risk of relapse according to the French COVAC cohort.[6]

The "large vessel" disease subset includes the larger vessels with more proximal disease. It is positive on angiography with cerebral infarcts, often bilaterally. Biopsy is frequently negative. Some of these patients may have a more rapidly progressive disease course and may have poor initial response to induction therapy.[4]

Medicine Department, University of Washington, MS 359860, 325 9th Avenue, Seattle, WA 98104, USA
E-mail address: alisonmb@uw.edu

Neuroimag Clin N Am 34 (2024) 23–29
https://doi.org/10.1016/j.nic.2023.07.008
1052-5149/24/© 2023 Elsevier Inc. All rights reserved.

Table 1
Differentiation of PCNSV by vessel size[4,12]

	Small Vessel Disease	Large Vessel Disease
Angiogram	Intracranial artery involvement or smaller vessel involvement. Angiography may be negative.	Intracranial internal carotid artery, vertebral artery, basilar artery, proximal anterior/middle/posterior cerebral arteries
MRI	May have leptomeningeal enhancement	No leptomeningeal enhancement
Brain biopsy, spinal cord biopsy	Biopsy often positive. May have ABRA	Biopsy may be negative
Infarcts	No infarcts	Infarcts, often bilateral
Disease course	Slowly progressive	Rapidly progressive
Response to treatment – induction	Better initial response to induction therapy	Poor response to induction therapy
Maintenance	Not always started on maintenance therapy	Often started on maintenance therapy
Relapse	Higher risk of relapse	May have lower risk of relapse

Abbreviations: ABRA, Aß-related angiitis; PCVNS, primary central nervous system vasculitis.

Due to the rarity of the disease, there are no randomized clinical trials for management of PCNSV. There are two phases of treatment, induction and maintenance. The modified Rankin scale (mRS) is a seven level measure used as an outcome in acute stroke trials has also been used to assess response to therapy.[7] Non-response is often defined by the lack of response after 6 months of treatment. Relapse has been defined by the worsening of prior symptoms or new neurologic symptoms after a period of inactive disease while the patient was on no medication or on a stable dose.[8,9] Long-term remission is the 1 year absence of manifestations of active PCNSV after the discontinuation of therapy.[8]

TREATMENT STRATEGIES

Treatment can be divided into induction and maintenance therapy (Fig. 1). Induction therapy may be more aggressive with high-dose IV steroids in patients deemed high risk or with a more aggressive disease course. Patients with large vessel disease often have worse response to induction therapy and should potentially be treated with IV glucocorticoids (GC) and cyclophosphamide (CYC). Cyclophosphamide for induction therapy for PCNSV was used in 45% of patients in the Mayo clinic cohort, 48% of patients in the All India Institute of Medical Sciences (AIIMS) cohort, 75% of a German cohort and 79% of the French COVAC cohort.[4,10–12]

An international survey of current practices surveying 185 physicians in Europe and Canada, reported that a combination of CYC and GC were the most frequently used induction medications with 84% of participants using this regimen in at least half of their patients. More than 75% of participants never used oral immunosuppressants such as azathioprine (AZA), mycophenolate mofetil (MMF) or methotrexate (MTX) for induction.[13]

Patients who fail induction therapy should be tried on another medication. There is some evidence for rituximab in patients who fail cyclophosphamide therapy or have contraindications to cyclophosphamide.[14] MMF has also been shown to have high rates of response when used as induction therapy.[15]

After induction therapy, maintenance therapy should be considered. In the past, not all patients were started on maintenance therapy, particularly those with small vessel disease who were thought to be less at risk of severe disease. There is growing evidence that maintenance therapy should be considered in all patients.[6] Maintenance was found to be associated with better long-term outcomes with respect to death and disability as well as lower relapse rates and should be considered in all patients regardless of disease severity.[8] Maintenance therapy is started at a median of 4 months after induction and the duration is approximately 24 months.[12] Medications for maintenance therapy varied widely but the most frequently used medication was AZA in the COVAC, Mayo and AIIMS cohorts.[4,6,10]

Relapse is common in PCNSV, with relapse rates of 12% in the AIIMS cohort, 30% in the Mayo clinic cohort, 34% in the COVAC cohort and 59% in the German cohort.[4,10–12] Relapses have been shown

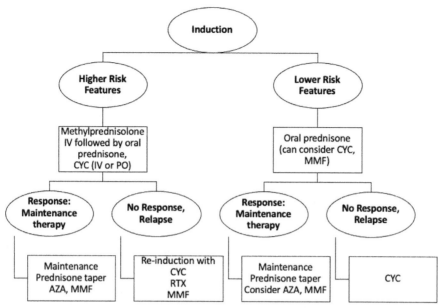

Fig. 1. Induction & maintenance therapy algorithm.

to occur up to 6 years after diagnosis.[11] Risk factors for relapse are contradictory, which may be due to differences in the cohorts or treatment strategies. Patients with seizures or meningeal enhancement at diagnosis were more likely to relapse in one study, though other studies have not confirmed these findings.[9] Higher relapse rates may also be seen in male patients.[11] Necrotizing and granulomatous patterns on brain biopsy may be associated with a worse course and higher likelihood of fatal outcome.[4] Patients treated with steroids alone or at lower steroid doses may be at higher risk of relapse.[4,11] Almost all patients who relapse were also given an increase in steroid dose in response to the relapse.[12] The overall median length of treatment time is longer in those with relapse compared to those without relapse (18 months vs 9 months).[4]

TREATMENT
Glucocorticoids

Steroids are prescribed for almost all patients. For more severe cases or those with high-risk features, methylprednisolone at a dose of 1000 mg intravenous (IV) is given daily for three to 5 days. Oral prednisone dose is started at 1 mg/kg/day, with a median dose of 60 mg per day and a maximum dose of 80 mg per day.[16] Steroids are tapered over time and a maintenance agent is often added. In some cases, especially with small artery vasculitis, steroids are historically the only treatment given, though it is now more common to use along with other immunosuppressants. The median length of prednisone therapy is

9 months in some groups and up to 24 months in other groups.[4,6] Increases in steroid doses are given with disease flares. Consideration for bone protective measures is important considering the bone loss effects of corticosteroids.[17]

Cyclophosphamide

Cyclophosphamide is an alkylating agent frequently used for the induction of PCNSV. Oral or IV administration can be used for induction, though there are no randomized trials comparing the two, and in one retrospective study, oral and IV cyclophosphamide induction therapies were equally effective in inducing remission.[8] Oral cyclophosphamide has been shown to result in less relapses in ANCA vasculitis,[18] however, for PCNSV, IV pulses are more often used in the literature than oral therapy,[12] and result in a lower lifetime cumulative cyclophosphamide dose. For ANCA vasculitis, the ACR clinical practice guidelines recommend up to 2 mg/kg/day orally for 3 to 6 months for induction or 15 mg/kg IV cyclophosphamide every 2 weeks for 3 doses followed by 15 mg/kg IV every 3 weeks for at least 3 doses.[16] Mesna is sometimes used for uroprotection but studies have not supported its use.[19]

Side effects include neutropenia, hemorrhagic cystitis, primary ovarian insufficiency, and bladder cancer. The risk of complications increases as the lifetime cumulative dose increases.[19] To prevent primary ovarian insufficiency, monthly gonadotropin-releasing hormone is recommended, such as leuprolide, in pre-menopausal women. Fertility preservation with sperm cryopreservation is recommended in men.[20]

Mycophenolate Mofetil and Mycophenolic Acid

MMF and MPA are medications used for maintenance therapy in many autoimmune diseases and induction in some diseases such as lupus nephritis. Though historically CYC has frequently been used as an induction agent, MMF is a reasonable alternative choice for induction as well as maintenance. Two recent studies have shown that MMF may be comparable or have better outcomes as an induction agent than CYC. The first was a retrospective cohort that compared the use of MMF to those treated with steroids and CYC; there was a trend toward a favorable response with MMF.[21] Additionally, a recent prospective study assessed MMF as both an induction and maintenance therapy in 26 patients and found that 96% of patients had a good clinical response to induction therapy with MMF. These patients were treated with 1g daily in two divided doses followed by 2 g daily for a minimum of 2 years with 12 months of follow up.[15] ACR clinical practice guidelines for ANCA vasculitis recommend up to 1500 mg oral twice per day.[16]

Side effects include gastrointestinal upset; MPA is coated and can be used when MMF is not tolerated. Bloodwork should be monitored for cytopenias as well as elevations in liver enzymes.

Azathioprine

Azathioprine is a purine antimetabolite that is commonly used as a maintenance therapy for a variety of autoimmune diseases. Azathioprine is the most often used medication for maintenance therapy.[8,12] ACR clinical practice guidelines for ANCA vasculitis recommend up to 2 mg/kg/day of azathioprine.[16] It is often started at 50 mg daily. Prior to starting azathioprine, a Thiopurine S-methyltransferase (TPMT) level should be obtained. Azathioprine should not be started in patients with a TMPT deficiency. Bloodwork should be monitored for liver abnormalities and cytopenias. Side effects include nausea and diarrhea. There is a seven-fold increase in myeloid neoplasm in patients exposed to azathioprine.[22]

Methotrexate

There is not much evidence in the literature for the use of methotrexate as a maintenance agent. However, it is used in clinical practice, though less commonly than AZA or MMF. Methotrexate can be used via oral or subcutaneous routes at a dose up to 25 mg per week.[16] Daily folic acid of 1 mg should be used to prevent side effects. Hepatotoxicity may occur with methotrexate and for that reason, administration is typically restricted to those patients without baseline liver disease and with normal liver enzymes.[23] Patients should be advised to limit alcohol intake. Side effects include GI upset, hair loss, and oral ulcers. After the initiation of methotrexate, labs including a complete blood count, liver transaminase levels and serum creatinine should be checked every 2 to 4 weeks after initiation for the first 3 months. For the following 3 to 6 months, it should be checked every 8 to 12 weeks. After the initial period, it can be checked every 6 months.[24]

Rituximab

Rituximab (RTX) is an anti-CD20 monoclonal antibody that has been successfully used in the treatment of ANCA vasculitides. American College of Rheumatology (ACR) clinical practice guidelines for ANCA vasculitis recommend 375 mg/m^2 IV weekly for 4 doses or 1000 mg on days 1 and 15 for induction.[16] For maintenance, doses of 500 mg IV every 6 months or 1000 g every 4 months have been used. One group published their findings on patient response to rituximab in six patients with PCNSV refractory to other immunosuppressive agents, showing that five out of six patients favorably responding to rituximab with the reduction in flares.[14] The AIIMS cohort used rituximab in 8.5% of their patients and did not find significant differences between treatment modality and outcome.[10] There is not as much evidence to use rituximab first-line for induction as there is for cyclophosphamide but it should be considered if patients fail first line therapy with cyclophosphamide, they have contraindications to cyclophosphamide or if there is disease relapse.

Major side effects include infusion reactions. Methylprednisolone 125 mg IV prior to the infusion is often used to reduce the chance of side effects. Patients should be monitored for neutropenia. Rituximab may increase the risk of hepatitis B reactivation and progressive multifocal encephalopathy.[25] Some patients on rituximab may develop hypogammaglobulinemia. If they have hypogammaglobulinemia and recurrent severe infections, immunoglobulin supplementation at replacement doses of 400 to 800 mg/kg/month should be considered.[16]

Anti-tumor Necrosis Factor Agents

Medications in the anti-TNF family include infliximab, adalimumab, etanercept, golimumab and certolizumab. There is limited data on using anti-TNF agents to treat PCNSV and it is not used for induction or maintenance as a first line of therapy.[26] There is a case report of two patients who were treated with anti-TNF therapy after failing other agents. One was treated with one dose of infliximab at 5 mg/kg and one was treated with etanercept 25 mg twice weekly for 20 months followed by 25 mg once weekly for 8 months.[27]

TNF inhibitors should be used with caution in patients with heart failure due to a black box warning. TNF inhibitors increase the risk of tuberculosis and screening is recommended prior to initiation.[24]

OTHER TREATMENT CONSIDERATIONS
Infectious Disease Testing

Prior to initiating therapy for other diseases, ACR clinical practice guidelines recommend testing all patients for infectious diseases, including Hepatitis B, hepatitis C, human immunodeficiency virus, and tuberculosis.[24]

Additional Therapy

Treatment with aspirin should be considered. Aspirin may be positively associated with long-term remission and there was no significant increase in the frequency of intracranial hemorrhage in patients treated with aspirin.[8] Aspirin use was not reported in all of the cohorts but published data shows aspirin use ranging from 15% of patients in the German cohort to 54% of the COVAC cohort.[11,12]

Prophylaxis

Prophylaxis to *P jiroveci* pneumonia is frequently incorporated in patients on cyclophosphamide with steroid therapy. It is also often given in patients on rituximab up to 6 months after the last dose of rituximab. It is sometimes included for patients on azathioprine and mycophenolate who are also on 20 mg or higher of prednisone.[16]

Vaccinations

Vaccination is important for patients on immunosuppression and should include influenza, pneumococcal, and zoster vaccinations. Live vaccines are typically not recommended in patients on immunosuppression. The ideal time for vaccination is prior to immunosuppression initiation, however this is not always practical. High-dose influenza vaccination is recommended over regular dose influenza vaccination and should still be given if the patient is on doses of prednisone 20 mg or more. Methotrexate should be held for 2 weeks after influenza vaccination if patient is at low risk of disease flare, while all other immunosuppression should be continued after vaccination. Other vaccines should be deferred until patients are on less than 20 mg of prednisone. Pneumococcal vaccination is strongly recommended for patients under 65 on immunosuppressive medications. Other vaccines to consider include human papilloma virus, hepatitis B, and COVID-19.[28]

Prior to rituximab, patients should get their vaccinations as they will not respond to vaccinations once rituximab therapy is started. If a patient is already on rituximab, vaccinations should be administered immediately before the next regularly scheduled dose of rituximab then rituximab should be delayed for next 2 weeks, if acceptablegiven the patient's disease activity. The influenza vaccine is the exception, which should be given on schedule, regardless of the last dose of rituximab.[24,28]

Pregnancy and Childbirth

For patients who are planning pregnancy, many medications are contraindicated. Azathioprine and prednisone are the only medications frequently used during pregnancy. Prednisone is known to be associated with low birth weight and an increased risk of pre-term delivery. In pregnancy, glucocorticoids should be tapered to 10 mg or less during pregnancy if clinically acceptable and adding a glucocorticoid sparing agent if necessary. For delivery, stress dose steroids are not necessary during a vaginal delivery but may be recommended for surgical (cesarean) delivery.[20]

It is recommended to taper prednisone to less than 20 mg per day prior to and during pregnancy. While breastfeeding, if the dose is higher than 20 mg, it is recommended to delay breastfeeding for 4 hours after taking the prednisone dose. Azathioprine is considered safe in women preconception, during pregnancy and has low transfer during breastfeeding. It can also be continued in men who are fathering a child.[20]

Cyclophosphamide, MMF/MPA and methotrexate are known teratogens and not compatible with pre-conception, pregnancy or breastfeeding. Cyclophosphamide should be discontinued 12 weeks prior to attempted conception in both men and women and fertility preservation should be offered to both men and women. MMF and MPA should be stopped at least 6 weeks prior to conception to assess disease activity but can be continued in men considering conceiving. Methotrexate should be stopped 1 to 3 months prior to conception in women and is not compatible with pregnancy. It can be continued in men who plan to conceive.[20]

Rituximab should be discontinued at conception in women, though exceptions may be made for life or organ-threatening disease during pregnancy. During the second half of pregnancy, the fetus is at risk for having minimal B cells at delivery.[20] Infants exposed to rituximab in utero should have live vaccines delayed until they are older than 6 months of age.[28]

LONG-TERM OUTCOMES

Studies showed good functional outcomes for approximately two-thirds of patients with modified Rankin Score (mRS) 0 to 2 in 63% of the COVAC cohort, 65% of the AIIMS cohort, and 66% of the German cohort.[10–12] A lymphocytic pattern on brain biopsy was associated with a good outcome.[4] Maintenance therapy is also associated with good outcome.[6] A soluble triggering receptor located on myeloid cells, sTREM2, may be an important biomarker for the severity of PCNSV. It is found in higher levels in both CSF and serum in patients with PCNSV. Higher levels in the CSF or in the blood are predictive of a good prognosis.[29]

Factors associated with high disability scores of mRS 4 to 6 were older age, large vessel involvement, and strokes. The AIIMS cohort found that delay in diagnosis and spinal cord involvement were associated with worse outcomes.[10] The COVAC cohort showed that higher disability scores and death were associated in patients found to have ABRA.[8]

Mortality rates ranged from 8% in the COVAC cohort to 9% in the German cohort.[11,12]

A necrotizing and/or granulomatous pattern on brain biopsy may be associated with a worse course and fatal outcome.[4] Other factors associated with increased mortality include older age, large vessel disease, and cerebral infarction.[4]

CLINICS CARE POINTS

- Definitive diagnosis for PCNSV may include angiography and brain biopsy.
- Induction therapy for PCNSV often includes steroids and cyclophosphamide.
- Maintenance therapy should be considered in all patients. Azathioprine is the most often used for maintenance.
- Relapse is common, and patients with relapse are often treated with higher doses of steroids and/or a change in therapy.
- Rituximab and mycophenolate may be good alternatives in patients who do not respond to initial therapy or those with relapse.
- When treating PCNSV, considerations that should be taken into account are fertility, vaccination, bone health, and prevention of infectious diseases.

DISCLOSURE

Genentech, United States funded a vascular ultrasound conference that I helped organize, Abbvie, United States funded a research fellow.

REFERENCES

1. Cravioto H, Feigin I. Noninfectious granulomatous angiitis with a predilection for the nervous system. Neurology 1959;9(9):599–609.
2. Newman W, Wolf A. Non-infectious granulomatous angiitis involving the central nervous system. Trans Am Neurol Assoc 1952;56:114–7.
3. Calabrese LH, Mallek JA. Primary angiitis of the central nervous system: Report of 8 new cases, review of the literature, and proposal for diagnostic criteria. Med (United States) 1988;67(1):20–39.
4. Salvarani C, Brown RD, Christianson T, et al. An Update of the Mayo Clinic Cohort of Patients with Adult Primary Central Nervous System Vasculitis. Med (United States) 2015;94(21):1–15.
5. Salvarani C, Brown RD, Hunder GG. Adult primary central nervous system vasculitis. Lancet 2012; 380(9843):767–77.
6. de Boysson H, Parienti JJ, Arquizan C, et al. Maintenance therapy is associated with better long-term outcomes in adult patients with primary angiitis of the central nervous system. Rheumatol (United Kingdom) 2017;56(10):1684–93.
7. Saver JL, Chaisinanunkul N, Campbell BCV, et al. Standardized Nomenclature for Modified Rankin Scale Global Disability Outcomes: Consensus Recommendations from Stroke Therapy Academic Industry Roundtable XI. Stroke 2021;52(9):3054–62.
8. Salvarani C, Brown RD, Christianson TJH, et al. Long-term remission, relapses and maintenance therapy in adult primary central nervous system vasculitis: A single-center 35-year experience. Autoimmun Rev 2020;19(4):102497.
9. De Boysson H, Zuber M, Naggara O, et al. Primary angiitis of the central nervous system: Description of the first fifty-two adults enrolled in the french cohort of patients with primary vasculitis of the central nervous system. Arthritis Rheumatol 2014;66(5): 1315–26.
10. Agarwal A, Sharma J, Srivastava MVP, et al. Primary CNS vasculitis (PCNSV): a cohort study. Sci Rep 2022;12(1):1–8.
11. Schuster S, Ozga AK, Stellmann JP, et al. Relapse rates and long-term outcome in primary angiitis of the central nervous system. J Neurol 2019;266(6): 1481–9.
12. De Boysson H, Arquizan C, Touzé E, et al. Treatment and long-term outcomes of primary central nervous system vasculitis updated results from the French registry. Stroke 2018;49(8):1946–52.

13. Nehme A, Lanthier S, Boulanger M, et al. Diagnosis and management of adult primary angiitis of the central nervous system: an international survey on current practices. J Neurol 2022;270(4):1989–98.

14. Salvarani C, Brown RD, Muratore F, et al. Rituximab therapy for primary central nervous system vasculitis: A 6 patient experience and review of the literature. Autoimmun Rev 2019;18(4):399–405.

15. Das S, Prosad R, Debanjali G, et al. Mycophenolate mofetil as induction and maintenance immunosuppressive therapy in adult primary central nervous system vasculitis : A prospective observational study. Clin Rheumatol 2023. 0123456789.

16. Chung SA, Langford CA, Maz M, et al. American College of Rheumatology/Vasculitis Foundation Guideline for the Management of Antineutrophil Cytoplasmic Antibody–Associated Vasculitis. Arthritis Care Res 2021;73(8):1088–105.

17. Buckley L, Guyatt G, Fink HA, et al. American College of Rheumatology Guideline for the Prevention and Treatment of Glucocorticoid-Induced Osteoporosis. Arthritis Rheumatol 2017;69(8):1521–37.

18. Harper L, Morgan MD, Walsh M, et al. Pulse versus daily oral cyclophosphamide for induction of remission in ANCA-associated vasculitis: Long-term follow-up. Ann Rheum Dis 2012;71(6):955–60.

19. Yilmaz N, Emmungil H, Gucenmez S, et al. Incidence of cyclophosphamide-induced urotoxicity and protective effect of mesna in rheumatic diseases. J Rheumatol 2015;42(9):1661–6.

20. Sammaritano LR, Bermas BL, Chakravarty EE, et al. American College of Rheumatology Guideline for the Management of Reproductive Health in Rheumatic and Musculoskeletal Diseases. Arthritis Rheumatol 2020;72(4):529–56.

21. Salvarani C, Brown RD, Christianson TJH, et al. Mycophenolate mofetil in primary central nervous system vasculitis. Semin Arthritis Rheum 2015;45(1):55–9.

22. Ertz-Archambault N, Kosiorek H, Taylor GE, et al. Association of therapy for autoimmune disease with myelodysplastic syndromes and acute myeloid leukemia. JAMA Oncol 2017;3(7):936–43.

23. Fraenkel L, Bathon JM, England BR, et al. American College of Rheumatology Guideline for the Treatment of Rheumatoid Arthritis. Arthritis Care Res 2021;73(7):924–39.

24. Singh JA, Saag KG, Jr SLB, et al. American College of Rheumatology Guideline for the Treatment of Rheumatoid Arthritis. Arthritis Rheumatol 2015. https://doi.org/10.1002/acr.22783.

25. Sharma K, Tolaymat S, Yu H, et al. Progressive multifocal leukoencephalopathy in anti-CD20 and other monoclonal antibody (mAb) therapies used in multiple sclerosis: A review. J Neurol Sci 2022;443(September):120459.

26. Salvarani C, Pipitone N, Hunder GG. Management of primary and secondary central nervous system vasculitis. Curr Opin Rheumatol 2016;28(1):21–8.

27. Salvarani C, Brown RD, Calamia KT, et al. Efficacy of tumor necrosis factor α blockade in primary central nervous system vasculitis resistant to immunosuppressive treatment. Arthritis Care Res 2008;59(2):291–6.

28. Bass AR, Chakravarty E, Akl EA, et al. 2022 American College of Rheumatology Guideline for Vaccinations in Patients With Rheumatic and Musculoskeletal Diseases. Arthritis Care Res 2023;75(3):449–64.

29. Guo T, Ma J, Sun J, et al. Soluble TREM2 is a potential biomarker for the severity of primary angiitis of the CNS. Front Immunol 2022;13:1–14.

Pathology of Primary Angiitis of the Central Nervous System

Selima Siala, MD[a,*], Nabil Rahoui, MD[b], Benjamin Cho, MD[b],
Carlos A. Zamora, MD, PhD[a]

KEYWORDS

• Primary angiitis of the central nervous system (PACNS) • Vasculitis • Diagnostic criteria • Biopsy

KEY POINTS

- Primary angiitis of the central nervous system (PACNS) is a rare and potentially severe form of vasculitis that is limited to the CNS and spinal cord.
- Unlike systemic vasculitis, the immunologic mechanisms underlying PACNS remain poorly understood, with some studies suggesting an antigen-specific immune response in cerebral arteries.
- Diagnostic criteria for PACNS include acquired unexplained neurologic symptoms, angiographic or histopathologic CNS angiitis findings, and no evidence of systemic vasculitis or similar conditions.
- To confirm vasculitis and exclude other diagnoses, brain biopsy is crucial despite its invasive nature, given the life-threatening nature of the disease.
- PACNS treatment involves potent immunosuppression, causing significant side effects, warranting cautious consideration before therapy initiation.

INTRODUCTION

Primary angiitis of the central nervous system (PACNS) is a rare and potentially severe form of vasculitis that is limited to the brain, meninges, and spinal cord. It is characterized by multifocal inflammation and destruction of the walls of small and medium-size blood vessels in the central nervous system (CNS).[1–3] The terms primary CNS vasculitis (PCNSV) and PACNS are often used interchangeably,[1] and we will refer to the latter for the remainder of this chapter. In the past, cases of PACNS have been reported under a variety of descriptive names, including noninfectious granulomatous angiitis of the nervous system, giant cell arteritis of the CNS, isolated angiitis of the CNS, and benign angiopathy of the CNS.[4–7] This heterogeneity reflects a poorly understood pathophysiology as well as diverse clinical, radiologic, and pathologic presentations.

PACNS has an estimated incidence of 2.4 per 1,000,000 person-years in North America.[2] It can occur at almost any age but most commonly affects middle aged adults, with half of affected patients between 40 and 60 years of age at the time of diagnosis. A variable gender distribution has been reported in different studies.[8,9]

The diagnosis of PACNS is challenging. Clinically, it presents with nonspecific neurologic symptoms ranging from simple headaches to seizures and marked cognitive impairment. Most patients have more than one manifestation during the disease. In addition to this clinical variability, there are no known biochemical, immunologic, or imaging investigations that are diagnostic of PACNS.

The diagnostic criteria of PACNS have varied over time and have been subject to debate. They were initially implemented in 1988 by Calabrese

[a] Department of Radiology, University of North Carolina School of Medicine, 101 Manning Drive, Chapel Hill, NC 27514, USA; [b] Department of Pathology and Laboratory Medicine, University of North Carolina School of Medicine, 101 Manning Drive, Chapel Hill, NC 27514, USA
* Corresponding author.
E-mail address: selima_siala@med.unc.edu

Neuroimag Clin N Am 34 (2024) 31–37
https://doi.org/10.1016/j.nic.2023.06.002
1052-5149/24/© 2023 Elsevier Inc. All rights reserved.

and Mallek[10] and were later modified to prevent misdiagnosis with PACNS's mimics and particularly reversible cerebral vasoconstriction syndrome (RCVS).[11,12] On imaging, although conventional MR imaging is highly sensitive for PACNS, findings are nonspecific and in some patients the study can be normal.[13]

Because the treatment of PACNS usually involves strong immunosuppressive therapy with potential significant side effects,[2,14] a high degree of suspicion for the disease must be established before initiation of therapy. To aid with the diagnosis, brain biopsy and tissue analysis are often required due to the lack of alternative methods of achieving a secure diagnosis.[10,12]

DISCUSSION
Diagnostic criteria

Diagnostic criteria for PACNS established by Calabrese and Mallek in 1988[10] are as follows: (1) history of acquired and otherwise unexplained neurologic or psychiatric symptoms such as headache, encephalopathy, or focal deficits; (2) presence of classic angiographic findings or histopathologic features of CNS angiitis; and (3) no evidence of systemic vasculitis or other disorder that could cause or mimic the angiographic or pathologic features of PACNS. These criteria have been widely used in clinical practice and research and are still applied in most recent studies.[15] Because of the nonspecificity of CNS angiography, a modification of these criteria was proposed by Birnbaum and Hellmann[12] to prevent misdiagnosis with RCVS. The proposed criteria are stratified by levels of diagnostic certainty as follows: (1) definite diagnosis of PACNS when there is histologic confirmation and (2)probable diagnosis in the absence of tissue confirmation with a high probability based on radiological findings and cerebrospinal fluid (CSF) profile consistent with PACNS. Rice and Scolding[11] have recently proposed a further modification of these criteria dividing into "definite" and "possible" PACNS. The authors propose abandoning the "probable" category given the low specificity of contrast angiography. They suggest that all suspected cases lacking histologic proof should be categorized as possible, and the role of angiography would therefore be restricted to rule out other specific disorders.[11]

CSF analysis

All patients suspected of PACNS undergo laboratory workup including a lumbar puncture.[15] CSF analysis is critical for the evaluation of patients with PACNS despite its reported variable sensitivity and low specificity.[12,15] The importance of CSF analysis resides in excluding malignant or infectious diseases as well as distinguishing PACNS from its angiographic mimics such as RCVS where the CSF studies are mostly normal. When positive, patients typically exhibit mild lymphocyte-predominant pleocytosis and elevated protein concentration with a normal glucose level.[16] In PACNS, lymphocyte values of more than 250 cells/μL are unusual and in such case an infectious etiology should be highly considered.

Brain biopsy

PACNS is the most common non-neoplastic indication for brain biopsy. It is performed to provide histologic proof of vasculitis and to identify alternative differential diagnoses.[17,18] Alternative diagnoses are often made during the workup of PACNS even in the presence of classic angiographic findings.[17] Despite its invasive nature, several studies have shown that brain biopsy is relatively safe and should be considered when PACNS is suspected given the life-threatening nature of the disease and the need for treatment if the diagnosis in confirmed.[11,19–21] Brain biopsy has a variable sensitivity between 50% and 75% in part owing to the focal and segmental distribution of histologic changes in PACNS.[10,15] To optimize the diagnostic yield, biopsy should target an area of imaging abnormalities when feasible (eg, areas of vascular enhancement on vessel wall MR imaging[22]) and should sample both leptomeninges and brain parenchyma.[1,18,23] This is preferable to untargeted biopsies that have a lower yield.[2]

Pathogenesis

The etiology and pathogenesis of PACNS are largely unknown. Although histopathologic findings have been extensively described, the underlying mechanisms remain unknown. Infectious agents have been proposed as triggers, in particular varicella zoster virus due to its well-known association with cerebral vasculitis.[1,2] Depending on the immunologic status of the patient, varicella zoster complications can manifest either as a large vessel arteritis (typically granulomatous) in immunocompetent subjects or as a small vessel encephalitis in immunocompromised patients.[24] These findings are evidenced by the presence of viral particles in the walls of affected vessels,[25] suggesting this entity to be a secondary vasculitis rather than PACNS. Other etiologic agents have been proposed including human immunodeficiency virus (HIV), with reported cases of HIV-associated CNS angiitis without any ongoing infectious, autoimmune, or neoplastic disease. The role of HIV in this setting is debated and some authors suggest an immune-mediated mechanism of the vasculitis whereas others consider a direct pathogenic cause of HIV.[26,27] Similarly, mycoplasma gallisepticum as well as West Nile virus have also been reported as potential etiologic agents.[28,29] Some authors have proposed an association between cerebral amyloid angiopathy and PACNS, suggesting a particular PACNS subset in this setting, characterized by transmural inflammation of the vessel walls.[30]

Little is known about the immunologic mechanisms involved in PACNS compared with systemic vasculitis. Some studies evaluated immunologic abnormalities in PACNS, mostly by analyzing CSF.[31–34] One study found evidence of deregulation of the alternative complement cascade in CSF of patients with PACNS compared with controls suggesting pathogenetic similarities between PACNS and antineutrophil cytoplasmic antibody-associated vasculitis.[33] However, a subsequent paper by Deb-Chatterji and colleagues[34] could not replicate these findings and thus, did not support this hypothesis. Other studies performed brain biopsy and histologic assessment.[35–38] A group of investigators examined the immunophenotype of a case of lymphocytic vasculitis involving small vessels, where immunohistochemical staining showed dominant infiltration by CD45R0+ T cells in and around the vessels, which would indicate involvement of memory T cells in the pathogenesis of vasculitis. These findings may hint that PACNS can be the result of an antigen-specific immune response occurring in the wall of cerebral arteries.[35] A recent study published by Salvarani and colleagues explored the gene expression profile of PACNS.[37] The authors performed RNA sequencing on brain biopsies from patients with different types of PACNS and compared them with normal brain tissue. They pointed out the genetic heterogeneity of the different histopathologic subtypes. In another histopathologic study, PACNS was shown to be characterized by MRP8-positive intermediate/late-activated macrophages.[38]

Histopathology

The hallmark biopsy finding in PACNS is transmural inflammation with damage of the vessel wall.[18] Although the histopathologic features can vary, there are 3 general histologic patterns: granulomatous inflammation, lymphocytic cellular infiltrates, and acute necrotizing vasculitis.[18,39]

Granulomatous vasculitis is the most common pattern described in the largest published cohort from the Mayo Clinic, representing 59% of cases.[16] It is characterized by destructive vasculocentric mononuclear inflammation with well-formed granulomas and/or multinucleated cells[1,2] (Fig. 1). Lymphocytic vasculitis is the second most common pattern and is seen in 22% of patients.[16] It is characterized by a predominance of lymphocytic infiltration with occasional plasma cells, typically in multiple layers and extending through the vascular wall causing distortion and/or destruction.[18] A marked lymphocytic infiltrate in the absence of significant parenchymal inflammation is required for the diagnosis, given the nonspecific nature of a lymphocytic infiltrate.[1] The third and least frequently seen pattern of injury in PACNS is necrotizing vasculitis (17%), characterized by transmural fibrinoid necrosis similar to that seen in polyarteritis nodosa and often acute inflammation.[1,2] This pattern involves predominantly small muscular arteries and is associated with disruption of the internal elastic lamina.[1,18] It commonly presents with hemorrhage. These 3 histologic patterns are typically not present in the same case and seem to remain stable over time suggesting that they do not represent different phases of the disease, with some authors suggesting that these subsets may represent more than one entity.[1,2]

It is noteworthy that the reported frequency of each subset differs between studies, and smaller cohorts have identified the lymphocytic pattern as the most prevalent subtype, followed by the granulomatous type.[9,40,41] This disparity may indicate interobserver variability in diagnosing lymphocytic vasculitis, as precise histologic criteria for "marked" lymphocytic inflammation and "distortion" of vascular walls have yet to be defined and pathologic characterization is challenging.

- Relationship to cerebral amyloid angiopathy

Cerebral amyloid angiopathy (CAA) is characterized by deposition of amyloid β in the media and adventitia of cortical and leptomeningeal vessels.[42] In a subset of patients with CAA, vascular inflammation may also be present with 2 described pathologic subtypes: one with a destructive transmural vascular inflammatory infiltrate, defined as amyloid β-related angiitis (ABRA),[43,44] and a second one, where amyloid deposition is associated with nondestructive perivascular inflammatory infiltration, known as CAA-related inflammation.[45,46]

The ABRA subtype is often seen with the granulomatous inflammation, which is reported in almost half of biopsy specimens, and is rarely seen with a nongranulomatous pattern[16] (Fig. 2). As this particular entity appears to have a distinct clinico-radiological presentation, it remains to be validated whether ABRA is better considered to be a definable subset of PACNS or an entirely separate disease.[30]

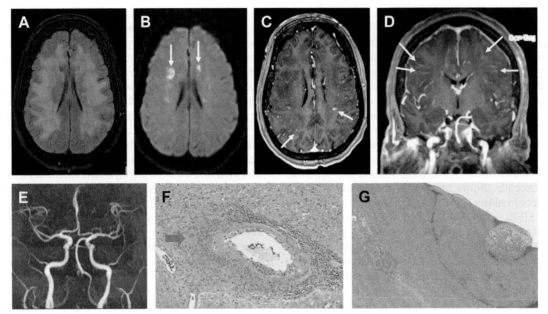

Fig. 1. Granulomatous angiitis of the central nervous system. (*A*) Axial FLAIR image shows extensive confluent signal abnormality of the bilateral white matter also involving both thalami and pons (not shown in this figure). (*B*) DWI sequence shows bilateral small acute infarcts in a watershed distribution. (*C, D*) Axial and coronal post-contrast T1 images show multiple bilateral foci of abnormal enhancement in a predominant perivascular distribution. (*E*) Time-of-flight MR angiography shows normal appearance of intracranial arteries. (*F, G*) Brain biopsy, H&E stain, 400× (*F*), 200× (*G*). In this case of granulomatous angiitis of the central nervous system, multiple arteries, variously located in the subarachnoid space, cerebral cortex, and cerebral white matter, show varying degrees of granulomatous inflammation characterized by epithelioid histiocytes and multinucleated giant cells (*blue arrow*). Lymphocytic perivascular inflammation is also present. Immunohistochemical staining for amyloid beta was negative (not shown in this figure). DWI, diffusion-weighted imaging; FLAIR, fluid attenuated inversion recovery.

Clinico-pathologic subsets

Some clinical and imaging presentations have been associated with histologic variants of PACNS which has led to identification of different clinico-pathologic subsets. However, it should be noted that these are not entirely specific or mutually exclusive, and there are varying degrees of overlap.

- Negative cerebral angiography and positive CNS biopsy: In these cases only very small arteries are affected that are too small to be detectable on angiography.[17] MR imaging is dominated by white matter changes from previous infarcts with or without enhancing abnormalities. In one study, these patients had a higher frequency of cognitive impairment along with higher white cell count and protein concentrations in the CSF compared with angiography-positive PACNS.[47]
- Prominent meningeal enhancement on MR imaging: The patients in this group also appear to have isolated involvement of small vessels with positive CNS biopsy and normal angiography. In a study with 8 patients from this subset with positive biopsy, 5 showed a granulomatous histologic pattern.[48]
- Amyloid deposits associated with granulomatous vasculitis: These patients are typically older than those with PACNS without amyloid deposits, are more likely to be male, and have a more acute onset with a higher frequency of cognitive impairment.[43]
- Rapidly progressive PACNS: Frequently associated with a fatal outcome, these patients typically present with large bilateral cerebrovascular lesions on angiography and multifocal bilateral cerebral infarctions on cross-sectional imaging. Biopsy usually reveals granulomatous or necrotizing patterns.[49]
- Spinal cord involvement: Present in about 5% of patients with the thoracic cord being predominantly involved. Of 5 documented cases with spinal cord involvement, 3 patients showed necrotizing vasculitis and 2 showed granulomatous subtype in CNS biopsy specimens.[50]
- Intracranial hemorrhage: Occurring in 12% of cases, these patients are less likely to have

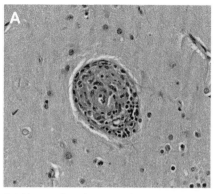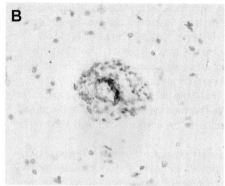

Fig. 2. Amyloid beta-related angiitis (ABRA). Brain biopsy: H&E stain, 600× (*A*), amyloid beta immunohistochemistry, 600× (*B*). In this case of amyloid beta-related angiitis, small vessels in the superficial cortex and leptomeninges are thickened and eosinophilic with varying degrees of perivascular chronic inflammation. The vessel on (*A*) shows associated non-necrotizing granulomatous inflammation. Amyloid beta immunohistochemistry is positive in the vessel wall (*B*).

cognitive dysfunction, a persistent neurologic deficit, or MR imaging evidence of cerebral infarction during the course of the disease compared with those without intracranial hemorrhage. Necrotizing vasculitis is the predominant histopathologic pattern associated with this group.[51]

SUMMARY

PACNS is a rare and potentially severe form of vasculitis limited to the CNS and meninges. Despite extensive research, the underlying etiology and pathogenesis of this disease remain unknown. PACNS is characterized by multifocal inflammation and destruction of the walls of blood vessels in the CNS, leading to cerebral ischemia with or without hemorrhage and a varied clinical presentation. Three primary histopathologic patterns have been identified, namely granulomatous inflammation, lymphocytic infiltrates, and necrotizing vasculitis, with the granulomatous subtype sometimes exhibiting amyloid β deposition. The well-established diagnostic criteria proposed by Calabrese and Mallek continue to be commonly used, although they have been modified to emphasize the critical role of cerebral tissue analysis for the definitive diagnosis of PACNS.

CLINICS CARE POINTS

- Diagnosing PACNS can be challenging as it manifests with nonspecific neurologic symptoms, and there are no specific biochemical, immunologic, or imaging tests for the disease.

- A biopsy is crucial not only to confirm vasculitis but also to exclude other potential diagnoses. Alternative diagnoses are often made even in the presence of classic angiographic findings of PACNS.

- To increase sensitivity, biopsy should target areas of imaging abnormalities when feasible and sample both leptomeninges and brain parenchyma.

- Despite its variable sensitivity and low specificity, CSF analysis is critical in evaluating patients with PACNS to exclude infectious or malignant disease and distinguish the condition from angiographic mimics such as RCVS.

- In biopsy-proven PACNS cases, it is worthwhile to review the pathology report to confirm that amyloid-β was assessed, as ABRA has distinct features.

DISCLOSURE

The authors have no relevant financial or nonfinancial interests to disclose.

REFERENCES

1. Giannini C, Salvarani C, Hunder G, et al. Primary central nervous system vasculitis: pathology and mechanisms. Acta Neuropathol 2012;123(6):759–72.
2. Salvarani C, Brown RD, Hunder GG. Adult primary central nervous system vasculitis. Lancet Lond Engl 2012;380(9843):767–77.
3. Beuker C, Schmidt A, Strunk D, et al. Primary angiitis of the central nervous system: diagnosis and treatment. Ther Adv Neurol Disord 2018;11. 1756286418785071.

4. Newman W, Wolf A. Non-infectious granulomatous angiitis involving the central nervous system. Trans Am Neurol Assoc 1952;56(77th Meeting):114–7.

5. McCormick HM, Neubuerger KT. Giant-Cell Arteritis Involving Small Meningeal and Intracerebral Vessels. J Neuropathol Exp Neurol 1958;17(3):471–8.

6. Cupps TR, Moore PM, Fauci AS. Isolated angiitis of the central nervous system. Prospective diagnostic and therapeutic experience. Am J Med 1983;74(1): 97–105.

7. Calabrese LH, Gragg LA, Furlan AJ. Benign angiopathy: a distinct subset of angiographically defined primary angiitis of the central nervous system. J Rheumatol 1993;20(12):2046–50.

8. Salvarani C, Brown RD, Calamia KT, et al. Primary central nervous system vasculitis: analysis of 101 patients. Ann Neurol 2007;62(5):442–51.

9. Agarwal A, Sharma J, Srivastava MVP, et al. Primary CNS vasculitis (PCNSV): a cohort study. Sci Rep 2022;12(1):13494.

10. Calabrese LH, Mallek JA. Primary angiitis of the central nervous system. Report of 8 new cases, review of the literature, and proposal for diagnostic criteria. Medicine (Baltim) 1988;67(1):20–39.

11. Rice CM, Scolding NJ. The diagnosis of primary central nervous system vasculitis. Pract Neurol 2020;20(2):109–14.

12. Birnbaum J, Hellmann DB. Primary angiitis of the central nervous system. Arch Neurol 2009;66(6): 704–9.

13. McVerry F, McCluskey G, McCarron P, et al. Diagnostic test results in primary CNS vasculitis: A systematic review of published cases. Neurol Clin Pract 2017;7(3):256–65.

14. Salvarani C, Brown RD, Christianson TJH, et al. Adult primary central nervous system vasculitis treatment and course: analysis of one hundred sixty-three patients. Arthritis Rheumatol Hoboken NJ 2015;67(6):1637–45.

15. Beuker C, Strunk D, Rawal R, et al. Primary Angiitis of the CNS: A Systematic Review and Meta-analysis. Neurol - Neuroimmunol Neuroinflammation. 2021; 8(6).

16. Salvarani C, Brown RDJ, Christianson T, et al. An Update of the Mayo Clinic Cohort of Patients With Adult Primary Central Nervous System Vasculitis: Description of 163 Patients. Medicine (Baltim) 2015;94(21):e738.

17. Kadkhodayan Y, Alreshaid A, Moran CJ, et al. Primary angiitis of the central nervous system at conventional angiography. Radiology 2004;233(3):878–82.

18. Miller DV, Salvarani C, Hunder GG, et al. Biopsy findings in primary angiitis of the central nervous system. Am J Surg Pathol 2009;33(1):35–43.

19. Rice CM, Gilkes CE, Teare E, et al. Brain biopsy in cryptogenic neurological disease. Br J Neurosurg 2011;25(5):614–20.

20. Alrawi A, Trobe JD, Blaivas M, et al. Brain biopsy in primary angiitis of the central nervous system. Neurology 1999;53(4):858–60.

21. Hall WA. The safety and efficacy of stereotactic biopsy for intracranial lesions. Cancer 1998;82(9): 1749–55.

22. Zeiler SR, Qiao Y, Pardo CA, et al. Vessel Wall MRI for Targeting Biopsies of Intracranial Vasculitis. AJNR Am J Neuroradiol 2018;39(11):2034–6.

23. Calabrese LH, Duna GF, Lie JT. Vasculitis in the central nervous system. Arthritis Rheum 1997;40(7): 1189–201.

24. Gilden DH, Kleinschmidt-DeMasters BK, LaGuardia JJ, et al. Neurologic complications of the reactivation of varicella-zoster virus. N Engl J Med 2000;342(9):635–45.

25. Nagel MA, Cohrs RJ, Mahalingam R, et al. The varicella zoster virus vasculopathies: clinical, CSF, imaging, and virologic features. Neurology 2008;70(11): 853–60.

26. Melica G, Brugieres P, Lascaux AS, et al. Primary vasculitis of the central nervous system in patients infected with HIV-1 in the HAART era. J Med Virol 2009;81(4):578–81.

27. Cheron J, Wyndham-Thomas C, Sadeghi N, et al. Response of Human Immunodeficiency Virus-Associated Cerebral Angiitis to the Combined Antiretroviral Therapy. Front Neurol 2017;8:95.

28. Harroud A, Almutlaq A, Pellerin D, et al. West Nile virus-associated vasculitis and intracranial hemorrhage. Neurol Neuroimmunol Neuroinflammation 2019;7(1):e641.

29. Arthur G, Margolis G. Mycoplasma-like structures in granulomatous angiitis of the central nervous system. Case reports with light and electron microscopic studies. Arch Pathol Lab Med 1977;101(7): 382–7.

30. Salvarani C, Hunder GG, Morris JM, et al. Aβ-related angiitis: Comparison with CAA without inflammation and primary CNS vasculitis. Neurology 2013;81(18): 1596–603.

31. Thom V, Schmid S, Gelderblom M, et al. IL-17 production by CSF lymphocytes as a biomarker for cerebral vasculitis. Neurol Neuroimmunol Neuroinflammation 2016;3(2):e214.

32. Strunk D, Schulte-Mecklenbeck A, Golombeck KS, et al. Immune cell profiling in the cerebrospinal fluid of patients with primary angiitis of the central nervous system reflects the heterogeneity of the disease. J Neuroimmunol 2018;321:109–16.

33. Mandel-Brehm C, Retallack H, Knudsen GM, et al. Exploratory proteomic analysis implicates the alternative complement cascade in primary CNS vasculitis. Neurology 2019;93(5):e433–44.

34. Deb-Chatterji M, Keller CW, Koch S, et al. Profiling Complement System Components in Primary CNS Vasculitis. Cells 2021;10(5):1139.

35. Iwase T, Ojika K, Mitake S, et al. Involvement of CD45RO+ T lymphocyte infiltration in a patient with primary angiitis of the central nervous system restricted to small vessels. Eur Neurol 2001;45(3): 184–5.

36. Melzer N, Harder A, Gross CC, et al. CD4(+) T cells predominate in cerebrospinal fluid and leptomeningeal and parenchymal infiltrates in cerebral amyloid β-related angiitis. Arch Neurol 2012;69(6):773–7.

37. Salvarani C, Paludo J, Hunder GG, et al. Exploring Gene Expression Profiles in Primary Central Nervous System Vasculitis. Ann Neurol 2022;93(1):120–30.

38. Mihm B, Bergmann M, Brück W, et al. The activation pattern of macrophages in giant cell (temporal) arteritis and primary angiitis of the central nervous system. Neuropathol Off J Jpn Soc Neuropathol 2014;34(3):236–42.

39. Lie JT. Primary (granulomatous) angiitis of the central nervous system: a clinicopathologic analysis of 15 new cases and a review of the literature. Hum Pathol 1992;23(2):164–71.

40. Sundaram S, Menon D, Khatri P, et al. Primary angiitis of the central nervous system: Clinical profiles and outcomes of 45 patients. Neurol India 2019; 67(1):105.

41. Oon S, Roberts C, Gorelik A, et al. Primary angiitis of the central nervous system: experience of a Victorian tertiary-referral hospital. Intern Med J 2013; 43(6):685–92.

42. Greenberg SM, Vonsattel JP. Diagnosis of cerebral amyloid angiopathy. Sensitivity and specificity of cortical biopsy. Stroke 1997;28(7):1418–22.

43. Salvarani C, Brown RD Jr, Calamia KT, et al. Primary central nervous system vasculitis: comparison of patients with and without cerebral amyloid angiopathy. Rheumatology 2008;47(11):1671–7.

44. Scolding NJ, Joseph F, Kirby PA, et al. Abeta-related angiitis: primary angiitis of the central nervous system associated with cerebral amyloid angiopathy. Brain J Neurol 2005;128(Pt 3):500–15.

45. Eng JA, Frosch MP, Choi K, et al. Clinical manifestations of cerebral amyloid angiopathy-related inflammation. Ann Neurol 2004;55(2):250–6.

46. Kinnecom C, Lev MH, Wendell L, et al. Course of cerebral amyloid angiopathy-related inflammation. Neurology 2007;68(17):1411–6.

47. Salvarani C, Brown RD, Calamia KT, et al. Angiography-negative primary central nervous system vasculitis: a syndrome involving small cerebral vessels. Medicine (Baltim) 2008;87(5):264–71.

48. Salvarani C, Brown RD, Calamia KT, et al. Primary central nervous system vasculitis with prominent leptomeningeal enhancement: a subset with a benign outcome. Arthritis Rheum 2008;58(2):595–603.

49. Salvarani C, Brown RD, Calamia KT, et al. Rapidly progressive primary central nervous system vasculitis. Rheumatol Oxf Engl 2011;50(2):349–58.

50. Salvarani C, Brown RD, Calamia KT, et al. Primary CNS vasculitis with spinal cord involvement. Neurology 2008;70(24 Pt 2):2394–400.

51. Salvarani C, Brown RD, Calamia KT, et al. Primary central nervous system vasculitis presenting with intracranial hemorrhage. Arthritis Rheum 2011; 63(11):3598–606.

Usefulness of Different Imaging Methods in the Diagnosis of Cerebral Vasculopathy

Carlos A. Zamora, MD, PhD[a],*, Mahmud Mossa-Basha, MD[b], Mauricio Castillo, MD, FACR[a]

KEYWORDS

• Vasculopathy • Vasculitis • Brain • Imaging • CTA • MRA • Vessel wall imaging • Utility

KEY POINTS

• Evaluation of vasculopathies is challenging due to overlapping clinical and imaging features, as well as limited sensitivity of most modalities for assessing small vessel disease.
• While conventional brain MRI has relatively high sensitivity in the diagnosis of vasculitis, findings are nonspecific and a small proportion of patients can have a normal scan.
• CTA and MRA are comparable diagnostic techniques which are largely based on depiction of the vessel lumen and provide limited assessment of the vessel wall.
• Conventional catheter-based cerebral angiography is the gold standard technique due to its exquisite spatial and temporal resolutions, but it is invasive and usually not the first-line imaging modality.
• VWI-MRI sequences offer further characterization of the vessel wall by providing images with high spatial resolution and suppression of CSF and arterial blood signal.

INTRODUCTION

Cerebral vasculopathies represent a diverse group of entities with varying pathophysiologies and clinical presentations. They may have a non-inflammatory basis or can be linked to different types of granulomatous or non-granulomatous inflammation, infection, or metabolic processes. In addition, vasculopathies can affect vessels of various sizes and may or may not be associated with systemic disease. As a result, diagnosis can pose a challenge due to overlapping features and normal imaging findings in many patients. This article assesses the usefulness of CT and MRI-based techniques as well as conventional catheter angiography in diagnosing cerebral vasculopathy, highlighting on the strengths and limitations of each method.

DISCUSSION

Computed Tomography Angiography

CTA is often the first-line imaging modality in the evaluation of cerebral vasculopathies due to its wide availability and ease of acquisition, particularly in the urgent and critical care setting. Diagnostic quality CTA requires adequate arterial contrast opacification while minimizing venous contamination. Several scanning methods are available to optimize arterial opacification, and their usage depends on institutional preference, as well as hardware and software capabilities.

1. Manual trigger: The operator initiates the scan manually when intravenous contrast is visible in the carotid or vertebral arteries. This method

[a] Division of Neuroradiology, Department of Radiology, University of North Carolina School of Medicine, CB 7510, Old Infirmary Building, 101 Manning Drive, Chapel Hill, NC 27599-7510, USA; [b] Department of Radiology, University of Washington, University of Washington School of Medicine, 1959 NE Pacific Street, Seattle, WA 98195, USA
* Corresponding author.
E-mail address: carlos_zamora@med.unc.edu

Neuroimag Clin N Am 34 (2024) 39–52
https://doi.org/10.1016/j.nic.2023.07.001

neuroimaging.theclinics.com

is operator dependent and prone to inconsistent arterial opacification between patients.

2. Fixed delay: The scan is initiated after a predetermined time delay from the start of contrast injection based on the expected time for contrast material to reach the target vessels, typically between 15 and 25 seconds. The selected time varies depending on scanner speed, number of detectors, and other technical factors. While this method eliminates operator dependency and provides more consistency than a manual trigger, it does not account for hemodynamic or age differences between patients.

3. Test bolus: involves injecting a small amount of contrast material to determine the time-to-peak enhancement in target vessels. The scan is then initiated after a fixed time delay from peak enhancement. This method can optimize the delivery of contrast material and may be tailored to decrease the total dose, although it requires more user involvement than the above techniques.

4. Automatic bolus tracking: This method involves monitoring the arrival of contrast material in a selected vessel (usually the aortic arch) using a low-dose preliminary scan. The full scan is initiated automatically after a predefined timed delay when the contrast material reaches a predetermined density threshold. This method eliminates operator dependency in timing of the acquisition.

All methods require high-flow injection, usually between 50 and 75 mL of non-ionic iodinated contrast material at 4 to 5 mL/second and preferably via a power injector. Injection of contrast material should be followed by a 50 to 100 mL saline chaser to flush dense contrast material from the venous system and minimize associated streak artifact.

Techniques with a fixed trigger delay do not take into account individual cardiovascular parameters such as blood circulation time, which can be problematic in patients with high or low cardiac output. For instance, in patients with high cardiac output, the delay may be too long and can lead to the scan missing the peak arterial enhancement. In patients with low cardiac output, the scan may be initiated too early and will terminate before peak enhancement is reached. Vascular tortuosity and severe stenoses are also factors that can contribute to delay in bolus arrival. Additionally, parameters in children are different and need to be optimized by patient age and body weight.

CTA can provide high spatial resolution depending on hardware and software capabilities, with routine collimation ranging between 0.625- and 1-mm. Actual slice thickness varies based on institutional preference, but 1 mm slice thickness is common for intracranial CTA. Thinner slices provide higher spatial resolution but also introduce noise. Regardless of the method used for scan triggering, some venous opacification will always be present on CTA as there is only a 5 to 6 second circulation time between arteries and veins.[1] This, among other factors mentioned later in the discussion, limits the utility of CTA for vasculopathies affecting the small vessels. As opposed to large vessel vasculitides, where CTA can show thickening of the vessel wall (particularly in the neck), the diagnosis of inflammatory vasculopathy on intracranial CTA is largely based on the evaluation and detection of luminal stenosis. Therefore, while CTA is useful for intracranial abnormalities that result in alterations of vascular morphology or luminal size, its use is limited for abnormalities of the vessel wall, except for the demonstration of calcified plaque, some dissection flaps, or significant mural thickening/hematoma. This is especially true for small artery vasculopathies affecting the perforator branches, including small artery vasculitis (lymphocytic and granulomatous angiitis), where on CTA absent branches or stenotic branches are not readily visible. This also applies to the evaluation of non-stenotic inflammatory vasculopathies. CTA is unable to depict inflammatory changes of the vessel wall due to a lack of contrast and spatial resolution and therefore the sensitivity for the diagnosis of cerebral vasculitis is low.

Another drawback of CTA is the difficulty of evaluating the lumen in vessels with heavily calcified plaque, due to artifacts resulting from the high linear attenuation coefficient of calcium. This can lead to the overestimation of the degree of luminal narrowing owing to average volume artifact, although it can be mitigated by optimizing the window width and level settings (**Fig. 1**).[2] There are no fixed width/level settings that will work on every scan, as they will ultimately depend on the degree of intraluminal contrast enhancement (and resultant intraluminal attenuation values) in a given CTA study. Beam hardening artifacts, resulting from a dense venous contrast bolus, hardware, or medical devices, can also limit the visualization of the vessel lumen.

Data obtained from CTA can be post-processed in different ways to facilitate interpretation. Maximum intensity projections (MIPs) are routinely performed based on the highest density pixels in the image series which are usually provided by intraluminal contrast, bone, and calcified plaque. MIPs increase the conspicuity of vascular structures while decreasing the contribution of

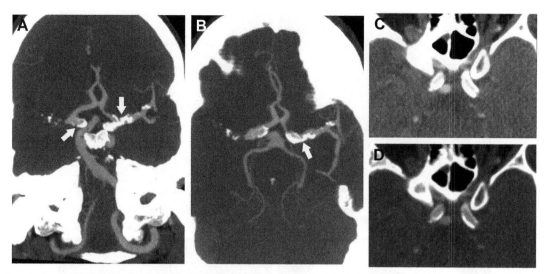

Fig. 1. Coronal (*A*) and axial (*B*) thick CTA MIP slabs in a patient with dolichoectatic vasculopathy and extensive vascular calcifications (*arrows*). The lumen is difficult to visualize with the default window settings (center 85, width 455) due to resultant artifact (*C*). A wider window width (center 250, width 800) is better able to separate the lumen from the calcified plaque (*D*). There are no universal window settings as these will vary depending on scanner parameters and concentration of intravenous contrast in a given scan.

surrounding tissues to the image, which works best with high-quality CTAs that have little venous contamination. Thick sliding slabs or volumetric reconstructions based on MIPs are also useful for presenting an overview of the vasculature and demonstrating segmental areas of stenosis. However, these become difficult to evaluate at the skull base due to the presence of adjacent bone. Nonetheless, there are several available techniques for bone removal that can improve the visualization of arteries at the skull base. These techniques include various software applications for manual or automatic bone removal on conventional scanners, as well as spectral differentiation using dual-energy CT that allows for the separation of iodine from calcium.[3] It is important to note that bone removal techniques may introduce artifacts at the vessel-wall interface and are more challenging to apply to heavily calcified vessels (**Fig. 2**). Also, the post-processing kernel is important for good delineation of the vessel margins. Softer kernels lead to blurry vascular margins, while kernels that are too sharp will introduce more noise (**Fig. 3**). Scanners typically offer various default or recommended kernels, which may require modification based on the radiologist's preference and the specific clinical application.

Conventional Magnetic Resonance Imaging of the Brain

The diagnosis of cerebral vasculopathies poses a significant challenge due to their variable and overlapping clinical manifestations. Brain MRI plays a critical role in supporting their diagnosis, distinguishing them from other intracranial pathologies, and guiding biopsy if necessary. Some pathologies associated with vasculopathy may demonstrate highly characteristic MRI patterns. For example, amyloid beta-related angiitis presents with lobar microhemorrhages, superficial siderosis, and asymmetric white matter hyperintensities representing vasogenic edema (**Fig. 4**).[4] Neurosarcoidosis may show characteristic "corkscrew" engorgement of deep medullary veins, leptomeningeal enhancement, and non-necrotizing basal and perivascular granulomas (**Fig. 5**).[5] Tuberculosis, an important cause of infectious vasculitis, may reveal a distinctive thick basal exudate with conglomerate enhancing rings representing caseating or liquefied granulomas (**Fig. 6**).[6] The characteristic MRI features of various vasculopathies will be described in more detail in their respective articles.

According to the American College of Radiology, MRI of the brain is an appropriate initial examination for patients suspected to have central nervous system (CNS) vasculitis.[7] Several studies suggest that MRI of the brain is highly sensitive for diagnosing CNS vasculitis, with a normal exam essentially ruling out the diagnosis.[8–10] In general, the combination of a normal MRI of the brain and negative CSF analysis has a high negative predictive value for CNS vasculitis, and such patients are likely to have a noninflammatory vasculopathy.[11] MRI findings of CNS vasculitis are

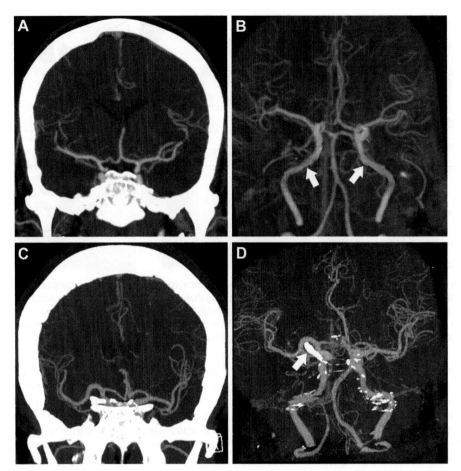

Fig. 2. Coronal thick CTA MIP slabs prior to (*A*, *C*) and following (*B*, *D*) bone removal in 2 different patients. Note edge artifacts on the bone removal images from the first patient (*arrows*). The post-processed images from the second patient (*D*) show scattered vascular calcifications along the carotid siphons. The arrow in (*D*) corresponds to a surgical aneurysm clip.

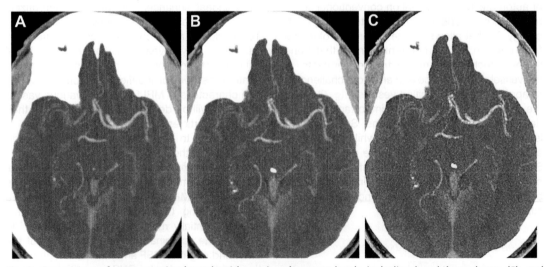

Fig. 3. Comparison of reconstruction kernels with varying sharpness levels, including low (*A*), moderate (*B*), and high (*C*). The reconstruction kernels in (*B*) and (*C*) exhibit progressively better vessel delineation compared to (*A*), albeit with a concomitant increase in image noise which is most pronounced with the sharpest kernel (*C*).

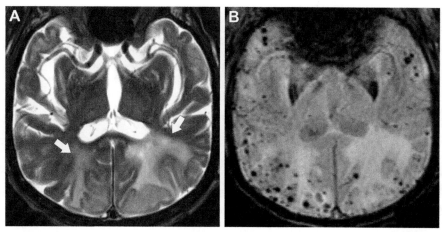

Fig. 4. Amyloid-beta related angiitis. Axial T2-weighted image (*A*) shows asymmetric white matter edema bilaterally (*arrows*). Axial SWI (*B*) demonstrates the characteristic lobar (cortical-subcortical) distribution of amyloid-related microhemorrhages.

nonspecific and may include chronic white matter changes, multiple infarcts (frequently of various ages and affecting different vascular territories), granulomatous masses, hemorrhage, and meningeal enhancement, among others (**Fig. 7**).[12] However, a more recent study found that some patients with CNS vasculitis (confirmed clinically and by catheter angiography) can have a normal conventional MRI of the brain, with a sensitivity of 87%.[13] Therefore, even though routine brain MRI has a relatively high sensitivity, patients with a working differential diagnosis of CNS vasculitis will likely benefit from more advanced imaging including angiographic and vessel wall sequences.

Magnetic Resonance Angiography

Several methods exist for performing MRA of the intracranial arteries, with or without intravenous contrast, each having its own strengths and limitations as described later in the discussion.

Time-of-flight Magnetic Resonance Angiography

This is the most utilized technique for noncontrast intracranial MRA and is based on the principle of flow-related enhancement. Typically, TOF-MRA can achieve a spatial resolution of around 0.5 to 1 mm depending on the MRI scanner and parameters, generally comparable to CTA. For image acquisition, multiple radiofrequency pulses are applied to the region of interest which saturate the spins and null their signal. As a result, unsaturated and fully magnetized flowing blood entering the field of interest appears as bright signal against a relatively dark background, providing high contrast. One drawback of TOF MRA is its lower sensitivity to

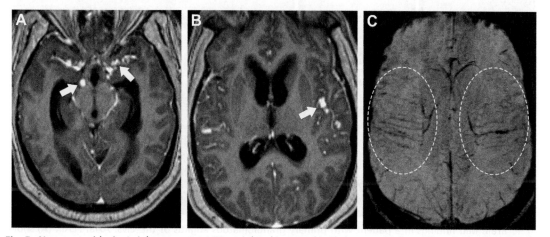

Fig. 5. Neurosarcoidosis. Axial postcontrast T1-weighted images (*A*, *B*) show multiple avidly enhancing nodules at the basal cisterns and sylvian fissures consistent with non-necrotizing granulomas (*arrows*). Axial SWI (*C*) shows enlarged deep medullary veins with a typical corkscrew appearance (ovals).

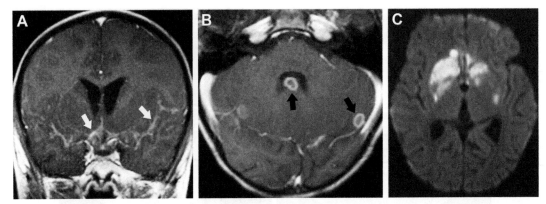

Fig. 6. CNS tuberculosis. Coronal (A) and axial (B) postcontrast T1-weighted images demonstrate an extensive enhancing exudate in the basal cisterns and sylvian fissures (*white arrows*). There are several ring enhancing lesions corresponding to caseating or liquefying granulomas (*black arrows*). DWI shows multiple striatocapsular infarcts (C) secondary to tuberculous vasculitis and/or reactive vasospasm. This constellation of findings is highly suggestive of CNS tuberculosis.

slow flow and in-plane flow as well as susceptibility to turbulent flow, which can lead to overestimation of the degree of stenosis or a misdiagnosis of occlusion (Fig. 8).[14,15] It can also result in underestimation or non-detection of aneurysms with turbulent or stagnant flow and underestimation of nidus size in arteriovenous malformations. Because TOF MRA is directional when a saturation band is applied to the superior sagittal sinus, it can provide a cleaner angiographic image with little to no venous contamination. It may also show areas where arterial flow is reversed, such as with subclavian steal syndrome.

2D-TOF MRA is based on the acquisition of multiple thin slices with a flow-compensated gradient echo sequence. In contrast, 3D-TOF MRA is based on simultaneous phase-encoding of a larger volume of tissue which leads to higher signal-to-noise ratio and spatial resolution. Both techniques are sensitive to motion which is usually more pronounced with 3D-TOF MRA, where it may corrupt the entire acquisition. Also, 3D-TOF MRA requires

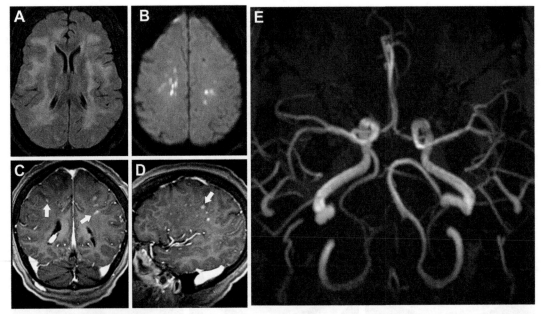

Fig. 7. Brain MRI findings in a patient with primary granulomatous angiitis of the CNS. Axial FLAIR (A) shows extensive confluent white matter signal abnormality bilaterally accompanied by numerous small infarcts on DWI (B). Coronal (C) and sagittal (D) post-contrast T1-weighted images demonstrate multiple small foci of enhancement along a perivascular distribution (*arrows*). TOF-MRA (E) was normal.

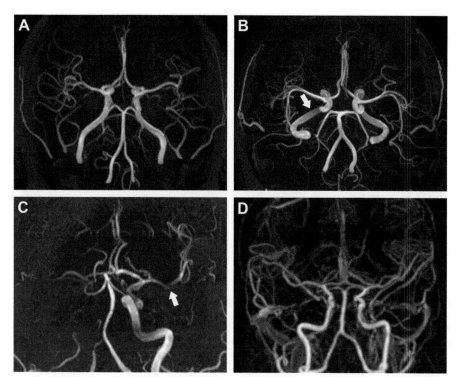

Fig. 8. 3D MIP TOF-MRA reformats in different patients (*A, B, C*). A normal study (*A*) shows excellent flow-related enhancement of the intracranial and extracranial vasculature. Figure (*B*) shows a different study with subtle in-plane signal loss in the cavernous internal carotid arteries (ICAs) due to spin saturation, more notably on the right (*arrow*). Figure (*C*) shows a different patient with more pronounced in-plane saturation artifact (*arrow*) mimicking a stenosis in the left middle cerebral artery (MCA). This patient also has an occluded right ICA with poor signal in right MCA branches. Figure (*D*) shows a normal CE-MRA in a different patient. CE-MRA is not susceptible to in-plane saturation artifacts but will have varying degrees of venous contamination as shown in this case.

longer scanning times. Finally, because the underlying sequences are T1-weighted, TOF techniques are susceptible to T1 shine-through artifact, and care must be taken not to confuse intrinsically bright material (such as a hematoma) with flow-related vascular enhancement (Fig. 9). As with CTA, MIPs may be helpful and rotational 3D reconstructions are also commonly performed. One caveat to keep in mind with MIPs and 3D reconstructions is that they can potentially exacerbate stenoses and artifactually introduce occlusions depending on how the postprocessing was performed. Therefore, any suspected narrowing on them should be confirmed on the source slices and ideally on multiple planes (Fig. 10). Also, susceptibility artifact is common adjacent to areas of dense bone and may mimic a stenosis, particularly at the point where the internal carotid artery enters the skull base (Fig. 11).

Phase-contrast Magnetic Resonance Angiography

Like TOF MRA, PC-MRA does not require intravenous contrast. This technique takes advantage of differences in the phase shift of spins in flowing blood versus spins in stationary tissues subjected to bipolar MR gradients. Such differences in phase shift are proportional to blood flow velocity and can provide quantifiable information about velocity and direction, in addition to vascular morphology.[16] Compared with TOF techniques, PC-MRA is better suited to visualize vessels with slow flow. It is also not affected by the T1 shine-through artifact that can be seen with TOF MRA and can thus be useful in the presence of hemorrhage. However, except for MR venography, this technique is not routinely utilized for intracranial angiography, primarily due to its long acquisition times and the availability of simpler techniques. Also, PC-MRA is more operator dependent than TOF techniques and requires accurate selection of velocity encoding (VENC) settings prior to scanning to prevent underestimation or overestimation of flow.

Contrast-enhanced Magnetic Resonance Angiography

This technique is analogous to CTA in that vascular contrast is provided by an intravenous

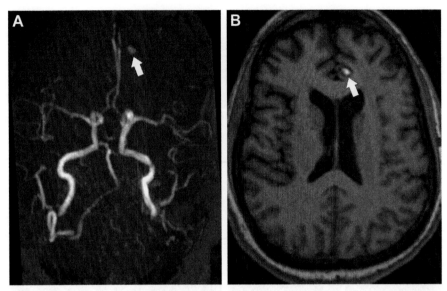

Fig. 9. 3D MIP TOF-MRA shows a bright focus adjacent to the left anterior cerebral artery which was initially misdiagnosed as a vascular lesion with flow related enhancement (*A*). Noncontrast T1-weighted image (*B*) shows this focus to represent a resolving hematoma with intrinsically bright signal due to methemoglobin (*arrow*). The finding in (*A*) is therefore consistent with T1 shine-through.

agent. CE-MRA is based on the paramagnetic properties of gadolinium which result in T1 shortening of flowing blood and increased vascular conspicuity. CE-MRA requires rapid injection of a compact bolus of a gadolinium-based contrast agent (GBCA), usually followed by a saline chaser. Injection can be performed manually or with a power injector. CE-MRA is generally based on a rapid 3D T1 spoiled gradient echo sequence. Similar to other MRA techniques, fat suppression is important to increase the utility of MIP reconstructions by nullifying bright signal from surrounding fatty tissues.

Unlike noncontrast MRA techniques, CE-MRA is not susceptible to flow-related artifacts such as those resulting from turbulence, slow flow, or directional flow (see Fig. 8). However, similar to CTA, single-phase CE-MRA requires careful timing for the scan to be performed when the contrast bolus reaches near peak concentration at the vessels of interest. To achieve this, vendors provide different software applications for bolus detection and scan triggering, frequently accompanied by some form of fluoroscopic MRI visualization.

In contrast to single-phase CE-MRA, time-resolved CE-MRA does not require precise estimation of contrast bolus arrival. This technique utilizes a rapid sequence of images to capture the movement of blood through the vessels over time. It relies on radial undersampling of the periphery combined with maximum sampling of the

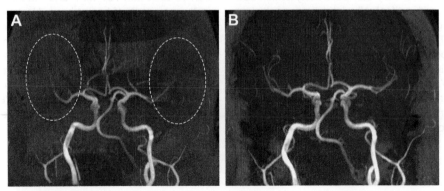

Fig. 10. 3D MIP TOF-MRA (*A*) shows artifactual tapering and truncation of M2 MCA branches bilaterally (ovals). Re-processed thick MIP slabs (*B*) show normal appearing vessels.

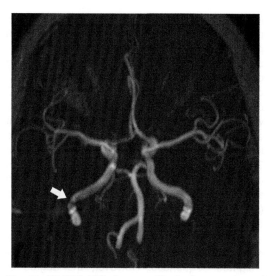

Fig. 11. 3D-TOF MIP shows artifactual narrowing of the proximal petrous ICAs (*arrow*) due to susceptibility effects as the vessel enters the skull base.

center of *k* space aimed at maintaining contrast resolution. The underlying principle is that stationary structures (ie, anatomic resolution) exhibit minimal changes, and thereby the technique temporally prioritizes contrast resolution. The temporal and spatial resolutions can be adjusted based on the degree of undersampling. The clinical use of time-resolved MRA techniques is mostly limited to pathologies that may benefit from non-invasive hemodynamic evaluation, such as arteriovenous malformations and dural arteriovenous fistulas.

In addition to a lack of flow-related artifacts, another advantage of CE-MRA is its high signal-to-noise ratio. However, similar to CTA, there will always be some degree of venous contamination even in optimally timed studies, which is a relative downside if the exam is performed to evaluate arterial vasculopathies. The technique also carries a small risk of adverse reactions related to the intravenous injection of a GBCA. While single phase CE-MRA is able to provide relatively high spatial resolution, there is a significant trade-off in time-resolved MRA between temporal and spatial resolution.

Balanced Steady-state Free Precession Magnetic Resonance Angiography

The bSSFP MRA technique uses gradient echo sequences that exploit the inherent T2/T1 relaxation properties of blood and surrounding tissues, resulting in images with a high contrast-to-noise ratio. Effective fat suppression is necessary as the T2/T1 ratio of fat is higher than that of arterial

blood. While commonly used for peripheral MRA, its usefulness for intracranial applications is limited for several reasons. First, the T2/T1 ratio of CSF is several times higher than that of arterial blood. This poses a challenge for arterial visualization and the creation of MIPs due to the technical difficulty of suppressing the bright CSF signal.[17] Second, bSSFP is sensitive to magnetic field inhomogeneities than can distort vascular anatomy near areas of air-tissue interface such as the paranasal sinuses and mastoid air cells. Third, this technique involves lengthy acquisition times that can lead to motion artifacts and further image degradation, although acceleration techniques may alleviate this issue.

Vessel Wall Magnetic Resonance Imaging

VW-MRI offers a distinct advantage over other angiographic techniques by enabling visualization and characterization of the structure and composition of the vessel wall. As a result, it has the potential to reveal pathology that may not be identifiable using modalities based on luminal enhancement. VW-MRI has become widely used in the evaluation of various vasculopathies. The pattern of vessel wall involvement identified by VW-MRI can provide valuable information to differentiate vasculitis from other pathologies such as atherosclerosis and Moyamoya disease.[18] It has also shown utility in differentiating atherosclerotic disease from reversible vasoconstrictive syndrome and infectious/inflammatory vasculopathies.[19] VW-MRI has also been used for the characterization of aneurysms and has shown potential utility as a biomarker of destabilizing mural changes that could lead to an increased risk of rupture.[20] Additionally, VW-MRI has demonstrated its utility in surgical guidance by increasing the yield of intracranial biopsy, which is otherwise associated with a high rate of false negatives.[21]

VW-MRI protocols vary between institutions depending on their hardware and software capabilities as well as radiologist preference and experience.[22] To optimize delineation of the vessel wall enhancement, VW-MRI generally requires sequences that offer high-resolution and signal-to-noise ratios, as well as effective suppression of intravascular and CSF signals. For 2D VW-MRI, typical voxel sizes are 2.0 x 0.4 × 0.4 mm, while for 3D-VWI, the voxel size ranges from 0.5 to 0.7 mm isotropic. It is worth noting that the normal thickness range of the middle cerebral and basilar arteries is between 0.2 and 0.3 mm.[23]

Several methods can be used to obtain "black blood" VW-MRI with suppressed arterial signal, including:

1. Spin echo: The tissue of interest is subjected to slice-selective 90° and 180° pulses. Spins in flowing blood are first subjected to the 90° pulse but have left the imaging slice by the time the 180° pulse is applied, and therefore do not generate signal. The signal from the stationary vascular wall, on the other hand, is preserved, resulting in a black blood image.

2. Spatial presaturation with inversion recovery (SPIR): This sequence involves the use of a spatially selective inversion pulse applied upstream of the imaging slice to null the signal from inflowing blood, resulting in a dark vessel lumen and bright vessel wall.

3. Double inversion recovery (DIR): This sequence is utilized for 2D VWI but is unable to adequately suppress flow in 3D acquisitions. It employs two inversion pulses with a time delay (TI) between them. The TI is adjusted to allow the spins from inflowing blood to lose signal and appear black against the background signal from stationary tissues. However, this necessary delay results in longer scanning times, which is a drawback of this technique and may make it difficult to image the vasculature with adequate spatial resolution. One additional disadvantage of DIR is the requirement for precise timing and maintaining a consistent difference in TI between pre- and post-contrast images. Other techniques such as quadruple inversion recovery may overcome some of these limitations but lead to longer scan times.[24]

4. Variable flip angle 3D turbo spin echo sequences (SPACE/CUBE/VISTA): These have intrinsic black blood effects primarily caused by intravoxel dephasing where spins within blood acquire phase at different velocities due to turbulent or laminar flow, leading to signal loss. However, being this a volumetric acquisition, a common issue is the presence of incomplete signal suppression along the vessel wall, which may be mistaken as enhancement. This is frequently exacerbated at points of in-plane, turbulent, or slow flow, similar to flow dephasing in TOF MRA.[25] Additional blood suppression techniques, such as flow-sensitive dephasing (MSDE) and Delay Alternating with Nutation for Tailored Excitation (DANTE), can be applied to suppress artifactual signal.[26] Disadvantages of MSDE include the reduction of signal-to-noise ratio and the introduction of T2 decay which limits the maximal achievable resolution. DANTE provides suppression of blood and CSF while maintaining native signal.

VW-MRI protocols include 2D and/or 3D pre- and postcontrast T1-weighted sequences. Multiple 2D images can be acquired in orthogonal planes and have the ability to provide excellent in plane resolution. However, one limitation of 2D sequences is their susceptibility to volume averaging due to the curvature and morphology of the intracranial vessels. Although cross-sectional 2D orthogonal images of a vessel can be obtained with high quality, this requires additional user input and scanning time, and the spatial coverage is limited.[27] Therefore, most centers favor isotropic 3D T1 sequences, which can provide whole brain coverage and the ability to reconstruct images in any plane after the scan has been completed (Fig. 12). Some centers prefer to use a combination of 2D and 3D acquisitions.

Proton density sequences offer a high signal-to-noise ratio and can be used as an alternative to T1-weighted sequences. However, the degree of contrast enhancement is not as pronounced as with T1-weighted sequences.[23] T2-weighted images can also be helpful for providing additional characterization of the vessel wall. While fat suppression techniques are important for nulling the bright signal of surrounding fat in the evaluation of extracranial arteries, this is not necessary for intracranial vascular assessment.

Digital Subtraction Angiography

Conventional digital subtraction angiography (DSA) via catheter injection remains the gold standard imaging modality for evaluating the vessel lumen. It offers the highest spatial resolution of clinically available techniques (up to 0.1–0.2 mm), making it more suitable for assessing small distal branches than CTA or MRA (Fig. 13).[28,29] DSA also provides very high temporal resolution, up to 0.25 seconds,[28] and is the most accurate technique for evaluating hemodynamic alterations. However, due to its invasive nature, DSA is seldom used as the initial imaging study for vasculopathies.

Although DSA can depict the vascular lumen in great detail, it is unable to show alterations of the vessel wall, and findings may remain undetected unless there an associated caliber change affecting large and medium-sized arterial branches. DSA may appear normal in vascular disease where there has been significant remodeling of the vessel lumen or the affected arteries are small perforator branches. Despite being considered more reliable than CTA and MRA, the sensitivity and specificity of DSA for diagnosing CNS vasculitis remains low.[30]

Computed Tomography and Magnetic Resonance Perfusion

Perfusion imaging can be a valuable tool in evaluating cerebrovascular diseases that may cause

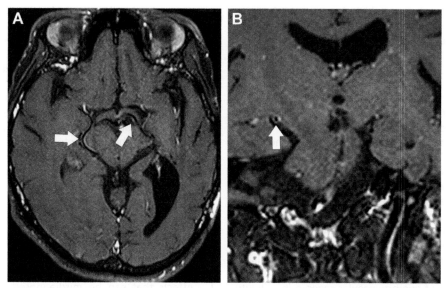

Fig. 12. Vessel wall imaging in a patient with lupus vasculitis. Axial post-contrast 3D T1-SPACE (*A*) shows segmental vessel wall enhancement involving the posterior cerebral arteries (PCAs) bilaterally (*arrows*). Oblique coronal reformat (*B*) shows a cross-section of the right PCA with a circumferential pattern of enhancement (*arrow*).

restricted intracranial blood flow. CT perfusion (CTP) is a useful technique that allows for the quantitative measurement of perfusion parameters such as cerebral blood flow, cerebral blood volume, and mean transit time. This is achieved through the linear relationship between CT attenuation and contrast concentration in the tissue of interest.[31] However, one of its drawbacks is the relatively high radiation dose compared to other CT techniques. In addition, CTP is associated with low signal-to-noise and contrast-to-noise ratios compared with DWI, which can lead to measurement errors.[32,33] In contrast, bolus-based MR perfusion (MRP) techniques do not allow for direct quantification and provide relative perfusion parameters.

There are 2 main bolus-based MRP techniques based on signal intensity-time curves obtained after intravenous administration of a GBCA. The first technique is dynamic susceptibility contrast (DSC) MRP, which relies on sequential T2 or T2* monitoring of the paramagnetic effects of the first pass of a GBCA bolus. The second technique, dynamic contrast enhanced (DCE) MRP, utilizes T1 relaxivity effects and offers a composite measurement of tissue permeability, perfusion, and fractional volumes of extravascular-extracellular and plasma spaces.[34,35]

Arterial spin labeling (ASL) is an additional MRP technique that does not require the use of intravenous contrast agents. This method employs the labeling of arterial blood water protons as an

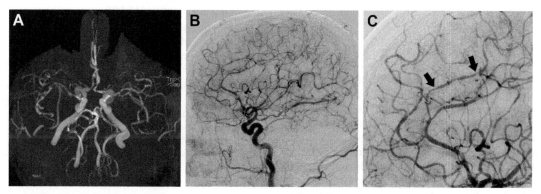

Fig. 13. 3D MIP TOF-MRA in a patient with primary angiitis of the CNS (*A*) shows extensive areas of stenosis and dilatation of the intracranial arteries with a beaded appearance. Lateral (*B*) and magnified (*C*) views from DSA provide a clearer depiction of the areas of stenosis involving middle and small size vessels (*arrows*).

endogenous tracer, which is accomplished by selectively inverting the magnetization of arterial blood entering the brain. As the labeled blood perfuses the tissue, the resulting images are used to estimate CBF. Compared to DSC and DCE perfusion, ASL perfusion has lower spatial resolution. However, it offers the advantage of not requiring the use of contrast agents and can provide quantification of CBF.

Other than evaluation of acute stroke and vasospasm, CTP and MRP techniques have a limited role in assessing cerebral vasculopathies. Studies have shown a possible utility of DCE perfusion in demonstrating increased permeability and capillary density in atherosclerotic plaque and increased permeability of aneurysm walls, although these applications have not gained widespread clinical use.[36–38] One area where perfusion techniques have shown potential utility is in the estimation of cerebrovascular reserve in patients with chronic ischemia due to stenosis, such as in moyamoya disease. Cerebrovascular reserve and reactivity can be evaluated with a hemodynamic stress test using a quantitative perfusion method such as CTP, ASL MRP, Technetium 99m hexamethylpropyleneamine oxime (HMPAO) SPECT, and ^{15}O-water PET techniques.[39,40] The test is frequently performed with acetazolamide, a vasodilator that causes increased CBF. The principle underlying this test is that the brain's ability to compensate for reduced blood flow caused by steno-occlusive disease depends on the reserve capacity of the cerebral vasculature. In patients with chronic hemodynamic stress, arterioles are already maximally dilated and will show a limited response to the acetazolamide challenge, while sites with normal vasculature will demonstrate increased CBF.[39] Other studies have shown more reliable measurements of cerebrovascular reactivity by utilizing blood oxygen level-dependent (BOLD) MRI during manipulation of arterial partial pressure of carbon dioxide via a rebreather.[41]

SUMMARY

Assessment of cerebral vasculopathies is challenging and can be facilitated by a comprehensive understanding of the available imaging methods and their utility. There are several angiographic techniques that can image the vessel lumen, each with unique advantages and disadvantages. Bolus-based angiographic methods such as CTA and CE-MRA require careful timing of a contrast bolus to enhance arterial conspicuity while minimizing venous enhancement. Non-contrast MRA techniques such as TOF and PC-MRA do not require contrast and are useful for showing arteries with high spatial resolution and little to no venous contamination. While digital subtraction angiography (DSA) remains the gold standard of angiographic techniques due to its exquisite spatial resolution, it is invasive and usually not the initial study of choice. In contrast to techniques that rely on depiction of the lumen, VW-MRI offers a noninvasive means of assessing vessel wall pathology and provide further characterization. In general, brain MRI offers relatively high sensitivity for the diagnosis of vasculitis and is useful in differentiating various non-inflammatory vasculopathies.

CLINICS CARE POINTS

- TOF MRA is susceptible to T1 shine-through effects that can be misdiagnosed as flow-related enhancement. This pitfall can be avoided by correlating with noncontrast T1 weighted images.

- TOF MRA is also prone to flow-related artifacts which may lead to overestimation of stenosis or a misdiagnosis of occlusion.

- While contrast-enhanced CTA or MRA can minimize flow-related artifacts, these techniques are accompanied by varying degrees of venous contamination even in optimally timed scans.

- CTA should be reconstructed using a kernel that is sufficiently sharp to delineate the vessel without introducing unnecessary noise. In addition, images should be viewed with optimal window width/level settings to avoid overestimating the degree of stenosis in patients with heavily calcified plaque.

- A normal CTA, MRA, or conventional catheter angiography does not rule out a diagnosis of vasculitis as the overall sensitivity is low. These patients may benefit from further characterization with VWI-MRI.

- Brain biopsy for vasculitis is associated with a high rate of false negatives, but the yield can be increased by utilizing VW-MRI for surgical guidance.

- Perfusion techniques have limited utility in evaluating vasculopathies outside of stroke and vasospasm. However, they can provide an estimation of cerebrovascular reactivity in patients with chronic steno-occlusive disease.

DISCLOSURE

The authors have nothing to disclose.

REFERENCES

1. Takhtani D. CT neuroangiography: a glance at the common pitfalls and their prevention. AJR Am J Roentgenol 2005;185(3):772–83.
2. Saba L, Mallarin G. Window settings for the study of calcified carotid plaques with multidetector CT angiography. AJNR Am J Neuroradiol 2009;30(7):1445–50.
3. van Straten M, Schaap M, Dijkshoorn ML, et al. Automated bone removal in CT angiography: comparison of methods based on single energy and dual energy scans. Med Phys 2011;38(11):6128–37.
4. Charidimou A, Boulouis G, Frosch MP, et al. The Boston criteria version 2.0 for cerebral amyloid angiopathy: a multicentre, retrospective, MRI-neuropathology diagnostic accuracy study. Lancet Neurol 2022;21(8):714–25.
5. Zamora C, Hung SC, Tomingas C, et al. Engorgement of Deep Medullary Veins in Neurosarcoidosis: A Common-Yet-Underrecognized Cerebrovascular Finding on SWI. AJNR Am J Neuroradiol 2018;39(11):2045–50.
6. Kim TK, Chang KH, Kim CJ, et al. Intracranial tuberculoma: comparison of MR with pathologic findings. AJNR Am J Neuroradiol 1995;16(9):1903–8.
7. ACR Appropriateness Criteria®—Cerebrovascular Diseases-Aneurysm VM, and Subarachnoid Hemorrhage. American College of Radiology. https://acsearch.acr.org/docs/3149013/Narrative/. Accessed 4/16/2023.
8. Greenan TJ, Grossman RI, Goldberg HI. Cerebral vasculitis: MR imaging and angiographic correlation. Radiology 1992;182(1):65–72.
9. Duna GF, Calabrese LH. Limitations of invasive modalities in the diagnosis of primary angiitis of the central nervous system. J Rheumatol 1995;22(4):662–7.
10. Harris KG, Tran DD, Sickels WJ, et al. Diagnosing intracranial vasculitis: the roles of MR and angiography. AJNR Am J Neuroradiol 1994;15(2):317–30.
11. Birnbaum J, Hellmann DB. Primary angiitis of the central nervous system. Arch Neurol 2009;66(6):704–9.
12. Suthiphosuwan S, Bharatha A, Hsu CC, et al. Tumefactive Primary Central Nervous System Vasculitis: Imaging Findings of a Rare and Underrecognized Neuroinflammatory Disease. AJNR Am J Neuroradiol 2020;41(11):2075–81.
13. Wasserman BA, Stone JH, Hellmann DB, et al. Reliability of normal findings on MR imaging for excluding the diagnosis of vasculitis of the central nervous system. AJR Am J Roentgenol 2001;177(2):455–9.
14. Stock KW, Wetzel S, Kirsch E, et al. Anatomic evaluation of the circle of Willis: MR angiography versus intraarterial digital subtraction angiography. AJNR Am J Neuroradiol 1996;17(8):1495–9.
15. Ishimaru H, Ochi M, Morikawa M, et al. Accuracy of pre- and postcontrast 3D time-of-flight MR angiography in patients with acute ischemic stroke: correlation with catheter angiography. AJNR Am J Neuroradiol 2007;28(5):923–6.
16. Van Goethem JW, van den Hauwe L, Ozsarlak O, et al. Phase-contrast magnetic resonance angiography. JBR-BTR. 2003;86(6):340–4.
17. Lu A, Brodsky E, Grist TM, et al. Rapid fat-suppressed isotropic steady-state free precession imaging using true 3D multiple-half-echo projection reconstruction. Magn Reson Med 2005;53(3):692–9.
18. Mossa-Basha M, de Havenon A, Becker KJ, et al. Added Value of Vessel Wall Magnetic Resonance Imaging in the Differentiation of Moyamoya Vasculopathies in a Non-Asian Cohort. Stroke 2016;47(7):1782–8.
19. Mossa-Basha M, Shibata DK, Hallam DK, et al. Added Value of Vessel Wall Magnetic Resonance Imaging for Differentiation of Nonocclusive Intracranial Vasculopathies. Stroke 2017;48(11):3026–33.
20. Larsen N, von der Brelie C, Trick D, et al. Vessel Wall Enhancement in Unruptured Intracranial Aneurysms: An Indicator for Higher Risk of Rupture? High-Resolution MR Imaging and Correlated Histologic Findings. AJNR Am J Neuroradiol 2018;39(9):1617–21.
21. Zeiler SR, Qiao Y, Pardo CA, et al. Vessel Wall MRI for Targeting Biopsies of Intracranial Vasculitis. AJNR Am J Neuroradiol 2018;39(11):2034–6.
22. Mossa-Basha M, Zhu C, Yuan C, et al. Survey of the American Society of Neuroradiology Membership on the Use and Value of Intracranial Vessel Wall MRI. AJNR Am J Neuroradiol 2022;43(7):951–7.
23. Mandell DM, Mossa-Basha M, Qiao Y, et al. Intracranial Vessel Wall MRI: Principles and Expert Consensus Recommendations of the American Society of Neuroradiology. AJNR Am J Neuroradiol 2017;38(2):218–29.
24. Yarnykh VL, Yuan C. T1-insensitive flow suppression using quadruple inversion-recovery. Magn Reson Med 2002;48(5):899–905.
25. Sannananja B, Zhu C, Colip CG, et al. Image-Quality Assessment of 3D Intracranial Vessel Wall MRI Using DANTE or DANTE-CAIPI for Blood Suppression and Imaging Acceleration. AJNR Am J Neuroradiol 2022;43(6):837–43.
26. Xie Y, Yang Q, Xie G, et al. Improved black-blood imaging using DANTE-SPACE for simultaneous carotid and intracranial vessel wall evaluation. Magn Reson Med 2016;75(6):2286–94.
27. Eiden S, Beck C, Venhoff N, et al. High-resolution contrast-enhanced vessel wall imaging in patients with suspected cerebral vasculitis: Prospective comparison of whole-brain 3D T1 SPACE versus 2D T1 black blood MRI at 3 Tesla. PLoS One 2019;14(3):e0213514.

28. Kaufmann TJ, Kallmes DF. Diagnostic cerebral angiography: archaic and complication-prone or here to stay for another 80 years? AJR Am J Roentgenol 2008;190(6):1435–7.

29. Pradilla G, Wicks RT, Hadelsberg U, et al. Accuracy of computed tomography angiography in the diagnosis of intracranial aneurysms. World Neurosurg 2013;80(6):845–52.

30. Rice CM, Scolding NJ. The diagnosis of primary central nervous system vasculitis. Pract Neurol 2020;20(2):109–14.

31. Hoeffner EG, Case I, Jain R, et al. Cerebral perfusion CT: technique and clinical applications. Radiology 2004;231(3):632–44.

32. Schaefer PW, Souza L, Kamalian S, et al. Limited reliability of computed tomographic perfusion acute infarct volume measurements compared with diffusion-weighted imaging in anterior circulation stroke. Stroke 2015;46(2):419–24.

33. Copen WA, Yoo AJ, Rost NS, et al. In patients with suspected acute stroke, CT perfusion-based cerebral blood flow maps cannot substitute for DWI in measuring the ischemic core. PLoS One 2017; 12(11):e0188891.

34. Essig M, Shiroishi MS, Nguyen TB, et al. Perfusion MRI: the five most frequently asked technical questions. AJR Am J Roentgenol 2013;200(1):24–34.

35. Jahng GH, Li KL, Ostergaard L, et al. Perfusion magnetic resonance imaging: a comprehensive update on principles and techniques. Korean J Radiol 2014;15(5):554–77.

36. Vakil P, Elmokadem AH, Syed FH, et al. Quantifying Intracranial Plaque Permeability with Dynamic Contrast-Enhanced MRI: A Pilot Study. AJNR Am J Neuroradiol 2017;38(2):243–9.

37. Taqueti VR, Di Carli MF, Jerosch-Herold M, et al. Increased microvascularization and vessel permeability associate with active inflammation in human atheromata. Circ Cardiovasc Imaging 2014;7(6):920–9.

38. Vakil P, Ansari SA, Cantrell CG, et al. Quantifying Intracranial Aneurysm Wall Permeability for Risk Assessment Using Dynamic Contrast-Enhanced MRI: A Pilot Study. AJNR Am J Neuroradiol 2015; 36(5):953–9.

39. Vagal AS, Leach JL, Fernandez-Ulloa M, et al. The acetazolamide challenge: techniques and applications in the evaluation of chronic cerebral ischemia. AJNR Am J Neuroradiol 2009;30(5):876–84.

40. Acker G, Lange C, Schatka I, et al. Brain Perfusion Imaging Under Acetazolamide Challenge for Detection of Impaired Cerebrovascular Reserve Capacity: Positive Findings with (15)O-Water PET in Patients with Negative (99m)Tc-HMPAO SPECT Findings. J Nucl Med 2018;59(2):294–8.

41. Sobczyk O, Crawley AP, Poublanc J, et al. Identifying Significant Changes in Cerebrovascular Reactivity to Carbon Dioxide. AJNR Am J Neuroradiol 2016;37(5):818–24.

Primary Large Vessel Vasculitis
Takayasu Arteritis and Giant Cell Arteritis

Griselda Romero-Sanchez, MD, MSc[a], Mona Dabiri, MD[b],
Mahmud Mossa-Basha, MD[c],*

KEYWORDS

- Large vessel vasculitis • Takayasu arteritis • Giant cell arteritis • MRA • Vessel wall MRI • CTA
- PET/CT

KEY POINTS

- Luminal imaging readily detects vasculitis complications, including aneurysmal dilation, dissection, or stenosis and may depict large artery wall thickening, but may be limited in the detection of early inflammatory changes.
- Vessel wall imaging (VWI) can identify early manifestations prior to the development of permanent sequela and allows for disease monitoring. 3D VWI improves image quality over 2D techniques.
- Ultrasound with imaging of the superficial temporal arteries is a first-line imaging tool in Giant cell arteritis.
- MRI/MRA is a first-line imaging modality for Takayasu arteritis.
- PET/CT detects mural inflammation and/or luminal changes in extracranial arteries to support the diagnosis of large vessel vasculitis.

INTRODUCTION

Takayasu arteritis (TA) and giant cell arteritis (GCA) are inflammatory autoimmune vasculopathies.[1,2] Both are considered large vessel vasculitides (LVV) with TA targeting the aorta and its branches, and GCA primarily targeting large and medium-sized arteries.[3–5] TA is seen most frequently in Eastern populations, with GCA occurring more commonly in Northern European descendants.[6,7] The mean age of onset for TA is in the third decade, whereas GCA tends to occur in more elderly individuals, being 20 times more common in the ninth than sixth decades.[7,8] Stroke or transient ischemic attack may be the first presentation of disease and are resultant from vascular complications and may lead to death in large-vessel vasculitis.[9]

The sequela of untreated LVV include chronic vessel stenosis, occlusion, aneurysm formation, blindness, and the harmful side-effects of over-treatment in later stage disease.[10] Unfortunately for TA, early detection has historically been difficult due to the vague clinical presentation, with most people presenting with nonspecific symptoms, including dizziness, syncope, and fatigue, and less than 20% presenting with fever during the active phase of disease.[1] In GCA, constitutional symptoms are common, with headache and visual impairment representing the most common symptoms. Vision loss is painless, and can be partial or complete, and unilateral or bilateral; once

[a] Department of Radiology, Instituto Nacional de Ciencias Medicas y Nutricion Salvador Zubiran, Textitlan 21 Casa 11, Santa Ursula Xitla, Tlalpan, Mexico City 14420, Mexico; [b] Department of Radiology, Children's Medical Center, Tehran University of Medical Sciences, Abi Avenue, Dolat St, Tehran 11369, Iran; [c] Department of Radiology, University of Washington School of Medicine, 1959 Northeast Pacific Street, Seattle, WA 98195, USA
* Corresponding author.
E-mail address: mmossab@uw.edu

Neuroimag Clin N Am 34 (2024) 53–65
https://doi.org/10.1016/j.nic.2023.07.002

established, it is irreversible.[11] Polymyalgia rheumatica presents in 40% to 60% of patients with GCA at the time of diagnosis.[12]

Early detection and diagnosis of large artery vasculitis such as TA is important because prompt initiation of treatment can prevent or delay the onset of permanent disease sequelae. Imaging plays a central role in establishing the presence of arterial wall inflammatory changes, detection of luminal changes, and detection of downstream complications. Longitudinal imaging is also an important component of assessing treatment response and disease recurrence. In this article, we discuss imaging modalities and approaches to LVV imaging, including the advantages and disadvantages of each.

DIAGNOSIS

In 1990, the American College of Rheumatology (ACR) developed criteria for the classification of TA and GCA.[13,14] They established six criteria for the classification of TA.[13] Five of these criteria are manifestations of stenosis, such as bruit, blood pressure difference between extremities, decreased pulse, claudication, and angiographic demonstration of vascular stenosis.[13] Although these criteria have high sensitivity and specificity (90% and 97%, respectively) for TA, they do not differentiate stenosis caused by active vessel wall inflammation versus post-inflammatory changes (eg, mural fibrosis). In addition, the criteria are not accurate in the detection of early disease prior to the development of stenosis, which is frequently irreversible and can lead to significant morbidity.

GCA criteria require the presence of 3 or more of the following: age at onset ≥50 years; new-onset headache; temporal artery abnormality, such as tenderness to palpation or decreased pulsation; erythrocyte sedimentation rate ≥50 mm/h; and abnormal artery biopsy showing vasculitis with mononuclear cells or granulomatous inflammation, and usually with giant cell infiltrates.[14] Temporal artery biopsy is the diagnostic gold standard for the confirmation of GCA, but it is invasive and lacks sensitivity, with false-negative test results in up to 60% of cases.[15] Performing a biopsy in TA is almost impossible in most cases due to the primary involvement of large extracranial arteries, including the common carotid and subclavian arteries, and the aorta.

Several studies have established that the diagnosis of LVV can be reliably confirmed by imaging, making imaging an important diagnostic test for the confirmation of GCA and TA, and a tool for treatment response evaluation.[16,17]

IMAGING MODALITIES

Different imaging modalities such as ultrasound, CTA, MRA/MRI, and FDG-PET/CT have been used for diagnosis, follow-up to monitor disease activity and outcome prediction. Imaging allows not only morphologic assessment, which includes lumen and vessel wall but also functional and molecular evaluation (Table 1 of typical imaging findings in LVV). Catheter-based imaging is rarely performed and is reserved for treatment purposes. Recommendations for using imaging in LVV in clinical practice were developed by the European League Against Rheumatism (EULAR).[18] EULAR recommends an early imaging test in patients with suspected LVV, with ultrasound and MRI being the first choices in GCA and TA, respectively. Contrast-enhanced CTA or PET/CT may be used alternatively. If the diagnosis is still in question after clinical examination and imaging, additional investigations, including temporal artery biopsy and/or additional imaging, can be performed.

ULTRASOUND/COLOR DOPPLER ULTRASOUND

Standardized ultrasound (US) and color Doppler ultrasound (CDUS) examinations in GCA should include at least the superficial temporal and axillary arteries. US is the most available imaging modality in the diagnosis of LVV. The "halo" and the "compression" signs are considered the most important ultrasound abnormalities for GCA. Abnormal vessels demonstrate a circumferential hypoechoic rim around the vessel lumen on transverse US view of the targeted artery, which is defined as the halo sign (Fig. 1), and the compression sign is described as the persistence of the hypoechoic halo during the compression of the vessel lumen.[19,20] Nielsen BD et al. reported that the sensitivity increased from 71% to 97% when adding carotid and axillary artery evaluation to the temporal artery ultrasound exam.[21] Another important ultrasound measure is the intimamedia thickness (IMT) measurement for superficial temporal and axillary arteries. The cut-off value for distinguishing normal from vasculitic arteries is 0.4 mm for temporal arteries and 1.0 mm for axillary arteries.[22]

US can accurately detect TA (Fig. 2), specifically for carotid, subclavian and axillary artery involvement. The "macaroni sign" is an ultrasound imaging sign for TA, and it is defined as characteristic circumferential arterial wall thickening of either one or both common carotid arteries.[23] In a recent meta-analysis, pooled sensitivity of ultrasound for

Table 1
Typical imaging findings of large-vessel vasculitis: Takayasu arteritis and giant cell arteritis at the diagnosis and follow-up

Imaging Modalities	Diagnosis Imaging Findings	Advantages	When to do it
US/CDUS	TA: Macaroni sign GCA: Halo and compression Signs TA and GCA: • Vascular stenosis/occlusion • IMT: > 0.4 mm for temporal arteries and 1.0 mm for axillary arteries	Widely accesible Lower cost than other imaging techniques	Initial diagnostic method and follow-up mainly in GCA Alternative diagnostic method for TA. Very limited in TA.
CTA	TA and GCA: • Circumferential wall thickening and enhancement of the vessel wall • Vascular stenosis, occlusion, ectasia, and aneurysm • Surrounding fat-stranding	Fast adquisition time Can assess the entire aorta and its main branches	Initial diagnostic method and follow-up in TA and GCA
MRA/MRI VWI	TA and GCA: • MRA- luminal stenosis/occlusion/ectasia and aneurysm • VWI Circumferential wall thickening and enhancement of the vessel wall GCA: VWI Circumferential wall thickening and enhancement of the vessel wall in smaller cranial arteries	No ionizing radiation exposure Improved lesion delineation and detection Allows the assessment of both cranial and extracranial arteries	Initial diagnostic method and follow-up in TA and GCA.çreferred diagnostic method for superficial extracranial arteries
PET/CT and PET/MR	TA and GCA: Vessel wall tracer uptake Vascular stenosis/occlusion/ectasia and aneurysm	Good overview of the aorta and its main branches Facilitates differentation between different pathologic entities.	The preferred diagnostic method in follow-up for both TA and GCA

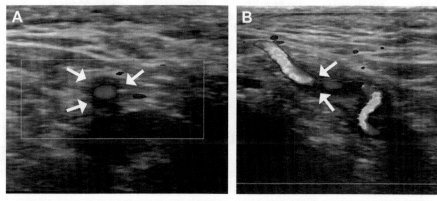

Fig. 1. 71-year-old woman with GCA. Temporal Artery Doppler mode ultrasound in transverse view (*A*) and longitudinal view (*B*) shows circumferential wall thickening corresponding to the 'halo sign' and a slight decrease in lumen caliber (*arrows*).

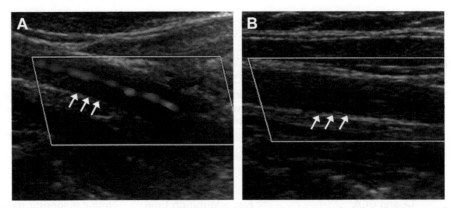

Fig. 2. 36-year-old woman was diagnosed with TA. Carotid Artery Doppler mode (*A*) and power mode (*B*) ultrasound showing a marked decreased caliber of the lumen vessel and circumferential wall thickening (*arrows*).

TA diagnosis was 81% (95% CI: 69%–89%), and specificity was greater than 90% relative to clinical diagnostic criteria.[24]

POSITRON EMISSION TOMOGRAPHY/ COMPUTED TOMOGRAPHY AND POSITRON EMISSION TOMOGRAPHY/MAGNETIC RESONANCE

According to EULAR recommendations, PET/CT may be used to detect mural inflammation and/or luminal changes in extracranial arteries to support the diagnosis of GCA with large artery involvement (Fig. 3), and can also be used to track treatment response (Fig. 4). PET/CT is not recommended for the assessment of inflammation of cranial arteries (superficial temporal arteries). PET/MR may

also be utilized to identify inflammatory relapse, progression, and aneurysm formation of large arteries. A pilot study demonstrated that hybrid FDG PET/MRI yielded highly comparable visual and quantitative results in relation to FDG PET/CT.[25]

There are some limitations of imaging, including PET/CT, for vasculitis assessment. Immunosuppression treatment can impact inflammatory activity of lesions, resulting in reduced presence of inflammatory cells. This issue is most significant after the first 3 days of glucocorticoid treatment, when the detection of inflammatory-related changes on PET/CT and vessel wall MRI is markedly limited.[26,27] Atherosclerosis can mimic inflammatory vasculopathies due to increased metabolic activity within lesions and similar appearance of

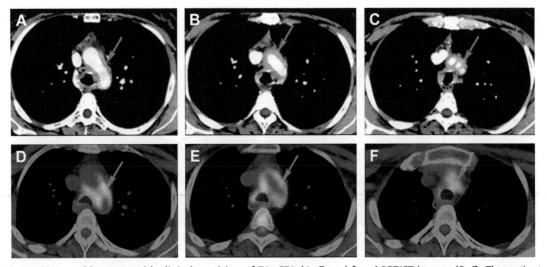

Fig. 3. 32-year-old woman with clinical suspicion of TA. CTA (*A–C*) and fused PET/CT images (*D–F*). The patient exhibited circumferential 18-FDG uptake along the walls of the aortic arch and the origin of the brachiocephalic trunk, left common carotid artery, and left subclavian artery (*arrows*).

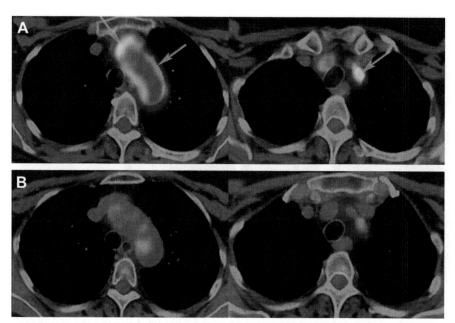

Fig. 4. 59-year-old woman with GCA and large vessel involvement. Fused PET/CT images at the level of the aortic arch and proximal great arteries (*A*) before therapy demonstrate 18-FDG uptake along the walls of the aortic arch and left subclavian artery (*arrows*). Fused PET/CT images at the same level as A (*B*) after the administration of corticosteroids and methotrexate demonstrate marked reduction in artery wall FDG uptake.

wall thickening. This is especially problematic for patients with GCA because atherosclerosis and GCA overlap in terms of age distribution. However, a differentiating feature in atherosclerosis is the less intense and more heterogeneous lesion activity when compared to inflammatory vasculopathies. The sensitivity of PET/CT for the diagnosis of GCA is 92%, and specificity is 85% with a high negative predictive value.[28] For detecting TA, the pooled sensitivity of FDG-PET/CT/CTA was 81% (95% CI, 69%–89%), and the pooled specificity was 74% (95% CI, 55%–86%).[24]

COMPUTED TOMOGRAPHY ANGIOGRAPHY

CTA is widely available, readily accessible, and can assess the entire aorta and its main branches with a single acquisition. Inflammatory vasculopathy imaging findings on CTA include circumferential vessel wall thickening and enhancement and perivascular fat-stranding (Fig. 5). CTA detects LVV complications, including aneurysmal dilation, dissection, or stenosis.[29,30] Lariviere and colleagues evaluated CTA in 24 patients with suspected GCA and found a sensitivity of 73% (95% CI 45%–92%) and a specificity of 78% (95% CI 40%–97%) using temporal artery biopsy and clinical diagnostic criteria of GCA after 6 months as the reference standard.[31] For the diagnosis of TA, Yamada and colleagues examined the role of CTA in 25 patients reporting a sensitivity of

100% (95% CI 76%–100%) and a specificity of 100% (95% CI 40%–100%) compared with conventional angiography in the evaluation of 200 arteries.[32]

MAGNETIC RESONANCE ANGIOGRAPHY// MAGNETIC RESONANCE IMAGING AND VESSEL WALL IMAGING

In primary LVV, MRA and MRI provide detailed information about arterial lumen and wall. In TA, MRA is a first-line diagnostic imaging modality, and in GCA, the EULAR recommends MRA/MRI, including vessel wall MRI (VWI) of cranial and extracranial arteries as an alternative if ultrasound is not available or inconclusive.[17] In recent years, VWI has brought about a shift in the imaging evaluation of vasculitis,[33] with increasing utilization in many vascular beds.[34] A recent survey of the ASNR indicated that LVV was the primary application for which institutions performed extracranial VWI.[35] Rather than focusing on changes in luminal caliber, VWI assesses vascular disease through the direct evaluation of vessel wall changes, including the presence or absence of active inflammation, wall edema, and thickening.[1,36–38] VWI can identify early vessel wall changes before developing luminal stenosis or occlusion.[1,36] A recent study evaluating 98 cases of biopsy-proven GCA demonstrated that VWI can provide an accurate diagnosis with an 88.7% sensitivity

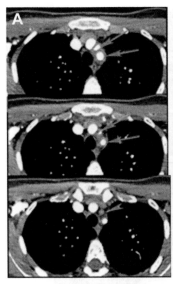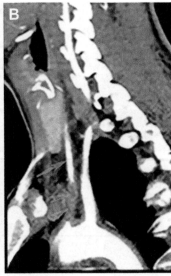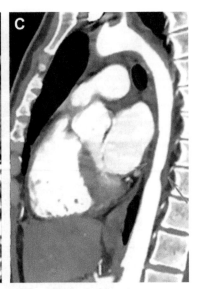

Fig. 5. 28-year-old male with TA. Axial CTA images (*A*) show concentric wall thickening of the left common carotid and left subclavian arteries (*arrows*). There is progressive tapering and subsequent occlusion of the left common carotid artery (*arrowhead*). Sagittal CTA image of aorta origins (*B*) shows the site of wall thickening with complete occlusion (*arrowheads*) and distal reconstitution of the left common carotid artery (*arrow*). Sagittal CTA image of thoracic aorta (*C*) shows wall thickening of the descending thoracic aorta with associated stenosis (*arrows*).

and 75% specificity for LVV.[38] The study emphasized the importance of early imaging, demonstrating that after approximately 5 days of corticosteroid treatment, the sensitivity of imaging markedly decreased.[38] VWI can be helpful in assessing treatment-related changes in LVV, helping to guide and modify immunomodulation regimens, indicating persistent active inflammation despite treatment versus inactive disease.[37,39] Wider availability of MRI scanners with the ability to perform VWI has made it a promising technique in diagnosing and monitoring LVV. Despite these clinical advantages, VWI has yet to find its way into standard clinical practice or established guidelines.

VESSEL WALL MAGNETIC RESONANCE IMAGING TECHNIQUE

For VWI, both 2-dimensional and 3-dimensional MRI techniques can be performed. 2-dimensional imaging of large arteries is typically performed in axial plane as the targeted large arteries (aorta and carotid arteries) course in a cranio-caudal direction and imaging in a plane perpendicular to the lumen achieves better wall assessment and blood signal suppression. An advantage of 2D imaging is that higher in-plane resolution may be achieved, blood suppression is better, and contrast resolution may be slightly better. A limitation of 2D imaging, however, is that it cannot be

reformatted in multiple planes as can be done with isotropic 3D acquisitions.

Consideration of blood suppression techniques is important to avoid flow-related artifacts that could be confused with vessel wall pathology. Double-inversion-recovery (DIR) is a technique that takes advantage of both blood flow and T1 blood signal characteristics for signal suppression and can be applied to 2-dimensional MRI sequences.[40] This technique employs a pair of 180-degree radiofrequency pulses in succession that result in slice magnetization alignment with the magnetic field. The inversion time (TI) is manually set to allow for inflowing spins to relax to the null point (point at which there is no signal), after which another radiofrequency pulse is applied that generates an echo for readout. Limitations of DIR include the prolongation of scan time, the potential need for cardiac or pulse gating, and accurate estimation of blood TI after contrast administration. Quadruple-inversion-recovery (QIR) can also be utilized, which negates the need to estimate blood TI post-contrast and cardiac gating.[41,42] Spin-echo techniques can be employed for blood suppression, although with slow flow or in-plane flow, blood suppression will be lost.

Recently, 3D VWI techniques have been developed and applied to VWI in an attempt to overcome some of the limitations specific to 2D VWI. Some of the potential advantages of 3D VWI include increased in-plane and through-plane resolution, significantly improved signal-to-noise and contrast-to-noise ratios of the vessel wall, improved blood suppression and overall image quality compared to 2D VWI.[43] Isotropic 3D acquisitions permit for multiplanar reconstructions, shortening scan times. This allows for coronal or sagittal plane scanning with axial reconstruction for the assessment of the arteries in short axis. This in combination with higher resolution optimizes imaging review and minimizes volume averaging effects. Variable refocusing flip angle techniques (VRFA) have received increased attention recently. These techniques have inherent dark blood characteristics from gradient moment-induced intravoxel dephasing and stimulated echo-induced intravoxel dephasing.[44] Additional blood signal suppression techniques can be employed with 3D imaging. One such technique is motion-sensitized driven equilibrium (MSDE), which uses flow-sensitive dephasing gradients to suppress flow; however, this technique results in T2 signal decay and overall signal loss. The delay alternating with nutation for tailored excitation (DANTE) pulse train is a series of low flip angle nonselective pulses interleaved with gradient pulses with short repetition times that can result in improved blood suppression without loss of signal or effects on tissue contrast.[44] Incorporation of DANTE pre-pulse significantly improves image quality, arterial and venous blood suppression, and enhances lesion conspicuity compared to conventional VRFA acquisitions.[44]

VWI offers considerable advantages over conventional MRI/MRA since it offers higher resolution, eliminates distracting signal and potential slow flow artifact from the luminal blood, and highlights vessel wall enhancement in areas of injury and inflammation. VWI can differentiate between stenosis secondary to active inflammation as compared to quiescent disease with scarred luminal stenoses as well as detect non-stenotic vessel wall disease.[36] However, the increased resolution and suppression of luminal blood is not without its cost. Although VWI offers flexible tissue contrast, high SNR, and is relatively insensitive to magnetic field inhomogeneities, due to longer scan times, it is vulnerable to motion artifacts and flow artifacts that may mimic wall lesions. As the scan time increases, so too does the likelihood of patient motion and resultant motion artifact.[45]

CLINICAL APPLICATION OF VESSEL WALL MAGNETIC RESONANCE IMAGING

VWI has shown clinical value in a number of applications, including the detection of early manifestations in pre-stenotic disease or before ischemic signs, monitoring disease changes/disease evolution, directing targeted biopsies of inflamed vessels, and avoiding potential artifacts that may arise if relying solely on standard MRI/MRA techniques.[1,10,36,38,39,46,47]

The imaging features seen with LVV include many of the same features in that of medium and small vessel vasculitis–smooth concentric vessel wall thickening, intense circumferential vessel wall enhancement, perivascular and vessel wall edema, and in later stages of the disease, luminal narrowing (Fig. 6).[36,38]

EARLY MANIFESTATIONS

Vessel wall imaging can corroborate clinical suspicion for active large vessel vasculitis even in the absence of ischemic signs or symptoms. Bley and colleagues, evaluated MRI findings (mural thickness, lumen diameter, and mural contrast enhancement) of superficial temporal arteries in 64 patients with suspected GCA; MR had a sensitivity of 80.6% and a specificity of 97.0% compared to ACR diagnostic criteria, and MR biopsy had a sensitivity of 90.5% and a specificity of 72.7% compared to temporal artery biopsy.[37] Wall thickness measurements of greater than 6 mm are usually considered pathologic. VWI can depict wall abnormalities prior to luminal changes in both GCA (Fig. 7) and TA (Fig. 8). Early manifestations of LVV are not detectable on luminal imaging. Delayed detection and diagnosis can lead to poor outcomes and permanent sequela, secondary to permanent arterial changes secondary to fibrotic wall changes in TA, leading to irreversible stenoses, occlusions and aneurysmal dilatation in TA, and permanent vision loss in GCA, that can manifest within a few days, due to ischemia.

DISEASE EVOLUTION

Vessel wall imaging can also be used to monitor for changes in disease status and to determine response to therapy. Bley, and colleagues demonstrated an excellent correlation between vascular inflammatory status (clinical symptoms and elevated inflammatory markers) with the degree of vessel enhancement in 17 patients with Giant Cell Arteritis.[39] Shortly after successful steroid therapy, normalization of symptoms and lab values was associated with a corresponding decrease/normalization in the degree of enhancement. Luminal imaging is limited in depicting changes in inflammatory disease activity, as luminal changes are permanent, and progression of inflammation, treatment response or quiescence of disease

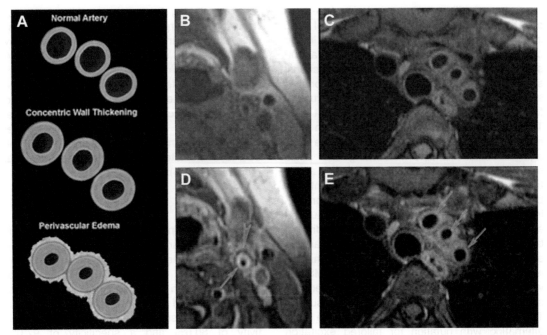

Fig. 6. Cartoon schematic of transverse view of arteries with three different conditions (*A*): normal vessel wall (top), arteries with concentric wall thickening (middle), and perivascular edema (bottom). Axial T1 pre- (*B* and *C*) and post-contrast (*D* and *E*) VWI, demonstrate circumferential wall thickening and enhancement (*arrows*) and perivascular edema (*arrowhead*) of multiple vessels, including the internal carotid artery and main aortic trunks.

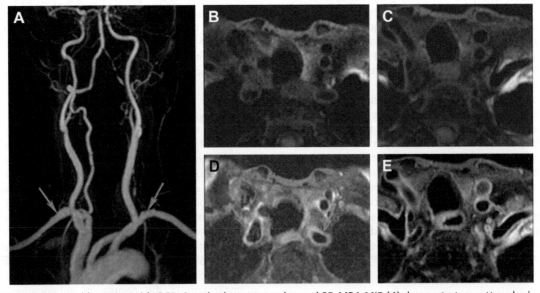

Fig. 7. 80-year-old woman with GCA. Standard contrast-enhanced 3D MRA MIP (*A*) demonstrates scattered minimal atherosclerotic stenoses (*arrows*), but no findings to suggest the presence of vasculitis. Axial T1 pre- (*B* and *C*) and post-contrast (*D* and *E*) VWI, demonstrates circumferential wall thickening and enhancement of multiple vessels, including the bilateral proximal common carotid and subclavian arteries (*arrows*), indicating multivessel inflammatory changes.

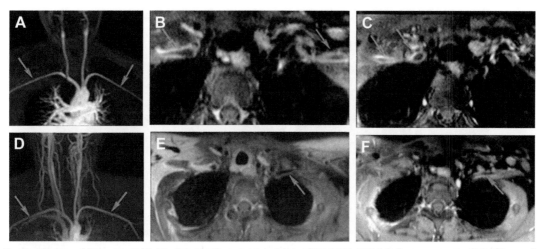

Fig. 8. 36-year-old woman with TA. Standard contrast-enhanced 3D MRA MIP (*A*) demonstrates mild diffuse sub-clavian narrowing (*arrows*), but no significant focal abnormalities. T1 post-contrast VWI (*B* and *C*), demonstrating marked circumferential wall thickening and enhancement of the great vessels and bilateral subclavian arteries, without significant luminal stenosis, indicating vessel wall inflammation. Follow-up after treatment with tocilizu-mab IV. Contrast-enhanced 3D MRA MIP (*D*) shows interval improvement in previously seen luminal narrowing of the bilateral subclavian arteries (*arrows*). T1 pre- (*E*) and post-contrast VWI (*F*) demonstrate decreased enhance-ment of the left subclavian artery (*arrows*).

may be difficult to differentiate. VWI can be contributory in this setting, specifically even if luminal findings are unchanged, direct assessment of the arterial wall permits inflammation assess-ment that might otherwise not be detectable (see Fig. 8; Figs. 9 and 10).

ADDITIONAL ADVANTAGES OF VESSEL WALL IMAGING

Standard MRI/MRA techniques may be limited due to potential artifacts that can mask vessel wall dis-ease. On post-contrast T1-weighted sequences,

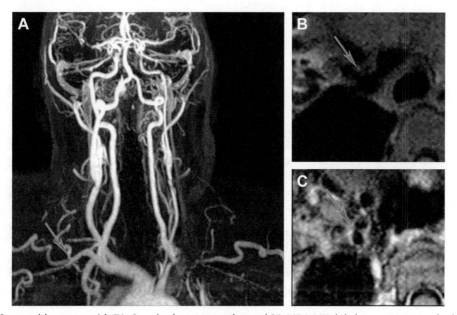

Fig. 9. 26-year-old woman with TA. Standard contrast-enhanced 3D MRA MIP (*A*) demonstrates marked stenosis/occlusion of the left greater than right subclavian arteries and the left common carotid artery with extensive collateral development. T1 pre- (*B*) and post-contrast VWI (*C*) performed as part of the same MRI scan demon-strate mild wall enhancement of the right common carotid artery and the subclavian artery suggestive of mild residual inflammation, and was stable compared to prior study (not shown).

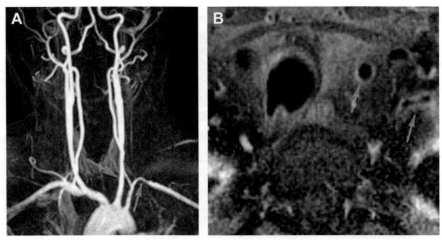

Fig. 10. 23-year-old male with TA who presented with fever and profound neutropenia. He was on long-term immunosuppression and had a marked interval increase in inflammatory markers (CRP 15.2 mg/L, ESR 101 mm/hr). Contrast-enhanced MRA MIP (*A*) demonstrates stenosis of the proximal left subclavian artery and mild irregularity of the left common carotid artery, stable from prior study. Post-contrast T1-weighted VWI (*B*) shows circumferential wall enhancement involving the areas of stenosis in the subclavian and common carotid arteries which had increased since the prior (not shown), indicating ongoing inflammation.

including 3D gradient-recalled echo techniques, inflammation-related intense arterial wall enhancement may match luminal signal and mask visualization of wall thickening and luminal stensosis (Fig. 11), which can be readily appreciated on VWI and first-past contrast-enhanced MRA. After intravenous contrast injection, the inversion time of blood will change compared to blood without contrast. Due to this effect, post-contrast T1-weighted sequences can have increased intraluminal signals

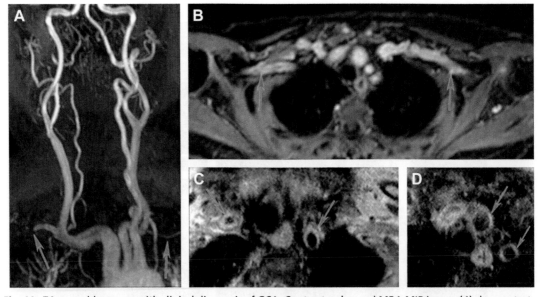

Fig. 11. 74-year-old woman with clinical diagnosis of GCA. Contrast-enhanced MRA MIP image (*A*) demonstrates occlusion of the proximal subclavian arteries (*arrows*). Axial post-contrast T1-weighed fat-suppressed gradient-recalled echo image (*B*) demonstrates apparent contrast filling the proximal subclavian arteries without evidence of stenosis (*arrows*). Double inversion T1-weighted post-contrast vessel wall sequences (*C* and *D*) demonstrate substantial vessel wall inflammatory change involving the brachiocephalic artery and left subclavian artery and luminal stenosis though with continued patency (*arrows*), providing clarifying information over the other MRI acquisitions.

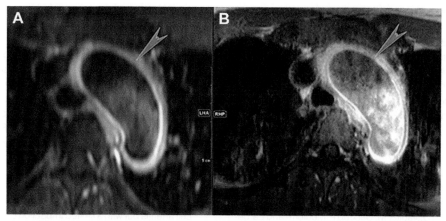

Fig. 12. 41-year-old woman with TA. 3D (*A*) and 2D VWI (*B*) of the aortic arch, with 3D VWI demonstrating better luminal suppression and improved conspicuity of the vessel wall abnormality (*arrowheads*).

that can mimic wall lesions. VWI with blood suppression can overcome these non-suppression artifacts (**Fig. 12**).

VESSEL WALL MAGNETIC RESONANCE IMAGING IN THE BIOPSY GUIDANCE

For a reliable diagnosis of GCA, a temporal artery biopsy is often required. One potential problem with blind biopsy is that oftentimes there can be skip lesions of affected vessels with intervening segments of normal uninvolved vessel and inflamed segments.[38] If the uninvolved vessel is biopsied, a false negative can result. Pre-biopsy evaluation with VWI may identify segments with active inflammation for biopsy targeting.[48] Using such images to help localize areas of involved vessels may improve the rate of successful biopsies and decrease false negative rates.

SUMMARY

In conclusion, imaging plays a central role in prompt diagnosis of large vessel vasculitis. Ultrasound is a first imaging choice for giant cell arteritis due to its high accuracy for the diagnosis and its accessibility, which is key due to the need for rapid diagnosis. VWI may play an increasingly greater role in both the diagnosis and follow-up of large vessel vasculitis. It helps guide treatment approaches and evaluate treatment response and confers a considerable advantage over luminal techniques such as DSA, CTA, and MRA. As the use of VWI widens, detection of pre-stenotic inflammation may help establish diagnosis earlier and improve patient outcomes with avoidance of late-stage disease complications, including blindness, stenosis, occlusion, and aneurysm formation.

CLINICS CARE POINTS

- Early diagnosis and appropriate treatment of large vessel vasculitis has a direct impact on patient outcomes.
- Rapid diagnosis of giant cell arteritis relies on a combination of MRA, CTA, ultrasound, vessel wall imaging, and/or superficial temporal artery biopsy.

DISCLOSURE

The authors have nothing to disclose.

REFERENCES

1. Jiang L, Li D, Yan F, et al. Evaluation of Takayasu arteritis activity by delayed contrast-enhanced magnetic resonance imaging. Int J Cardiol 2012;155(2): 262–7.
2. Boes CJ. Bayard Horton's clinicopathological description of giant cell (temporal) arteritis. Cephalalgia 2007;27(1):68–75.
3. Kerr GS. Takayasu's arteritis. Rheum Dis Clin North Am 1995;21(4):1041–58.
4. Salvarani C, Cantini F, Hunder GG. Polymyalgia rheumatica and giant-cell arteritis. Lancet 2008; 372(9634):234–45.
5. Weyand CM, Goronzy JJ. Clinical practice. Giant-cell arteritis and polymyalgia rheumatica. N Engl J Med 2014;371(1):50–7.
6. Sueyoshi E, Sakamoto I, Uetani M. MRI of Takayasu's arteritis: typical appearances and complications. AJR Am J Roentgenol 2006;187(6):W569–75.

7. Bhatti MT, Tabandeh H. Giant cell arteritis: diagnosis and management. Curr Opin Ophthalmol 2001; 12(6):393–9.

8. Johnston SL, Lock RJ, Gompels MM. Takayasu arteritis: a review. J Clin Pathol 2002;55(7):481–6.

9. Vautier M, Dupont A, de Boysson H, et al. Prognosis of large vessel involvement in large vessel vasculitis. J Autoimmun 2020;108:102419.

10. Borg FA, Dasgupta B. Treatment and outcomes of large vessel arteritis. Best Pract Res Clin Rheumatol 2009;23(3):325–37.

11. Vodopivec I, Rizzo JF 3rd. Ophthalmic manifestations of giant cell arteritis. Rheumatology 2018; 57(suppl_2):ii63–72.

12. Saadoun D, Vautier M, Cacoub P. Medium- and Large-Vessel Vasculitis. Circulation 2021;143(3):267–82.

13. Arend WP, Michel BA, Bloch DA, et al. The American College of Rheumatology 1990 criteria for the classification of Takayasu arteritis. Arthritis Rheum 1990; 33(8):1129–34.

14. Hunder GG, Bloch DA, Michel BA, et al. The American College of Rheumatology 1990 criteria for the classification of giant cell arteritis. Arthritis Rheum 1990;33(8):1122–8.

15. Gribbons KB, Ponte C, Carette S, et al. Patterns of Arterial Disease in Takayasu Arteritis and Giant Cell Arteritis. Arthritis Care Res 2020;72(11):1615–24.

16. Furuta S, Cousins C, Chaudhry A, et al. Clinical Features and Radiological Findings in Large Vessel Vasculitis: Are Takayasu Arteritis and Giant Cell Arteritis 2 Different Diseases or a Single Entity? J Rheumatol 2015;42(2):300–8.

17. Schäfer VS, Jin L, Schmidt WA. Imaging for Diagnosis, Monitoring, and Outcome Prediction of Large Vessel Vasculitides. Curr Rheumatol Rep 2020; 22(11):76.

18. Dejaco C, Ramiro S, Duftner C, et al. EULAR recommendations for the use of imaging in large vessel vasculitis in clinical practice. Ann Rheum Dis 2018; 77(5):636–43.

19. Schmidt WA, Kraft HE, Vorpahl K, et al. Color duplex ultrasonography in the diagnosis of temporal arteritis. N Engl J Med 1997;337(19):1336–42.

20. Aschwanden M, Daikeler T, Kesten F, et al. Temporal artery compression sign–a novel ultrasound finding for the diagnosis of giant cell arteritis. Ultraschall der Med 2013;34(1):47–50.

21. Nielsen BD, Hansen IT, Keller KK, et al. Diagnostic accuracy of ultrasound for detecting large-vessel giant cell arteritis using FDG PET/CT as the reference. Rheumatology 2020;59(8):2062–73.

22. Schäfer VS, Juche A, Ramiro S, et al. Ultrasound cut-off values for intima-media thickness of temporal, facial and axillary arteries in giant cell arteritis. Rheumatology 2017;56(9):1479–83.

23. Maeda H, Handa N, Matsumoto M, et al. Carotid lesions detected by B-mode ultrasonography in Takayasu's arteritis: "macaroni sign" as an indicator of the disease. Ultrasound Med Biol 1991;17(7): 695–701.

24. Barra L, Kanji T, Malette J, et al. Imaging modalities for the diagnosis and disease activity assessment of Takayasu's arteritis: A systematic review and meta-analysis. Autoimmun Rev 2018;17(2):175–87.

25. Einspieler I, Thürmel K, Pyka T, et al. Imaging large vessel vasculitis with fully integrated PET/MRI: a pilot study. Eur J Nucl Med Mol Imaging 2015; 42(7):1012–24.

26. Nielsen BD, Gormsen LC, Hansen IT, et al. Three days of high-dose glucocorticoid treatment attenuates large-vessel 18F-FDG uptake in large-vessel giant cell arteritis but with a limited impact on diagnostic accuracy. Eur J Nucl Med Mol Imag 2018;45(7):1119–28.

27. Aghayev A, Steigner ML. Systemic vasculitides and the role of multitechnique imaging in the diagnosis. Clin Radiol 2021;76(7):488–501.

28. Sammel AM, Hsiao E, Schembri G, et al. Diagnostic Accuracy of Positron Emission Tomography/Computed Tomography of the Head, Neck, and Chest for Giant Cell Arteritis: A Prospective, Double-Blind, Cross-Sectional Study. Arthritis Rheumatol 2019;71(8): 1319–28.

29. Weinrich JM, Lenz A, Adam G, et al. Radiologic Imaging in Large and Medium Vessel Vasculitis. Radiol Clin North Am 2020;58(4):765–79.

30. García-Martínez A, Arguis P, Prieto-González S, et al. Prospective long term follow-up of a cohort of patients with giant cell arteritis screened for aortic structural damage (aneurysm or dilatation). Ann Rheum Dis 2014;73(10):1826–32.

31. Lariviere D, Benali K, Coustet B, et al. Positron emission tomography and computed tomography angiography for the diagnosis of giant cell arteritis: A real-life prospective study. Medicine (Baltim) 2016; 95(30):e4146.

32. Yamada I, Nakagawa T, Himeno Y, et al. Takayasu arteritis: evaluation of the thoracic aorta with CT angiography. Radiology 1998;209(1):103–9.

33. Guevara ME, Lin W, Mossa-Basha M. FRI0247 Black Blood Mri/A for Diagnosis of Large Vessel Vasculitis. Ann Rheum Dis 2014;73(Suppl 2):472–3.

34. Mossa-Basha M, Zhu C, Yuan C, et al. Survey of the American Society of Neuroradiology Membership on the Use and Value of Intracranial Vessel Wall MRI. AJNR Am J Neuroradiol 2022;43(7):951–7.

35. Mossa-Basha M, Yuan C, Wasserman BA, et al. Survey of the American Society of Neuroradiology Membership on the Use and Value of Extracranial Carotid Vessel Wall MRI. AJNR Am J Neuroradiol 2022; 43(12):1756–61.

36. Choe YH, Han BK, Koh EM, et al. Takayasu's arteritis: assessment of disease activity with contrast-enhanced MR imaging. AJR Am J Roentgenol 2000;175(2):505–11.

37. Bley TA, Uhl M, Carew J, et al. Diagnostic value of high-resolution MR imaging in giant cell arteritis. AJNR Am J Neuroradiol 2007;28(9):1722–7.

38. Klink T, Geiger J, Both M, et al. Giant cell arteritis: diagnostic accuracy of MR imaging of superficial cranial arteries in initial diagnosis-results from a multicenter trial. Radiology 2014;273(3):844–52.

39. Bley TA, Markl M, Schelp M, et al. Mural inflammatory hyperenhancement in MRI of giant cell (temporal) arteritis resolves under corticosteroid treatment. Rheumatology 2008;47(1):65–7.

40. Mandell DM, Mossa-Basha M, Qiao Y, et al. Intracranial Vessel Wall MRI: Principles and Expert Consensus Recommendations of the American Society of Neuroradiology. AJNR Am J Neuroradiol 2017;38(2):218–29.

41. Saba L, Yuan C, Hatsukami TS, et al. Carotid Artery Wall Imaging: Perspective and Guidelines from the ASNR Vessel Wall Imaging Study Group and Expert Consensus Recommendations of the American Society of Neuroradiology. AJNR Am J Neuroradiol 2018;39(2):E9–31.

42. Coolen BF, Calcagno C, van Ooij P, et al. Vessel wall characterization using quantitative MRI: what's in a number? Magma 2018;31(1):201–22.

43. Mossa-Basha M, Alexander MA, Maki JH, et al. Exploring other vascular Dimensions: Comparison of 3-dimensional and 2-dimensional vessel wall imaging techniques for the assessment of large artery vasculopathies. Singapore: International Society of Magnetic Resonance in Medicine; 2016. Paper presented at.

44. Sannananja B, Zhu C, Colip CG, et al. Image-Quality Assessment of 3D Intracranial Vessel Wall MRI Using DANTE or DANTE-CAIPI for Blood Suppression and Imaging Acceleration. AJNR Am J Neuroradiol 2022;43(6):837–43.

45. Vranic JE, Cross NM, Wang Y, et al. Compressed Sensing-Sensitivity Encoding (CS-SENSE) Accelerated Brain Imaging: Reduced Scan Time without Reduced Image Quality. AJNR Am J Neuroradiol 2019;40(1):92–8.

46. Khan A, Dasgupta B. Imaging in Giant Cell Arteritis. Curr Rheumatol Rep 2015;17(8):52.

47. Ammirati E, Moroni F, Pedrotti P, et al. Non-invasive imaging of vascular inflammation. Front Immunol 2014;5:399.

48. Zeiler SR, Qiao Y, Pardo CA, et al. Vessel Wall MRI for Targeting Biopsies of Intracranial Vasculitis. AJNR Am J Neuroradiol 2018;39(11):2034–6.

Imaging of Small Artery Vasculitis

Omar Hamam, MD, Samuel C. Cartmell, MD, Javier M. Romero, MD*

KEYWORDS

- Stroke • Vasculitis • Vessel wall imaging (VWI) • MR angiography • CT angiography

KEY POINTS

- Small artery vasculitis is a multifaceted medical condition distinguished by inflammation and subsequent flow impairment of the small blood vessels.
- The diagnostic algorithm for small artery vasculitis involves a combination of clinical, laboratory, and imaging findings.
- Understanding the diagnostic limitations and advantages of multiple diagnostic exams, such as biopsy, angiography, or other imaging modalities, is essential for accurate diagnosis.
- Proper utilization of medical imaging techniques is necessary for the appropriate evaluation of small artery vasculitis.

INTRODUCTION

Small artery vasculitis of the central nervous system (CNS) comprises a collection of rare and serious conditions characterized by the inflammation of the blood vessels within the brain and spinal cord.[1] There are two well-defined groups of small artery vasculitis determined by the presence or absence of immunoglobulin complex deposition in the vessel wall. Small artery vasculitis with immune complex deposition includes anti-glomerular basement membrane disease, cryoglobulinemic vasculitis, and IgA vasculitis.[2] The absence of immune complex deposition in the vessel wall is generally associated with anti-neutrophil cytoplasmic antibody (ANCA) and includes microscopic polyangiitis, granulomatosis with polyangiitis, eosinophilic granulomatosis with polyangiitis, and primary angiitis of the CNS (PACNS). The events triggering the immunologic cascade and the molecular mechanisms for PACNS are unknown and this entity frequently presents a diagnostic challenge in which imaging plays a crucial role. This article will explore the clinical and imaging features of small artery vasculitis with special attention to recent imaging techniques that can provide insight into this important collection of diseases.

TYPES OF SMALL ARTERY VASCULITIS
Primary Angiitis of the Central Nervous System

PACNS primarily affects small and medium-sized arteries in the CNS, leading to various neurologic symptoms.[3] This condition poses significant diagnostic and therapeutic challenges due to its nonspecific clinical presentation and the potential for severe complications.[4]

The history of CNS angiitis can be traced back to the early 20th century when it was first recognized as a distinct clinical entity.[5] Initially, it was often misdiagnosed as other neurologic disorders, making accurate estimation of its incidence and prevalence difficult. Difficulties in determining its true prevalence persist, although a recent study estimated that 2.4 individuals for every million people are affected. With advances in diagnostic techniques and increased awareness among physicians, the recognition and diagnosis of PACNS have improved over time.[6]

PACNS can affect both the leptomeningeal and parenchymal arteries.[7] As a result, there is a broad

Neurovascular Laboratory R.H Ackerman, Radiology, Mass General Brigham, 55 Fruit street, Boston, MA, 02115, USA
* Corresponding author.
E-mail address: jmromero@mgh.harvard.edu

Neuroimag Clin N Am 34 (2024) 67–79
https://doi.org/10.1016/j.nic.2023.07.009

manifestation of disease including headaches, stroke, hemorrhage, cognitive impairment, seizures, and focal neurologic deficits.[8]

The exact pathogenesis of PACNS remains incompletely understood. However, it is believed to involve an autoimmune-mediated inflammatory response targeting the blood vessels of the CNS.[9] It is hypothesized that an abnormal immune response triggers an inflammatory cascade leading to endothelial cell activation and infiltration of immune cells into the vessel walls.[10] This immune cell infiltration results in vascular damage, disruption of the blood-brain barrier, and subsequent tissue injury.

Histopathological examination of brain tissue from individuals with PACNS reveals distinct findings consistent with vasculitis.[11] The characteristic histopathological feature is fibrinoid necrosis, which refers to the destruction of the vessel wall leading to the formation of a fibrin-rich necrotic material occurring in the media and adventitia layers of the affected arteries.[12] In addition to fibrinoid necrosis, immunohistochemical studies have demonstrated the presence of various immune cells consisting of lymphocytes, plasma cells, and macrophages within and around the affected vessel walls, further supporting the autoimmune nature of the disease.[13]

The presence of these immune cells suggests an ongoing immune response and highlights the importance of the adaptive immune system in the pathogenesis of PACNS.[14] Corticosteroids and cytotoxic agents represent the current mainstays of treatment for small artery vasculitis.

IgA Arteritis

IgA arteritis, also known as Henoch-Schönlein purpura (HSP) represents the most common type of vasculitis in children.[15] PACNS primarily involves the inflammation of the blood vessels within the CNS, while HSP is characterized by the inflammation of small blood vessel in various organs such as the skin, joints, gastrointestinal tract, and kidneys and rarely the nervous system.[16]

PACNS and HSP are distinct clinical entities with different manifestations, underlying pathologies, and affected vascular beds. PACNS specifically targets the arteries in the brain and spinal cord, leading to neurologic symptoms.[17] On the other hand; HSP is a systemic vasculitis that primarily affects gastrointestinal symptoms such as stomach pain and hematochezia, purpura, and nephritis.[16]

Microscopic Polyangiitis (Microscopic Polyarteritis)

Microscopic polyarteritis (MPA) is another form of vasculitis characterized by the inflammation of small- and medium-sized blood vessels,[17] particularly in the kidneys, lungs, and peripheral nerves.[18] MPA is a type of ANCA-associated vasculitis linked to myeloperoxidase (MPO).[19] Involvement of the CNS is less frequently described and generally consists of intracerebral or subarachnoid hemorrhage, pachymeningitis, and ischemic strokes.[20,21]

When PACNS coexists with MPA, it may contribute to the development of additional neurologic manifestations in patients with MPA. These manifestations can include stroke-like symptoms, cranial neuropathies, or other CNS complications.[22]

Granulomatosis with Polyangiitis

Granulomatosis with polyangiitis (GPA), formerly known as Wegener's granulomatosis, is a systemic vasculitis characterized by granulomatous inflammation and necrotizing vasculitis that predominantly affects the upper and lower respiratory tracts, kidneys, and other organs.[23] In contrast to the affinity to produce peripheral nerve inflammation, CNS involvement is extremely rare, representing only 7% to 11% of GPA. Three different histologic patterns of CNS involvement have been described in GPA[24]: CNS vasculitis of the small vessels of the brain or spinal cord, contiguous granulomatous invasion from extracranial sites, and isolated intracranial (cerebral or meningeal) granulomatous lesions.[25]

Eosinophilic Granulomatosis with Polyangiitis

Eosinophilic granulomatosis with polyangiitis (EGPA), formerly known as Churg-Strauss syndrome, is a rare systemic vasculitis characterized by eosinophilic inflammation and necrotizing vasculitis that can affect multiple organ systems.[26,27]

Neurologic complications in EGPA can include peripheral neuropathies, mononeuritis multiplex, and rarely, CNS involvement.[28] In a recent trial by Liu and colleagues, ischemic lesions were the most common manifestations, accounting for 63.2%, followed by posterior reversible encephalopathy syndrome (36.8%), spinal cord involvement (15.8%), medulla oblongata involvement (15.8%), and intracranial hemorrhages (15.8%).[29]

DIAGNOSTIC WORKUP
Inflammatory Biomarkers

The diagnosis and monitoring of small artery vasculitis and PACNS rely heavily on the utilization of inflammatory biomarkers (Table 1). The most frequently studied inflammatory biomarkers linked

Table 1
Findings in the diagnostic workup of suspected small artery vasculitis[30]

Diagnostic Test/Procedure	Findings
Clinical Evaluation	Intense thunderclap headache, cognitive impairment, stroke-like events, and seizures
Laboratory Tests	Elevated erythrocyte sedimentation rate (ESR), C-reactive protein (CRP), and/or autoantibodies (eg, ANCA, ANA)
Cerebrospinal Fluid (CSF) Analysis	Lymphocytic pleocytosis, elevated protein levels, presence of oligoclonal bands
Imaging Studies	
Magnetic Resonance Imaging (MRI)	Bilateral T2 or FLAIR abnormalities in the cortex, deep gray and white matter, multifocal stenoses and dilatations in small vessels, ischemic and hemorrhagic lesions
Magnetic Resonance Angiography (MRA)	Multifocal segmental artery narrowing macro- and micro-arteries
Routine contrast-enhanced MRI	Focal punctate parenchymal enhancement indicating inflammatory changes of perforating vessels.
High-Resolution MRI (black blood vessel wall imaging)	Direct characterization of vessel wall abnormalities including concentric patterns of wall thickening and wall enhancement
Brain Biopsy	Transmural inflammation, granulomatous or lymphocytic cellular infiltrates, necrotizing vasculitis, neointimal proliferation, thromboses, intimal fibrosis

Abbreviations: CSF, cerebrospinal fluid; DSA, digital subtraction angiography; MRI, magnetic resonance tomography; PACNS, primary angiitis of the central nervous system.

to small artery vasculitis will be discussed later in discussion.

Increased concentrations of CRP are suggestive of systemic inflammation and are detectable in individuals with small artery vasculitis. Nevertheless, the diagnostic efficacy of CRP levels alone is restricted, as PACNS may not invariably exhibit a significant elevation of such levels. Similar to CRP, ESR exhibits limited specificity for PACNS and can be affected by various other factors.[31]

ANCAs are among the most promising and specific biomarkers and an area of active investigation. Although research is ongoing, recent results suggest that ANCA subtype, and specifically the presence of myeloperoxidase or proteinase-3-ANCA, may be more valuable for prognosis and therapeutic response than clinical presentation. It is possible to observe an elevation in the WBC or an increase in the levels of particular subtypes of WBCs, such as neutrophils and lymphocytes. Nevertheless, these observations are not exclusive to PACNS and are also evident in other inflammatory or infectious ailments.[32]

Studies have reported increased levels of proinflammatory cytokines, interleukin-6 (IL-6), tumor necrosis factor-alpha (TNF-α), and interferon-gamma (IFN-γ), in cases of PACNS. Cytokines play a contributory role in the recruitment and activation of immune cells, thereby intensifying the inflammatory process in PACNS.[33]

Elevated levels of vascular endothelial growth factor (VEGF) have been detected in patients with PACNS and are believed to play a role in the pathogenesis of angiogenesis and impairment of the blood-brain barrier.[34]

Cerebrospinal Fluid Findings

The analysis of CSF is a pivotal component in the diagnostic evaluation of small artery vasculitis. CSF findings are variable; however, lymphocytic pleocytosis, elevated protein levels, and oligoclonal bands are common.[35] The term lymphocytic pleocytosis denotes an elevation in the number of lymphocytes present in the CSF, which serves as an indicator of inflammation in the CNS.[36] Disruption or breakdown of the blood-brain barrier may result in increased protein levels.[37] Oligoclonal bands are composed of immunoglobulins and indicate an adaptive immune response within the CNS.[38] CSF analysis, in conjunction with clinical and neuroimaging assessments, serves to substantiate the diagnosis of PACNS and distinguish it from alternative neurologic disorders.[11]

DIFFERENTIAL DIAGNOSIS
Reversible Cerebral Vasoconstriction Syndromes

Distinguishing between RCVS and PACNS can be challenging due to their clinical and radiological similarities. Both illnesses involve the inflammation of the blood vessels of the CNS and can result in similar symptoms. Nonetheless, their causes, treatments, and natural histories differ. The hallmark of RCVS is an acute thunderclap headache, often described as the worst the patient has ever experienced. Visual abnormalities, seizures, and focal impairments may also coexist. Notably, RCVS symptoms usually resolve within weeks.[11,39] In contrast, PACNS symptoms, such as headaches, cognitive impairment, stroke-like events, and epileptic seizures, typically worsen without treatment.

Intracranial Atherosclerotic Diseases

Differentiation between PACNS and ICAD can pose a significant diagnostic challenge. Although both conditions may exhibit comparable symptoms such as headaches and stroke-like events, PACNS and other types of small artery vasculitis are distinguished by the segmental concentric inflammation of the blood vessels, whereas atheromatous disease is primarily associated with focal, eccentric plaque accumulation.[40] Achieving accurate differentiation may require the use of diagnostic imaging and biopsy, which can help establish the concentric versus eccentric patterns described above.

Cerebral Autosomal Dominant Arteriopathy with Subcortical Infarcts and Leukoencephalopathy

While both conditions can present with similar clinical features such as cognitive impairment and stroke-like events, PACNS involves inflammatory changes in the blood vessels and can manifest throughout the CNS, whereas CADASIL is a genetic disorder characterized by progressive small vessel disease often within characteristic territories. Genetic testing and neuroimaging can aid in the differential diagnosis.[40] MRI imaging of CADASIL is characterized by white matter involvement of the anterior temporal lobes and external capsules.

Mitochondrial Encephalomyopathy, Lactic Acidosis, and Stroke-Like Episodes

MELAS is typified by a distinct clinical triad comprising stroke-like episodes, lactic acidosis, and mitochondrial dysfunction. It typically occurs in children and young adults, with nearly 90% of cases presenting before the age of 40. In contrast to small artery vasculitis, adult patients with MELAS present with basal ganglia calcification and infarcts preferentially involving the parieto-occipital lobes, although both conditions can cause headaches, cognitive impairment, and stroke-like events.[41]

Moya Moya Disease

Moya Moya disease is characterized by a gradual constriction of the cerebral vasculature in part due to fibrocellular proliferation within the intima. It primarily affects the terminal intracranial segment of the internal carotid arteries and proximal middle cerebral arteries, which can result in either ischemic infarctions or hemorrhagic events. In contrast, PACNS is a primary inflammatory condition affecting smaller vessels and only occasionally involving larger arteries. As a result, the angiographic and neuroimaging appearance of these two conditions is distinct and imaging plays a crucial role in distinguishing between them.[42]

Radiation Vasculitis

Radiation vasculitis manifests as a delayed sequela of radiation therapy and exhibits parenchymal microhemorrhages, infarcts and less frequently large parenchymal hemorrhages. These manifestations are similar to those in small artery vasculitis, hence a comprehensive clinical assessment, thorough the investigation of any prior history of radiation, and careful analysis of imaging results are imperative for a precise diagnosis.[43] Clinically, small artery vasculitis has an acute inflammatory presentation associated with headaches and elevated inflammatory biomarkers whereas radiation vasculitis may be more insidious in onset.

Imaging

Computed tomography
Non-contrast computed tomography (CT) is often the first imaging tool used to evaluate patients with a suspected intracranial process. While it is sensitive for the evaluation of intracranial hemorrhage including vasculitis-related hemorrhage, it is relatively insensitive for the detection of small infarcts, particularly in comparison with MRI (Fig. 1). Absence of findings on CT should not preclude

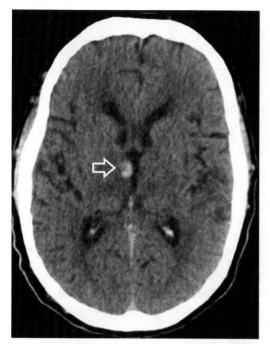

Fig. 1. Non-contrast CT of the head demonstrates significant periventricular white matter hypoattenuation and a small right ventral thalamic hemorrhage (*arrow*).

evaluation with MRI if there is clinical suspicion of vasculitis or other acute ischemic process.[44]

Magnetic resonance imaging

Conventional magnetic resonance imaging (MRI) is highly sensitive and plays an important role in the diagnosis of PACNS. The majority of patients show MRI abnormalities, although findings are not specific and must be carefully differentiated from other potential diagnoses. The initial MRI sequences should include T1-weighted, T2-weighted, fluid-attenuated inversion-recovery (FLAIR), apparent diffusion coefficient maps, diffusion, and gradient echo sequences, with and without gadolinium administration. Typical findings of PACNS include bilateral T2 or FLAIR abnormalities involving the cortex, deep gray and white matter (Figs. 2 and 3) coexisting with multifocal stenoses and dilatations of medium and small vessels.[45]

Ischemic lesions may be accompanied by subarachnoid and intraparenchymal hemorrhage (Figs. 4 and 5). Mass lesions resembling tumors or abscesses can also be observed, and gadolinium enhancement may be present in parenchymal lesions and in the leptomeninges.[46]

Angiography

In cases of suspected small artery vasculitis and PACNS, it is recommended to use angiographic techniques such as computed tomography angiography (CTA), magnetic resonance angiography (MRA) (Fig. 6), and digital subtraction angiography (DSA) (see Fig. 4; Fig. 7) to visualize intracranial vessels for detecting stenosis and dilatation, known as "vessel beading." Although these findings are often seen in small vessel vasculitis and PACNS, they are not specific and can also occur in other non-inflammatory vasculopathies and non-vasculitic conditions, such as atherosclerosis, radiation-induced changes, neurofibromatosis, infections, and vasospasm. Therefore, relying solely on angiographic findings may not be sufficient to confirm the diagnosis of PACNS.[47] The different modalities will be discussed later in discussion.

Computed tomography angiography

CTA is a powerful tool for the evaluation of the intracranial circulation. It is widely available, rapid, provides detailed information about vessel morphology, and can be used to evaluate luminal abnormalities in PACNS. However, CTA has some notable limitations, especially in comparison to DSA and MRI/MRA. Specifically, the spatial resolution of DSA remains superior to that of CTA, making it more sensitive to irregularities in small distal vessels.[47] Similarly, the contrast resolution of MRI is superior to CTA, providing better depiction of abnormalities of the vessel wall.[48]

Magnetic resonance angiography

MRA is another valuable tool for the non-invasive assessment of the intracranial circulation, although is generally inferior to CTA in terms of spatial resolution and sensitivity to motion. Nonetheless, MRA can readily demonstrate abnormalities of the vessel lumen, including stenoses, dilations, and occlusions, particularly within proximal vessels. When it comes to detecting lesions in the posterior circulation and distal arteries, MRA generally performs less well than other modalities, particularly DSA.[49] MRA is often used in conjunction with MRI-based vessel wall imaging (VWI, discussed later in discussion) in cases of suspected or confirmed vasculitis. In such cases, it can become a powerful adjunct that is well suited to monitor disease progression.

Digital subtraction angiography

DSA, sometimes also referred to as conventional cerebral angiography, is an invasive procedure requiring the insertion of a catheter into the blood vessels and injection of contrast material, followed by the acquisition of real-time fluoroscopic images. DSA offers superior temporal and spatial resolution over other techniques and as a result is still considered the gold standard for detecting

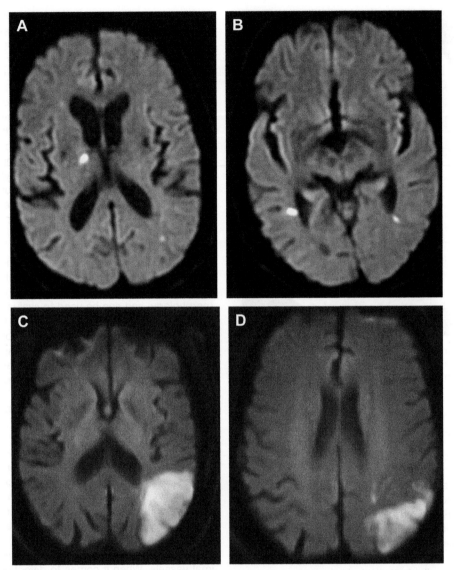

Fig. 2. MRI of the brain with diffusion weighted images shows multiple foci of restricted diffusion in the deep gray matter (*A*) and periventricular white matter (*B*) likely representing infarcts of perforating vascular territories. (*C, D*) Wedge-shaped area of acute infarction in the left parietal-occipital lobe, likely reflecting involvement of an MCA branch.

abnormalities of the vessel lumen, both in PACNS and other cerebrovascular conditions.[31]

As in CTA and MRA, features indicative of primary CNS vasculitis may include multiple segments of narrowing and dilatation, multifocal occlusions of intracranial vessels, fusiform arterial dilatations, development of collateral circulation, and delayed contrast enhancement.[50]

Despite DSA's superior spatial and temporal resolution, the study may appear normal when inflammatory changes do not alter the vessel lumen (ie, no dilation, stenosis, or intimal injury) or when they involve arteries smaller than 500 μm in diameter. Focal involvement can also be missed and result in a false negative test. The overall sensitivity and specificity of conventional angiography has been reported in the range of 25%–35%.[51] Thus, even in the presence of normal or inconclusive DSA results, a brain biopsy should be considered when there is a high clinical suspicion of PACNS. Conversely, even in the presence of classic angiographic findings, biopsy may yield an alternative diagnosis.[51]

Lastly, there are inherent risks associated with any invasive procedure, including the potential for vascular injury, bleeding, and allergic reactions

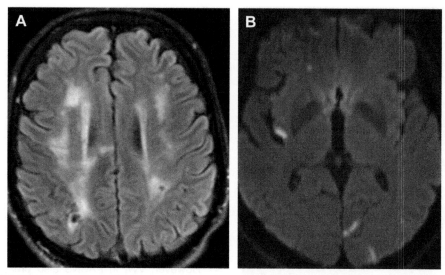

Fig. 3. (*A*) FLAIR image of the brain demonstrates patchy and confluent periventricular hyperintensities. (*B*) Multiple foci of acute cortical infarctions in a patient with eosinophilic granulomatosis with polyangiitis.

to the contrast material, and DSA is no exception, although it is generally safe.[51]

Vessel Wall Imaging

VWI plays a crucial role in the evaluation and diagnosis of small artery vasculitis and PACNS as it helps distinguish inflammatory vasculopathies from non-inflammatory disorders such as atherosclerosis and other conditions that may share similar clinical and radiological features with PACNS.[52]

Various approaches can be employed for vascular imaging in PACNS, high-resolution contrast-enhanced MRI (HR-MRI) "black blood" techniques being the most common. These protocols generally consist of a 3D T1-weighted sequence with sub-centimeter isotropic voxels

and an inversion pulse to null the signal within the intracranial vessels. Images are obtained before and after the administration of gadolinium contrast. MRA is often performed concurrently to assess for corresponding luminal abnormalities.[53] Please refer to a separate article in this issue regarding further technical details and usefulness of different angiographic techniques.

HR-MRI can assess the presence of features such as wall thickening, wall enhancement, morphology, and pathologic findings in and around the walls of intracranial vessels.[54] (Figs. 8 and 9). The combination of these features can strongly suggest the presence of vasculitis and differentiate it from other disorders.[55] The primary differentiating feature of small artery vasculitis is the pattern of mural enhancement. Whereas vasculitis tends to produce concentric mural

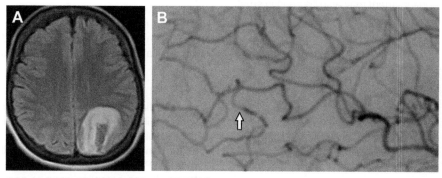

Fig. 4. 56-year-old female with sudden onset headache. (*A*) MRI-FLAIR shows an intraparenchymal hemorrhage in the left parietal lobe with surrounding edema. (*B*) Conventional angiogram demonstrates a beaded appearance of branches of the posterior cerebral artery (*arrow*), characteristic of small artery vasculitis of the CNS.

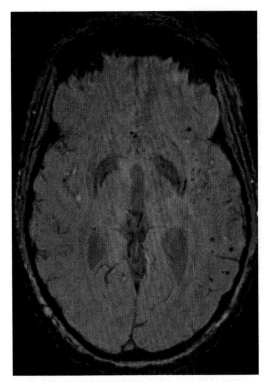

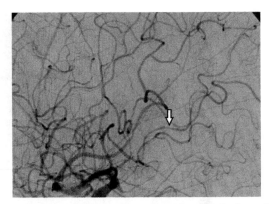

Fig. 7. Conventional angiogram with multiple sites of segmental narrowing and beaded appearance representing vasculitis in a patient with PACNS (*arrow*).

Fig. 5. MRI susceptibility weighted image of the brain shows multiple foci of low signal intensity, likely representing microhemorrhages of the subcortical white matter, in a patient with PACNS.

However, VWI in PACNS also presents challenges and limitations. Interpreting the imaging results requires expertise and knowledge of the typical features of PACNS. Technical constraints, such as the small size of intracranial vessels, can impact image quality and diagnostic accuracy. Additionally, access to advanced imaging techniques may be limited in some health care settings. Further advances in this noninvasive technique may mitigate some of these issues and hold promise for future diagnostic perspectives.[55]

enhancement of the intracranial vessels, ICAD produces abnormalities eccentric to the vessel lumen (Fig. 10). Widespread mural enhancement is especially suggestive of PACNS or other small artery vasculitis, particularly if distant from sites of parenchymal signal abnormality (eg, ACA concentric mural enhancement in the presence of posterior circulation infarcts). Other findings, such as wall thickening or enhancement within the adjacent parenchyma can be supportive but tend not be as informative. Parenchymal punctate and radial enhancement may also be seen in small artery vasculitis (Fig. 11).

Other Modalities

While MRI, CT, and catheter angiography constitute the most important imaging modalities to diagnose small artery vasculitis in current clinical practice, other approaches are under active investigation. These include tools from nuclear medicine such as positron emission tomography with [11C]-PK11195, a marker of microglial activation. These studies have shown potential for detecting vascular inflammatory activity in patients with large vessel vasculitis. Implementing these tools could be beneficial for diagnosing PACNS in cases where MRI results are inconclusive. The specific choice of imaging technique may vary depending on the availability, expertise, and individual patient factors.[56]

Brain biopsy

PACNS is diagnosed by brain biopsy when imaging tests fail. The morbidity and invasive nature of a brain biopsy is a major drawback; bleeding, infection, and structural damage are all possible outcomes. PACNS occurs in focal and segmental patterns, hence sampling error is another major concern, and a negative biopsy does not exclude the diagnosis. In addition, infections, neoplasms

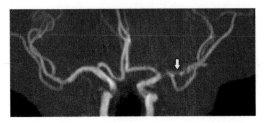

Fig. 6. MRA of the head demonstrates multifocal segmental narrowing of left MCA branches in a patient with Henoch Schonlein purpura (*arrow*).

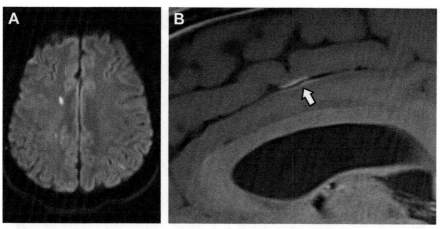

Fig. 8. 22-year-old with nephropathy and stroke. (A) Punctate foci of restricted diffusion in the right centrum semiovale, representing acute infarction. (B) MRI-VWI shows concentric enhancement of the anterior cerebral artery, likely representing vasculitis in a patient with IgG vasculitis (arrow).

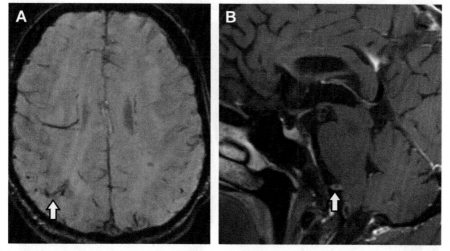

Fig. 9. 59-year-old male with headaches, focal neurologic deficit, and eosinophilic granulomatosis with polyangiitis. (A) Susceptibility weighted images demonstrate linear blooming in the bilateral parietal lobes, representing superficial siderosis (arrow). (B) MRI-VWI shows concentric enhancement of the vertebral arteries (arrow).

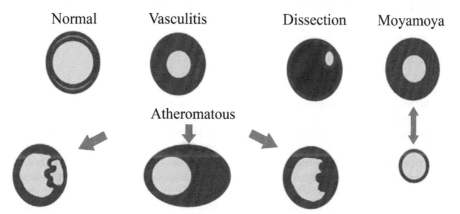

Fig. 10. Graph depicts morphologic abnormalities on MRI-VWI of dissection, vasculitis, Moya Moya and atheromatous disease.

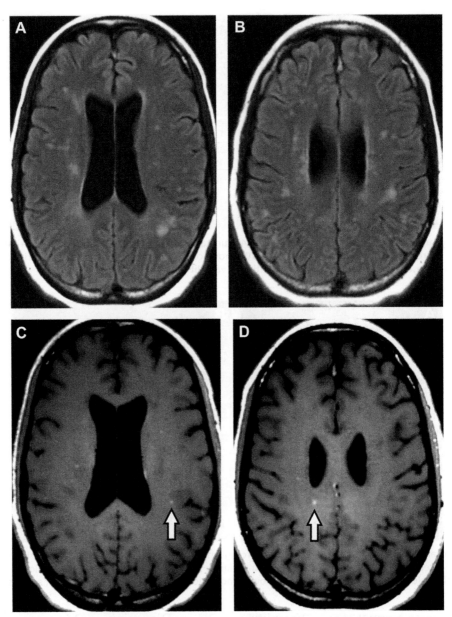

Fig. 11. 26-year-old male with severe migraines. (*A, B*) FLAIR-MRI of the brain shows multiple white matter hyperintensities. (*C, D*) Post contrast T1 weighted images demonstrate multiple punctate foci of parenchymal enhancement in a patient with granulomatosis with polyangiitis (*arrows*).

(especially lymphoma), and degenerative diseases can mimic PACNS upon histologic analysis. Targeting brain biopsy to areas of imaging abnormalities can boost diagnostic yield to above 80%. If surgery cannot reach the lesions, a biopsy of the non-dominant frontal lobe and leptomeningeal tissue is recommended, in these situations, the sensitivity of brain biopsy is probably in the range of 50%. PACNS is characterized histologically by transmural inflammation causing vessel wall destruction, in which granulomatous inflammation,

lymphocytic infiltrates, or acute necrotizing vasculitis are typically seen. Granulomatous vasculitis, comprising 56% of patients with PACNS, is often associated with beta-A4 amyloid deposition. Lymphocytic vasculitis causes inflammation with lymphocytes, plasma cells, histiocytes, neutrophils, and eosinophils. Necrotizing vasculitis causes acute necrosis, inflammation, and bleeding. Intimal fibrosis indicates healing, but neointimal development and thromboses are poor prognostic signs.[57]

SUMMARY

Small-vessel vasculitis can have a wide range of signs and symptoms, making clinical diagnosis challenging. Imaging has emerged as a valuable tool for characterizing different types of vasculitis based on the involved vascular bed. Pathologic and angiographic findings have shown limited sensitivity and specificity for diagnosing small artery vasculitis, which may be improved with the use of high-resolution vessel wall imaging.

CLINICS CARE POINTS

- Small-vessel vasculitis may sometimes involve medium-sized and large-vessels.
- Systemic involvement of the lungs, kidneys and skin is critical for differentiating the subtypes of small artery vasculitis.
- The current mainstays of treatment for small artery vasculitis are corticosteroids and cytotoxic agents.

DISCLOSURE

None of the authors have significant disclosures.

REFERENCES

1. Ekkert A, Šaulytė M, Jatužis D. Inflammatory disorders of the central nervous system vessels: narrative review. Medicina 2022;58(10):1446.
2. Henry P, Perry AJ, Mackenzie DP. Recurrent ulcerative necrotising stomatitis in two dogs with concurrent steroid-responsive chronic rhinitis and suspected underlying oral vasculitis. Vet Rec Case Rep 2022;10:e488.
3. Mansueto G, Lanza G, Fisicaro F, et al. Central and Peripheral Nervous System Complications of Vasculitis Syndromes From Pathology to Bedside: Part 1—Central Nervous System. Curr Neurol Neurosci Rep 2022;22:47–69.
4. Cho Tracey A. Ann Jones. CNS vasculopathies: Challenging mimickers of primary angiitis of the central nervous system. Best Pract Res Clin Rheumatol 2020; 34(4). https://doi.org/10.1016/j.berh.2020.101569.
5. Byram K, Hajj-Ali RA, Calabrese L. CNS Vasculitis: an Approach to Differential Diagnosis and Management. Curr Rheumatol Rep 2018;20(6):37.
6. Miao X, Shao T, Wang Y, et al. The value of convolutional neural networks-based deep learning model in differential diagnosis of space-occupying brain diseases. Front Neurol 2023;14:1107957. https://doi.
org/10.3389/fneur.2023.1107957. Published 2023 Feb 2.
7. Li Y, Shang K, Cheng X, et al. Cerebral Vasculitis. In: Li H, Wang J, Zhang X, editors. Radiol. Infect. Dis 2023;1. https://doi.org/10.1007/978-981-99-0039-8_19.
8. Li D, Qin W, Guo Y, et al. Clinical, laboratory, and radiological features of cerebral amyloid angiopathy-related inflammation (CAA-ri): retrospective, observational experience of a single centre. Neurol Sci 2023;44:631–8.
9. Filippi M, Rocca MA. Primary CNS Vasculitides. In: White matter diseases. Cham: Springer; 2020.
10. Beuker C, Strunk D, Rawal R, et al. Primary angiitis of the CNS: a systematic review and meta-analysis. Neurology-Neuroimmunology Neuroinflammation 2021; 8(6). https://doi.org/10.1212/NXI.0000000000001093.
11. Hajj-Ali RA, Younger DS, Calabrese LH. Central Nervous System Vasculitis and Reversible Cerebral Vasoconstriction Syndrome. In: Stone JH, editor. A clinician's pearls & myths in rheumatology. Cham (Switzerland): Springer; 2023. p. 465–72.
12. Sundaram S, Sylaja PN. Primary Angiitis of the Central Nervous System - Diagnosis and Management. Ann Indian Acad Neurol 2022;25(6):1009–18. https://doi.org/10.4103/aian.aian_368_22.
13. Younger DS. Overview of primary and secondary vasculitides. Vasculitides 2019;15.
14. Ruland T, Wolbert J, Gottschalk MG, et al. Cerebrospinal Fluid Concentrations of Neuronal Proteins Are Reduced in Primary Angiitis of the Central Nervous System. Front Neurol 2018;9:407. https://doi.org/10.3389/fneur.2018.00407.
15. Strunk D, Schmidt-Pogoda A, Beuker C, et al. Biomarkers in Vasculitides of the Nervous System. Front Neurol 2019;10:591. https://doi.org/10.3389/fneur.2019.00591.
16. Sivakumar, T. A CASE REPORT ON HENOCH-SCHONLEIN PURPURA.2020.
17. Tamaki H, Hajj-Ali RA. Central Nervous System Vasculitis. In: Cho T, Bhattacharyya S, Helfgott S, editors. Neurorheumatology. Cham: Springer; 2019. https://doi.org/10.1007/978-3-030-16928-2_12.
18. Antoine Hankard, Puéchal Xavier, Martin Silva Nicolas, et al. Characteristics of ANCA-associated vasculitis with aneurysms: Case series and review of the literature. Autoimmun Rev 2023;22(5). https://doi.org/10.1016/j.autrev.2023.103293.
19. Hecker Constantin, Tobias Welponer, Herold Manfred, et al. Update on treatment strategies for vasculitis affecting the central nervous system. Drug Discov Today 2022;27(4):1142–55.
20. Litak J, Mazurek M, Kulesza B, et al. Cerebral Small Vessel Disease. Int J Mol Sci 2020;21(24):9729.
21. Gill CM, Piquet AL, Cho TA. Central Nervous System Vasculitis. In: Piquet AL, Alvarez E, editors. Neuroimmunol. Cham: Springer; 2021.

22. Mitoma H, Manto M, Gandini J. Central Nervous System Vasculitis and Related Diseases. In: Mitoma H, Manto M, editors. Neuroimmune diseases. Clin. Neurosci. Res. Cham: Springer; 2019.

23. Padoan Roberto, Campaniello Debora, Gatto Mariele, et al. Current clinical and therapeutic approach to tumour-like mass lesions in granulomatosis with polyangiitis. Autoimmun Rev 2022;21(3). https://doi.org/10.1016/j.autrev.2021.103018.

24. Callen Andrew, Narvid Jared, Chen Xiaolin, et al. Chapter 14 - Neurovascular disease, diagnosis, and therapy: Cervical and intracranial atherosclerosis, vasculitis, and vasculopathy, Handb. Clin. Neurol. Elsevier 2021;176:249–66.

25. Phillips Regina Miecznikoski. Vasculitis: Complex, Challenging, and Dangerous. Journal of Radiology Nursing, Radiol. Nurs 2023;42(1):90–4.

26. Romero Gómez Carlos, Halbert Hernández Negrín, María del Mar Ayala Gutiérrez. Eosinophilic granulomatosis with polyangiitis. Med Clin 2023;160(7):310–7.

27. Egan AC, Kronbichler A, Neumann I, et al. The Sound of Interconnectivity; The European Vasculitis Society 2022 Report. Kidney Int. Rep 2022. https://doi.org/10.1016/j.ekir.2022.05.018.

28. Zhang Z, Liu S, Guo L, et al. Clinical characteristics of peripheral neuropathy in eosinophilic granulomatosis with polyangiitis: a retrospective single-center study in China. J. Immunol. Res 2020;2020:1–10.

29. Liu S, Guo L, Fan X, et al. Clinical features of central nervous system involvement in patients with eosinophilic granulomatosis with polyangiitis: a retrospective cohort study in China. Orphanet J Rare Dis 2021;16:152.

30. Sarti C, Picchioni A, Telese R, et al. "When should primary angiitis of the central nervous system (PACNS) be suspected?": literature review and proposal of a preliminary screening algorithm. Neurol Sci 2020;41:3135–48.

31. Beuker C, Schmidt A, Strunk D, et al. Primary angiitis of the central nervous system: diagnosis and treatment. Ther Adv Neurol Disord 2018;11. https://doi.org/10.1177/1756286418785071. 1756286418785071.

32. Strunk D, Schulte-Mecklenbeck A, Golombeck KS, et al. Immune cell profiling in the cerebrospinal fluid of patients with primary angiitis of the central nervous system reflects the heterogeneity of the disease. J Neuroimmunol 2018;321:109–16. https://doi.org/10.1016/j.jneuroim.2018.06.004.

33. Hagman S, Mäkinen A, Ylä-Outinen L, et al. Effects of inflammatory cytokines IFN-γ, TNF-α and IL-6 on the viability and functionality of human pluripotent stem cell-derived neural cells. J Neuroimmunol 2019;331:36–45. https://doi.org/10.1016/j.jneuroim.2018.07.010.

34. Zhan H, Li H, Liu C, et al. Association of Circulating Vascular Endothelial Growth Factor Levels With Autoimmune Diseases: A Systematic Review and Meta-Analysis. Front Immunol 2021;12:674343. https://doi.org/10.3389/fimmu.2021.674343.

35. Kalashnikova LA, Dobrynina LA, Legenko MS. [Primary central nervous system vasculitis]. Zh. Nevrol 2019;119(8):113–23.

36. Rose Jeppesen and others. Cerebrospinal fluid and blood biomarkers of neuroinflammation and blood-brain barrier in psychotic disorders and individually matched healthy controls. Schizophr Bull 2022;48(6):1206–16.

37. Guilmot A, Slootjes SM, Duprez T, et al. Focal status epilepticus may trigger relapse of primary angiitis of the CNS. Epileptic Disord 2022;24(1):203–7.

38. Tiu Vlad Eugen, Popescu Bogdan Ovidiu, Iulian Ion Enache, Tiu Cristina, et al. Serum and CSF Biomarkers Predict Active Early Cognitive Decline Rather Than Established Cognitive Impairment at the Moment of RRMS Diagnosis. Diagnostics 2022;12(11):25–71.

39. Isin Unal-Cevik MD. Doruk Arslan. Similarities and differences between migraine and other types of headaches: migraine mimics. Neurol. Perspect. J 2023. https://doi.org/10.1016/j.neurop.2023.100122.

40. Pescini F, Torricelli S, Squitieri M, et al. Intravenous thrombolysis in CADASIL: report of two cases and a systematic review. Neurol Sci 2023;44:491–8.

41. Ekker MS, Verhoeven JI, Schellekens MM, et al. Risk Factors and Causes of Ischemic Stroke in 1322 Young Adults. Stroke 2023;54(2):439–47.

42. Berlit P. Diagnosis and treatment of vasculitis. Eur Neurol 2022;26.

43. Yang W, Krakauer JW, Wasserman BA. Radiation-induced intracranial vasculitis on high-resolution vessel wall MRI. J Neurol 2022;269:483–5.

44. Erhart DK, Ludolph AC, Althaus K. Cerebral infarctions following an increase in corticosteroids: an atypical case of reversible cerebral vasoconstriction syndrome. J Neurol 2022;269:5655–9.

45. Wang LL, Mahammedi A, Vagal AS. Imaging of Headache Attributed to Vascular Disorders. Neurol Clin 2022;40(3):507–30.

46. Wahed LA, Cho TA. Imaging of Central Nervous System Autoimmune, Paraneoplastic, and Neurorheumatologic Disorders. Minneap Minn 2023;29(1):255–91.

47. Elsebaie Nermeen, Ahmed A, Gamaleldin O. Atypical intracranial aneurysms: spectrum of imaging findings in computed tomography and magnetic resonance imaging. Clin. Imaging 2022;83:1–10.

48. Li X, Liu C, Zhu L, et al. The Role of High-Resolution Magnetic Resonance Imaging in Cerebrovascular Disease: A Narrative Review. Brain Sci 2023;3(4):677.

49. Hedjoudje A, Darcourt J, Bonneville F, et al. The Use of Intracranial Vessel Wall Imaging in Clinical Practice. Radiologic Clinics 2023;61(3):521–33.

50. Davis AJ. Imaging of the Neurovasculitides. In: Saba L, Raz E, editors. Neurovascular imaging. New York, NY: Springer; 2016.

51. Yang Wenjie, Bruce A, Wasserman. Central nervous system vasculitis. Advances in Magnetic Resonance Technology and Applications 2023;9:305–19. Academic Press.

52. Amin M, Uchino K, Hajj-Ali RA. Central nervous system vasculitis: primary angiitis of the central nervous system and central nervous system manifestations of systemic vasculitis. Rheum Dis Clin 2023.

53. Kim D, Heo YJ, Jeong HW, et al. Compressed sensing time-of-flight magnetic resonance angiography with high spatial resolution for evaluating intracranial aneurysms: comparison with digital subtraction angiography. NeuroRadiol J 2021;34(3):213–21. https://doi.org/10.1177/1971400920988099.

54. Ronen JA, Nguyen A, Mueller JN, et al. Intracranial Atherosclerosis Versus Primary Angiitis of the Central Nervous System: a Case Report. Cureus 2018;10(7):e3031.

55. Sundaram S, Kumar PN, Sharma DP, et al. High-Resolution Vessel Wall Imaging in Primary Angiitis of Central Nervous System. Ann Indian Acad Neurol 2021;24(4):524–30.

56. Deb-Chatterji M, Schuster S, Haeussler V, et al. Primary Angiitis of the Central Nervous System: New Potential Imaging Techniques and Biomarkers in Blood and Cerebrospinal Fluid. Front Neurol 2019;10:568.

57. Farag S, El-Dien HZ, Abdelazeem Y, et al. Value of vessel wall magnetic resonance imaging in the diagnosis of cerebrovascular diseases. Egypt J Neurol Psychiatry Neurosurg 2020;56:114.

Imaging of Vasculitis Associated with Systemic Disease

Igor Gomes Padilha, MD[a,b,c,d,1], Ahmad Nehme, MD, MSc[e,f,1],
Hubert de Boysson, MD, PhD[e,g], Laurent Létourneau-Guillon, MD, MSc[d,h,*]

KEYWORDS

- Vasculitis • Central nervous system • Neuroimaging • Stroke • Systemic lupus erythematosus
- Rheumatoid arthritis • Sjögren's syndrome

KEY POINTS

- Multiple systemic diseases can lead to central nervous system vasculitis. However, vasculitis is a rare event with many potential mimickers.
- Vasculitis should be distinguished from complications related to a systemic disease or its treatment, including opportunistic infections.
- Neuroimaging has a key role in suggesting the possibility of vasculitis and can provide clues of an underlying systemic disease.

INTRODUCTION

The vasculitides are defined by inflammation of the vessel wall and can be differentiated according to their clinical and paraclinical findings, the type, size and distribution of the involved vessels, their histologic features, and the presence of associated conditions.[1] As defined in the 2012 Chapel Hill Consensus, vasculitis can occur as a primary process or be secondary to a systemic disease or probable etiology.[2] In patients with systemic diseases, vasculitis can affect nearly all organs.[3,4] Central nervous system (CNS) vasculitis in systemic diseases is rare but is generally associated with increased morbidity and mortality.[4,5]

Systemic diseases associated with CNS vasculitis include connective tissue disorders (eg, systemic lupus erythematosus [SLE],[4] Sjögren's syndrome [SS]),[3] rheumatoid arthritis (RA),[6] sarcoidosis,[7] and other rarer entities. Systemic diseases have a wide range of pathophysiological mechanisms and target organs. Consequently, CNS involvement in a systemic disease is more likely to result from other mechanisms than vasculitis, including meningoencephalitis or opportunistic infections in the setting of immunosuppression.[8] Biopsy-positive CNS vasculitis in patients with systemic diseases is mainly documented in case reports.[9–11] Without a positive biopsy, the diagnosis of CNS vasculitis is often uncertain but is supported by markers of intracranial vascular disease (eg, brain infarcts or intracranial stenoses) and CNS inflammation (eg, abnormal cerebrospinal fluid or nonischemic parenchymal and leptomeningeal gadolinium enhancement).[12]

[a] Division of Neuroradiology, Diagnósticos da América SA – DASA, São Paulo, São Paulo, Brazil; [b] Division of Neuroradiology, Santa Casa de São Paulo School of Medical Sciences, São Paulo, São Paulo, Brazil; [c] Division of Neuroradiology, United Health Group, São Paulo, São Paulo, Brazil; [d] Radiology Department, Centre Hospitalier de l'Université de Montréal (CHUM), Université de Montréal, Montreal, Quebec, Canada; [e] Normandie University, Caen, France; [f] Department of Neurology, Caen University Hospital, Caen, France; [g] Department of Internal Medicine, Caen University Hospital, Caen, France; [h] Imaging and Engineering Axis, Centre de Recherche du Centre Hospitalier de l'Université de Montréal (CRCHUM), Montreal, Quebec, Canada
[1] Authors contributed equally as first authors.
* Corresponding author. Department of Radiology, Centre Hospitalier de l'Université de Montréal (CHUM), Montreal, Quebec H2X 0C1, Canada.
E-mail address: laurent.letourneau-guillon.1@umontreal.ca

Neuroimag Clin N Am 34 (2024) 81–92
https://doi.org/10.1016/j.nic.2023.07.010
1052-5149/24/© 2023 Elsevier Inc. All rights reserved.

CNS vasculitis in systemic diseases can involve variable-sized vessels, but small vessel disease is more common.[13] Clinical manifestations of CNS vasculitis are protean and vary according to the size of the involved vessels. Small vessel CNS vasculitis is more likely to lead to seizures and cognitive impairment, whereas medium vessel CNS vasculitis more frequently presents with focal neurologic symptoms.[12] The disease course is frequently subacute but acute presentations with rapidly successive infarcts and chronic presentations with aseptic meningitis are possible.

Rapid identification and treatment of vasculitis are necessary in patients with systemic diseases to improve outcomes.[13] However, misdiagnosing vasculitis can lead to treatment escalation with potential adverse events. Although an intracranial biopsy remains the gold standard for the definite diagnosis of CNS vasculitis, the latter is not always obtained.[14] However, contrary to primary angiitis of the CNS, specific markers or extra-CNS tissue biopsy can support the diagnosis of CNS vasculitis associated with a systemic disease.

NEUROIMAGING ROLE IN CENTRAL NERVOUS SYSTEM VASCULITIS DIAGNOSIS

Neuroimaging has a key role in suggesting the possibility of vasculitis and can provide clues of an underlying systemic disease (eg, pachymeningitis in RA and sarcoidosis,[15–17] salivary gland involvement in SS[15]).

Box 1
Selected imaging manifestations in systemic lupus erythematosus

- White matter lesions (subcortical, deep, and periventricular)
- Brain volume loss (global and regional)
- Intracranial calcifications (basal ganglia, cerebral white matter, cerebellum)
- Infarcts (including large territorial, lacunar, borderzone, localized cortical, all associated with antiphospholipid antibodies)
- Intracerebral or subarachnoid hemorrhage
- Microbleeds
- Posterior reversible encephalopathy syndrome (related to the disease, its complications [eg, hypertension, renal failure] or its treatment)[31,32]
- Coexisting autoimmune demyelinating disorders (eg, neuromyelitis optica spectrum disorder)

Imaging manifestations of CNS vasculitis are related to the various consequences of inflammation and vessel wall disruption, producing ischemic or hemorrhagic complications and blood–brain disruption, the latter causing secondary vasogenic edema and gadolinium enhancement.[18] Conventional brain MR imaging findings include infarcts, microbleeds, intracranial hemorrhage, white matter hyperintensities, and parenchymal or leptomeningeal gadolinium enhancement, but often remain nonspecific.[18] MR angiography (MRA) can show focal or multifocal arterial narrowing or dilations but has low sensitivity and remains of limited specificity to differentiate vasculitis from other arteriopathies (eg, intracranial atherosclerosis or reversible cerebral vasoconstriction syndrome).[19] In combination with suggestive clinical and laboratory findings, MR imaging may support the possibility of vasculitis and prompt the recommendation for further investigations. In addition, extra-CNS imaging findings can suggest the presence of a systemic disease (eg, polyarthritis in RA, hilar/mediastinal lymphadenopathy in sarcoidosis).

Vessel wall imaging (VWI)-MR imaging can help detect and characterize arterial lesions. In the appropriate setting and combined with other findings, VWI can support the diagnosis of CNS vasculitis.[20] One potential caveat of VWI is pseudoenhancement related to incomplete blood flow suppression, which can mimic vasculitis.[21] The authors refer the reader to a dedicated chapter published in this issue regarding VWI-MR imaging use in vasculitis diagnosis.

SYSTEMIC LUPUS ERYTHEMATOSUS

SLE is a multiple-organ relapsing-remitting autoimmune disorder with a higher incidence in women, Black, Asian, and Hispanic populations.

Neurologic or psychiatric complications related to SLE are grouped under the term neuropsychiatric SLE (NPSLE), which may occur in approximately half of SLE patients.[22,23] The American College of Rheumatology nomenclature describes 19 NPSLE syndromes involving the central and peripheral nervous system.[24] Other neurologic syndromes that can occur in SLE and that are not captured by this classification include posterior reversible encephalopathy syndrome and coexisting neuromyelitis optica spectrum disorder (NMOSD).[22] Predictors of neurologic involvement in SLE include antiphospholipid antibody positivity and disease activity.[25]

The pathogenesis of NPSLE is related to both ischemic and neuroinflammatory mechanisms.[22,23] The ischemic pathway is thought to

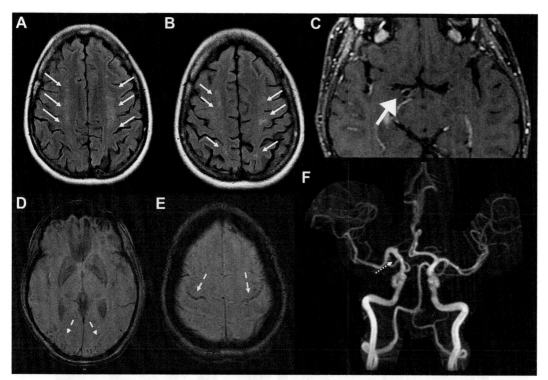

Fig. 1. Systemic lupus erythematosus: A 32-year-old woman with a 3-year history of SLE presented with psychosis and progressive cognitive impairment despite medical management. Axial fluid-attenuated inversion recovery MR images (*A, B*) demonstrated white matter hyperintensities in the centrum semiovale (*white arrows*), suggesting chronic watershed infarcts. Diffusion-weighted imaging was negative at the time of presentation (not shown). Axial susceptibility weighted imaging sequences (*D, E*) identified multiple foci of susceptibility (*dashed white arrows*). The time-of-flight MR-angiogram revealed mild narrowing and irregularity of the right internal carotid artery terminus (*dotted arrow* in *F*) with concentric wall enhancement on post-contrast T1 TSE vessel wall imaging (*white arrow* in *C*). Vasculitis was confirmed after a brain biopsy. (*Courtesy of* F Pacheco, MD PhD, and A da Rocha MD PhD, São Paulo, Brazil.)

contribute primarily to focal neurologic diseases, such as stroke and seizures.[22,23] SLE is associated with a twofold increased risk of stroke.[26,27] The ischemic pathway is mediated by

> **Box 2**
> **Neuroimaging manifestations in Sjögren's syndrome**
>
> - White matter lesions
> - Microbleeds
> - Rare cases of recurrent infarcts and intracranial stenoses
> - Rare cases of necrotizing arteritis and spinal subarachnoid hemorrhage
> - Head and neck: involvement of salivary and lacrimal glands
> - Coexisting autoimmune demyelinating disorders (eg, neuromyelitis optica spectrum disorder)

antiendothelial cell antibodies and complement, which are likely key factors in the production of vasculopathy and vasculitis.[26] Endothelial cell proliferation and microthrombi are more frequent than vasculitis,[26] which is generally considered uncommon. However, a recent autopsy series questioned this assumption, with vasculitis present in approximately 30% of patients with NPSLE.[26]

Compared with the ischemic pathway, the neuroinflammatory pathway refers to a different mechanism leading to more diffuse neurologic manifestations such as cognitive impairment.[13,22] This pathway involves autoimmune-mediated neuroinflammation, which results in blood–brain barrier disruption and migration of autoantibodies with downstream CNS alterations.[22,23]

Antiphospholipid syndrome (APS) is another important cause of neurologic manifestations in SLE and may mimic vasculitis. APS is defined by arterial, venous or microvascular thrombotic and obstetric events occurring in patients with persistent antiphospholipid antibodies (anticardiolipin

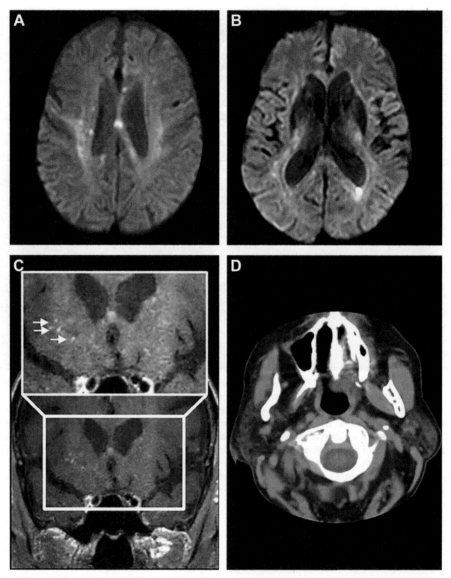

Fig. 2. Sjögren's syndrome: A 77-year-old woman with a previous history of antiphospholipid syndrome and mitral valve prolapse presented with acute onset cognitive impairment and bilateral hyperacusis. Antiphospholipid syndrome was adequately anticoagulated with warfarin. Axial diffused-weighted imaging (*A, B*) revealed multi-territorial punctate acute infarcts. Coronal T1 post-gadolinium (*C*) shows deep foci of punctate enhancement (*arrows*). Axial non-contrast head CT (*D*) demonstrates heterogeneous parotid glands. Cerebrospinal fluid analysis showed an inflammatory profile (white blood cells: 5 per mm³, protein level: 2.59 g/L). Anti-Ro/SSA and anti-La/SSB antibodies were significantly elevated in serum. The paraclinical findings were compatible with an autoimmune rather than a thrombotic process. The patient was diagnosed with cerebral vasculitis secondary to extraglandular Sjögren's syndrome.

antibodies, anti-β2-glycoprotein I, and/or lupus anticoagulant).[28] The most frequent arterial thrombotic manifestations are transient ischemic attack and ischemic stroke.[28] Additional nonthrombotic manifestations include cognitive dysfunction, valve vegetations, and livedo.[28] APS is often associated with systemic diseases, including SLE, SS, and RA, but can also occur in isolation (primary APS).[28] Antiphospholipid antibodies can trigger the activation of inflammatory and endothelial cells, promote coagulation, and ultimately result in vasculopathy and thrombosis.[34] In one study evaluating patients with SLE, abnormal MR imaging findings were more frequent in the presence of APS. These included a higher prevalence of infarcts, with sizes ranging from large and territorial to lacunar. Contrarily, white matter lesions were not associated with APS.[29] Intracranial stenoses or occlusions can be identified in APS but result from thrombosis and non-inflammatory vasculopathy rather than vasculitis.[29,30]

Box 1 lists the conventional imaging findings described in SLE. NPSLE has a poor correlation between clinical and radiological findings.[33] Approximately half of the patients with NPSLE have no abnormalities on conventional brain MR imaging.[29,35,36] An autopsy study revealed that most small vessel injuries identified on histopathology remained undetected on 7T MR imaging studies performed on ex vivo specimens.[26]

The most common finding in NPSLE is cerebral white matter lesions, ranging from 60% to almost 90% of patients.[23,35,37] Brain volume loss is described in less than 20% of patients with NPSLE.[35,37] More advanced MR imaging techniques, including magnetization transfer, diffusion tensor, spectroscopy, functional MR imaging, and brain volumetry, have been studied in NPSLE.[33,38] Still, these techniques need to be validated in the clinical setting to support management decisions.

Acute hemorrhagic complications are rare, estimated at less than 5%[39,40] (**Fig. 1**). Most hemorrhagic events occur intracranially[39] with rare reports of spinal subarachnoid hemorrhage (SAH).[41,42] These events can occur in stable or active SLE.[39] Compared with the general population, patients with SLE have a three times higher risk of intracerebral hemorrhage and a four times higher risk of SAH.[43] Three imaging patterns have been identified in SLE-associated SAH: distal fusiform aneurysms, multiple saccular aneurysms, and angiographically negative SAH.[39,40,44] Few cases with histopathological correlation revealed transmural angiitis as the source of ruptured aneurysms.[45,46] However, in another report of a ruptured pseudoaneurysm, vasculitis was not found,[44] highlighting the complex pathophysiology of this disease and the potential contribution of different mechanisms leading to cerebrovascular events in SLE.

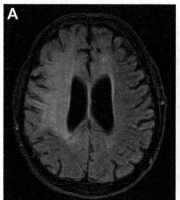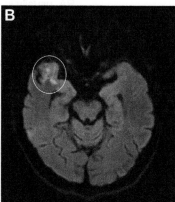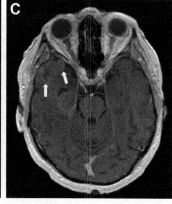

Fig. 3. Rheumatoid arthritis. A 65-year-old man with a 10-year history of rheumatoid arthritis presented with subacute onset cognitive impairment. His rheumatoid arthritis was previously well controlled on etanercept (a TNF-alpha inhibitor), oral methotrexate and prednisone. Axial fluid-attenuated inversion recovery MR images (*A*) showed asymmetric right more than left white matter hyperintensities. Axial diffusion-weighted imaging (*B*) identified right temporal foci of diffusion restriction (*circle*, apparent diffusion coefficient not shown). Axial gadolinium-enhanced T1-weighted imaging (*C*) revealed right temporal cortical enhancement (*arrows*). Susceptibility weighted and MR-angiogram images were normal (not shown). An infectious workup was negative. A stereotaxic right temporal biopsy was obtained and identified lymphocytic vasculitis. The patient was diagnosed with CNS vasculitis, which could be secondary to rheumatoid arthritis and/or the TNF-alpha inhibitor. (Neurology Unit of chambéry, France.)

SJÖGREN'S SYNDROME

SS is a chronic autoimmune disease that predominantly affects the salivary and lacrimal glands, leading to dry eyes and mouth (sicca syndrome). Additional findings required for the diagnosis include objective evidence of ocular and oral dryness (eg, Schirmer test) or glandular parenchymal damage (eg, lymphoplasmacytic infiltration of exocrine glands or suggestive anomalies on salivary gland imaging), as well as markers of underlying autoimmunity (eg, anti-Ro/SSA [Sjögren syndrome type A] and anti-La/SSB [Sjögren syndrome type B] antibodies).[47] SS can occur as a primary disorder or in association with other conditions such as SLE and RA. Extraglandular manifestations can develop in all organs, with various reported mechanisms (eg, epithelitis, immune complex deposition, lymphoproliferation). Primary SS increases the risk of developing non-Hodgkin lymphoma, typically mucosa-associated lymphoid tissue lymphoma.[48]

Neurologic involvement in SS is more common in the peripheral than the central nervous system.[49] Similar to SLE, NMOSD should be ruled out before establishing a diagnosis of Neuro-Sjögren.[50] Vasculitis occurs in less than 10% of patients with primary SS, more often in the presence of hypocomplementemia or cryoglobulinemia.[5,49]

Similar to SLE, a broad range of neuroimaging findings have been reported in SS (Box 2). The most common are white matter T2 hyperintensities[51,52] (Fig. 2). Rare presentations include recurrent infarcts with intracranial stenoses and necrotizing vasculitis with spinal aneurysms and SAH.[53,54–56] Ancillary imaging findings to support the diagnosis of SS include salivary and lacrimal gland involvement.[15] Parotid gland changes are easiest to evaluate on MR imaging. Findings include an early phase of homogeneous enlargement, an intermediate phase of heterogeneity (cysts and solid masses, with a salt-and-pepper appearance), and a chronic phase of end-stage atrophy.[57]

RHEUMATOID ARTHRITIS

RA is a chronic autoimmune condition characterized by polyarticular and usually symmetric synovitis, which can progress to joint narrowing and bony erosion. In patients with a compatible clinical presentation, the diagnosis of RA is supported by the presence of rheumatoid factors and anti-citrullinated peptide antibodies. Rheumatoid vasculitis occurs in less than 1% of patients with RA, usually in the setting of long-standing and severe disease.[58] The incidence of rheumatoid vasculitis is decreasing due to improvements in the treatment of RA. Among neurologic manifestations of RA, carpal tunnel syndrome, subluxation of cervical vertebrae with spinal cord compression and peripheral neuropathy are more frequent than cerebral involvement, which includes pachymeningitis, rheumatoid nodules, and vasculitis. Tumor necrosis factor (TNF)-alpha inhibitors are associated with an increased risk of CNS inflammatory events, particularly in patients with RA.[59] In a patient with RA treated with a TNF-alpha inhibitor, both the underlying disease and the drug may be associated with vasculitis.[60–62]

CNS rheumatoid vasculitis is rare and mostly affects small vessels.[63] Predictors of vasculitis in patients with RA include smoking and disease severity.[64] The few reports of CNS vasculitis in RA are in patients with nodular destructive disease and high levels of rheumatoid factors. Although the pathogenetic processes that cause clinically relevant systemic vasculitis are unknown, immune complexes are thought to play a significant role.

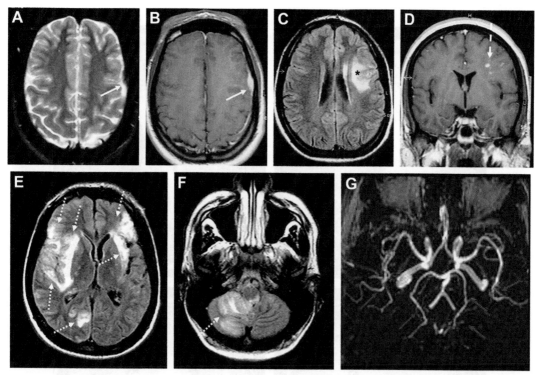

Fig. 4. Sarcoidosis: A 40-year-old woman with a 6-year history of biopsy-proven mediastinal sarcoidosis presented with headaches. Axial T2 (*A*) and post-contrast T1-weighted imaging (*B*) demonstrated focal T2 hypointense pachymeningeal thickening with associated enhancement (*white arrows*). The headaches were attributed to pachymeningitis. The patient had been treated with methotrexate since the diagnosis of sarcoidosis. Three years later, the patient presented with progressive cognitive impairment and worsening headaches. Axial fluid-attenuated inversion recovery MR images (FLAIR) (*C*) identified vasogenic edema (*asterisk*). Diffusion-weighted imaging (not shown) was normal. Coronal post-contrast T1-weighted imaging depicted enhancement in the left corona radiata (*dashed white arrow* in *D*). One year later, the patient developed multiple infarcts in both the anterior and posterior circulations (*dotted white arrows* in *E* and *F*: axial FLAIR), associated with arterial irregularities of bilateral M3 and P2/P3 branches (*red arrows* in *G*: time-of-flight MR-angiogram). The patient was diagnosed with medium vessel vasculitis associated with neurosarcoidosis. (*Courtesy of* F Pacheco, MD PhD, and A da Rocha MD PhD, São Paulo, Brazil.)

The risk of stroke is higher in patients with RA than in the general population, with a stronger association in young adults.[65] This increased risk is thought to result from chronic inflammation and premature atherosclerosis. Consequently, intracranial stenoses in a patient with RA are more likely to result from atherosclerosis than vasculitis, particularly if other vascular risk factors are present.[65]

The neuroimaging appearance of CNS vasculitis in RA is comparable to other CNS vasculitides with ischemic and/or hemorrhagic lesions and multifocal intracranial stenoses[9,63] (Box 3). Other intracranial manifestations of RA include rheumatoid meningitis, demonstrated by pachymeningeal or leptomeningeal enhancement, and dural rheumatoid nodules[15,63] (Fig. 3).

SARCOIDOSIS

Sarcoidosis is an inflammatory granulomatous disease that is more commonly observed in Black

individuals and females. It primarily affects the lungs, lymph nodes, eyes, and skin and is characterized histologically by the presence of noncaseating granulomas. Clinical neurologic involvement occurs in approximately 5% of patients with sarcoidosis. Among those with neurosarcoidosis, 10% have isolated CNS involvement.[66] Cranial neuropathies are among the most common presentations and typically involve the optic, facial, and cochleovestibular nerves.[67]

Sarcoidosis is associated with an increased risk of stroke,[68] which usually results from small vessel/perforator disease[17] and can present with perivascular enhancement.[69] Silent lacunar infarcts can also be identified.[17] Other than vasculitis, the reported mechanisms of ischemic stroke in sarcoidosis include compression of intracranial arteries by a mass lesion and cardiogenic events due to heart involvement. In addition, intracerebral hemorrhage can result from sarcoid-associated cerebral venous thrombosis.

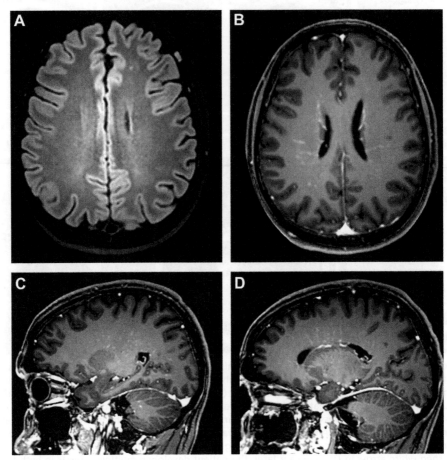

Fig. 5. Inflammatory bowel disease: A 45-year-old man with a previous history of well-controlled ulcerative colitis presented with subacute onset vertigo and ataxia. Axial fluid-attenuated inversion recovery MR images (A) revealed mild hyperintensities within the deep periventricular white matter (in addition to scattered focal hyperintensities). Diffusion-weighted imaging (not shown) was normal. Axial (B) and sagittal (C, D) post-contrast T1-weighted imaging revealed radially oriented linear enhancement. A brain biopsy showed granulomatous vasculitis. The patient was diagnosed with cerebral vasculitis associated with inflammatory bowel disease. A similar imaging pattern has been described in autoimmune glial fibrillary acidic protein (GFAP) astrocytopathy.

A list of potential neuroimaging findings in sarcoidosis is described in Box 4.

Sarcoidosis-associated CNS vasculitis must be suspected in patients with recurrent hemorrhages or infarcts if they are young, have no alternative stroke mechanism, and exhibit additional imaging findings that may suggest neurosarcoidosis, such as pituitary, hypothalamic, basal meningeal, and spinal cord involvement.[17,70] Small vessel arterial and venous granulomatous vasculitis is more common, resulting in negative angiographic studies.[17,69] In neurosarcoidosis, medium vessel disease is rare and does not always lead to stroke. As a result, infarcts are more often lacunar than territorial in neurosarcoidosis[7,17] (Fig. 4). Recent studies have also shown tortuosity and engorgement of the deep medullary veins in approximately

one-third of patients with neurosarcoidosis, although the underlying mechanism is not completely understood.[7]

MISCELLANEOUS
Inflammatory Bowel Disease

Extraintestinal manifestations of inflammatory bowel disease (IBD) can result from nutritional deficiencies, a prothrombotic state that can lead to arterial and venous events, autoimmunity, or treatment-related adverse events.[71] Primary systemic vasculitides are reported to co-occur with IBD, but isolated CNS vasculitis is only described in case reports.[11,72] In patients with IBD and primary vasculitis, the diagnosis of IBD usually preceded that of vasculitis by many years. Interestingly,

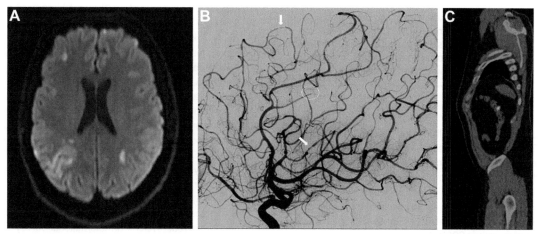

Fig. 6. Paraneoplastic CNS vasculitis: A 38-year-old man presented with headache and cognitive impairment. Axial diffusion-weighted imagingl (*A*) revealed multi-territorial acute infarcts. The lumbar puncture revealed cerebrospinal fluid inflammation. Digital subtraction angiogram (*B*) identified multiple intracranial stenoses (*arrows*) and occlusions (*circle*). A whole-body fluorodeoxyglucose-positron emission tomography (*C*) scan identified focal hypermetabolism within the proximal descending colon, which was biopsied and confirmed to be an adenocarcinoma. The patient was diagnosed with paraneoplastic cerebral vasculitis. (*Courtesy of* Ophélie Osman MD, Marseille, France.)

most reported cases of primary vasculitis occurred during a quiescent stage of IBD.[73] This raises the hypothesis that vasculitis in patients with IBD results from a higher susceptibility to autoimmunity rather than IBD itself. The reported imaging findings are similar to other CNS vasculitides[71] (**Fig. 5**).

Paraneoplastic Central Nervous System Vasculitis

Paraneoplastic granulomatous CNS vasculitis is associated with lymphoma, particularly Hodgkin's lymphoma.[74] Predictors of lymphoma in patients with otherwise unexplained CNS vasculitis include male sex and leptomeningeal enhancement.[74] Isolated reports have associated solid tumors with CNS lymphocytic vasculitis.[75,76] In most patients, the primary tumor is discovered during the vasculitis workup. However, in patients with cancer, other CNS disease mechanisms are more common than vasculitis (eg, parenchymal or meningeal metastases, stroke due to hypercoagulability, disseminated intravascular coagulation or nonbacterial thrombotic endocarditis, paraneoplastic encephalitis, and treatment-related adverse events) (**Fig. 6**).

SUMMARY

Neurologic involvement in systemic diseases can arise from various causes and presents with a diverse range of symptoms. CNS vasculitis is a rare manifestation of systemic diseases and can be mimicked by many other conditions. When faced with neuroimaging features suggestive of vasculitis in patients with a systemic disease, it is crucial to thoroughly exclude other complications related to the disease or its treatment. Conversely, in patients with possible primary CNS vasculitis, it is important to conduct a careful evaluation for imaging markers of an underlying systemic disease. Although often nonspecific in isolation, imaging findings, combined with clinical information, may narrow the differential diagnosis and aid in patient management.

CLINICS CARE POINTS

- Vasculitis is a rare mechanism of central nervous system involvement in patients with systemic diseases.

- In patients with systemic diseases, central nervous system vasculitis should be suspected in the presence of intracranial vascular disease and markers of central nervous system inflammation.

- In patients with systemic diseases, central nervous system vasculitis can occur as a result of the underlying disease or its treatment (eg, varicella zoster vasculitis in the setting of immunosuppression).

- Systemic diseases are associated with premature atherosclerosis and an increased risk of stroke. Intracranial atherosclerosis is an important mimic of central nervous system vasculitis.

- Systemic diseases can co-exist with other neurological syndromes that can mimic central nervous system vasculitis (eg, posterior reversible encephalopathy syndrome, neuromyelitis optica spectrum disorder).

FUNDING

L. Letourneau-Guillon has received a Clinical Research Scholarship—Junior 1 Salary Award (number 311203) from the Fonds de Recherche du Quebec en Sante (FRQ-S) and Fondation de l'Association des Radiologistes du Quebec (FARQ). A. Nehme is supported by a Fonds de Recherche du Quebec - Sante (FRQ-S) training grant (number 296911).

CONFLICTS OF INTEREST

The authors have no relevant conflict of interest to declare.

REFERENCES

1. Ball GV, Fessler BJ, Bridges SL. Oxford textbook of vasculitis. 3rd edition. Oxford, UK: Oxford University Press; 2014.
2. Jennette JC, Falk RJ, Bacon PA, et al. 2012 Revised International Chapel Hill Consensus Conference Nomenclature of Vasculitides. Arthritis Rheum 2013;65(1):1–11.
3. Scofield RH. Vasculitis in Sjögren's Syndrome. Curr Rheumatol Rep 2011;13(6):482–8.
4. Drenkard C, Villa AR, Reyes E, et al. Vasculitis in systemic lupus erythematosus. Lupus 1997;6(3):235–42.
5. Brito-Zerón P, Ramos-Casals M, Bove A, et al. Predicting adverse outcomes in primary Sjogren's syndrome: identification of prognostic factors. Rheumatology 2007;46(8):1359–62.
6. Genta MS, Genta RM, Gabay C. Systemic rheumatoid vasculitis: a review. Semin Arthritis Rheum 2006;36(2):88–98.
7. Bathla G, Abdel-Wahed L, Agarwal A, et al. Vascular Involvement in Neurosarcoidosis: Early Experiences From Intracranial Vessel Wall Imaging. Neurol Neuroimmunol Neuroinflamm 2021;8(6):e1063.
8. Devinsky O, Petito CK, Alonso DR. Clinical and neuropathological findings in systemic lupus erythematosus: the role of vasculitis, heart emboli, and thrombotic thrombocytopenic purpura. Ann Neurol 1988;23(4):380–4.
9. Spath NB, Amft N, Farquhar D. Cerebral vasculitis in rheumatoid arthritis. QJM 2014;107(12):1027–9.
10. Rowshani AT, Remans P, Rozemuller A, et al. Cerebral vasculitis as a primary manifestation of systemic lupus erythematosus. Ann Rheum Dis 2005;64(5):784–6.
11. Raj N, Arkebauer M, Waters B, et al. A Case of Cerebral Vasculitis Associated with Ulcerative Colitis. Case Rep Rheumatol 2015;2015:598273.
12. Nehme A, Boulanger M, Aouba A, et al. Diagnostic and therapeutic approach to adult central nervous system vasculitis. Rev Neurol 2022;178(10):1041–54.
13. Mama-Larbi N, Tlili-Graiess K, Askri A, et al. Vasculitis Associated with Connective Tissue Disease In Lotfi H, Stanson AW, M. Bouhaouala H, Joffre F, eds. "Systemic Vasculitis." Medical Radiology, 2012. Springer Berlin, Germany.
14. Nehme A, Lanthier S, Boulanger M, et al. Diagnosis and management of adult primary angiitis of the central nervous system: an international survey on current practices. J Neurol 2023;270(4):1989–98.
15. Abdel Razek AAK, Alvarez H, Bagg S, et al. Imaging Spectrum of CNS Vasculitis. Radiographics 2014;34(4):873–94.
16. Paci R, Giuffrida CM, Marangolo M, et al. Neuroradiologic picture of cerebral vasculitis in rheumatoid arthritis. Neuroradiology 1983;25(5):343–5.
17. Bathla G, Watal P, Gupta S, et al. Cerebrovascular Manifestations of Neurosarcoidosis: An Underrecognized Aspect of the Imaging Spectrum. AJNR Am J Neuroradiol 2018;39(7):1194–200.
18. Boulouis G, de Boysson H, Zuber M, et al. Primary Angiitis of the Central Nervous System: Magnetic Resonance Imaging Spectrum of Parenchymal, Meningeal, and Vascular Lesions at Baseline. Stroke 2017;48(5):1248–55.
19. Harris KG, Tran DD, Sickels WJ, et al. Diagnosing intracranial vasculitis: the roles of MR and angiography. AJNR Am J Neuroradiol 1994;15(2):317–30.
20. Eiden S, Beck C, Venhoff N, et al. High-resolution contrast-enhanced vessel wall imaging in patients with suspected cerebral vasculitis: Prospective comparison of whole-brain 3D T1 SPACE versus 2D T1 black blood MRI at 3 Tesla. West J. PLoS One 2019;14(3):e0213514.
21. Kang N, Qiao Y, Wasserman BA. Essentials for Interpreting Intracranial Vessel Wall MRI Results: State of the Art. Radiology 2021;300(3):492–505.
22. Govoni M, Hanly JG. The management of neuropsychiatric lupus in the 21st century: still so many unmet needs? Rheumatology 2020;59(Supplement_5):v52–62.
23. Ota Y, Srinivasan A, Capizzano AA, et al. Central Nervous System Systemic Lupus Erythematosus: Pathophysiologic, Clinical, and Imaging Features. Radiographics 2022;42(1):212–32.
24. C COMMITTEE ON NEUROPSYCHIATRIC LUPUS NOMENCLATURE. The American College of Rheumatology nomenclature and case definitions for neuropsychiatric lupus syndromes. Arthritis Rheum 1999;42(4):599–608.

25. Ahn GY, Kim D, Won S, et al. Prevalence, risk factors, and impact on mortality of neuropsychiatric lupus: a prospective, single-center study. Lupus 2018;27(8):1338–47.

26. Cohen D, Rijnink EC, Nabuurs RJA, et al. Brain histopathology in patients with systemic lupus erythematosus: identification of lesions associated with clinical neuropsychiatric lupus syndromes and the role of complement. Rheumatology 2017;56(1):77–86.

27. Hanly JG, Li Q, Su L, et al. Cerebrovascular Events in Systemic Lupus Erythematosus: Results From an International Inception Cohort Study. Arthritis Care Res 2018;70(10):1478–87.

28. Garcia D, Erkan D. Diagnosis and management of the antiphospholipid syndrome. N Engl J Med 2018;378:2010–21. Longo DL, ed.

29. Kaichi Y, Kakeda S, Moriya J, et al. Brain MR findings in patients with systemic lupus erythematosus with and without antiphospholipid antibody syndrome. AJNR Am J Neuroradiol 2014;35(1):100–5.

30. Provenzale JM, Barboriak DP, Allen NB, et al. Antiphospholipid antibodies: findings at arteriography. AJNR Am J Neuroradiol 1998;19(4):611–6.

31. Gatla N, Annapureddy N, Sequeira W, et al. Posterior Reversible Encephalopathy Syndrome in Systemic Lupus Erythematosus. J Clin Rheumatol 2013;19(6):334–40.

32. Liu B, Zhang X, Zhang FC, et al. Posterior reversible encephalopathy syndrome could be an underestimated variant of "reversible neurological deficits" in Systemic Lupus Erythematosus. BMC Neurol 2012;12(1):152.

33. Appenzeller S, Pike GB, Clarke AE. Magnetic Resonance Imaging in the Evaluation of Central Nervous System Manifestations in Systemic Lupus Erythematosus. Clinic Rev Allerg Immunol 2008;34(3):361–6.

34. Arinuma Y, Kikuchi H, Wada T, et al. Brain MRI in patients with diffuse psychiatric/neuropsychological syndromes in systemic lupus erythematosus. Lupus Sci Med 2014;1(1):e000050.

35. Postal M, Lapa AT, Reis F, et al. Magnetic resonance imaging in neuropsychiatric systemic lupus erythematosus: current state of the art and novel approaches. Lupus 2017;26(5):517–21.

36. Luyendijk J, Steens SCA, Ouwendijk WJN, et al. Neuropsychiatric systemic lupus erythematosus: Lessons learned from magnetic resonance imaging. Arthritis Rheum 2011;63(3):722–32.

37. Sarbu N, Alobeidi F, Toledano P, et al. Brain abnormalities in newly diagnosed neuropsychiatric lupus: Systematic MRI approach and correlation with clinical and laboratory data in a large multicenter cohort. Autoimmun Rev 2015;14(2):153–9.

38. Kandemirli SG, Bathla G. Neuroimaging findings in rheumatologic disorders. J Neurol Sci 2021;427:117531.

39. Gao N, Wang ZL, Li MT, et al. Clinical characteristics and risk factors of intracranial hemorrhage in systemic lupus erythematosus. Lupus 2013;22(5):453–60.

40. Mimori A, Suzuki T, Hashimoto M, et al. Subarachnoid hemorrhage and systemic lupus erythematosus. Lupus 2000;9(7):521–6.

41. Harriott A, Faye EC, Abreu N, et al. Aneurysmal Subarachnoid and Spinal Hemorrhage Associated With Systemic Lupus Erythematosus. Stroke 2016;47(3). https://doi.org/10.1161/STROKEAHA.115.012373.

42. Yang X, Richard SA, Liu J, et al. Systemic Lupus Erythematosus Flare up as Acute Spinal Subarachnoid Hemorrhage with Bilateral Lower Limb Paralysis. Clinics and Practice 2018;8(2):1069.

43. Holmqvist M, Simard JF, Asplund K, et al. Stroke in systemic lupus erythematosus: a meta-analysis of population-based cohort studies. RMD Open 2015;1(1):e000168.

44. Torné R, Rodríguez-Hernández A, Bernard T, et al. Subarachnoid hemorrhage in systemic lupus erythematosus: Systematic review and report of three cases. Clin Neurol Neurosurg 2015;128:17–24.

45. Kelley RE. Cerebral Transmural Angiitis and Ruptured Aneurysm: A Complication of Systemic Lupus Erythematosus. Arch Neurol 1980;37(8):526.

46. Sakaki T, Morimoto T, Utsumi S. Cerebral transmural angiitis and ruptured cerebral aneurysms in patients with systemic lupus erythematosus. Minim Invasive Neurosurg 1990;33(04):132–5.

47. Vitali C, Del Papa N. Classification Criteria for Sjögren's Syndrome. In: Sjogren's syndrome. Elsevier; 2016. p. 47–60.

48. Van Ginkel MS, Glaudemans AWJM, Van Der Vegt B, et al. Imaging in Primary Sjögren's Syndrome. JCM 2020;9(8):2492.

49. Carvajal Alegria G, Guellec D, Mariette X, et al. Epidemiology of neurological manifestations in Sjögren's syndrome: data from the French ASSESS Cohort. RMD Open 2016;2(1):e000179.

50. Pittock SJ, Lennon VA, de Seze J, et al. Neuromyelitis optica and non organ-specific autoimmunity. Arch Neurol 2008;65(1):78–83.

51. Soliotis FC. Central nervous system involvement in Sjogren's syndrome. Ann Rheum Dis 2004;63(6):616–20.

52. Akasbi M, Berenguer J, Saiz A, et al. White matter abnormalities in primary Sjogren syndrome. QJM 2012;105(5):433–43.

53. Alexander EL, Craft C, Dorsch C, et al. Necrotizing arteritis and spinal subarachnoid hemorrhage in Sjögren syndrome: Spinal Arteritis in Sjögren Syndrome. Ann Neurol 1982;11(6):632–5.

54. Sakata H, Fujimura M, Sato K, et al. Efficacy of Extracranial–Intracranial Bypass for Progressive Middle Cerebral Artery Occlusion Associated with

Active Sjögren's Syndrome: Case Report. J Stroke Cerebrovasc Dis 2014;23(8):e399–402.

55. Li JA, Meng HM, Cui ZT, et al. Recurrent Cerebral Infarctions in Primary Sjögren Syndrome: A Case Report and Literature Review. Front Neurol 2018;9: 865.

56. Klingler JH, Gläsker S, Shah MJ, et al. Rupture of a spinal artery aneurysm attributable to exacerbated Sjögren syndrome: case report. Neurosurgery 2009;64(5):E1010–1.

57. Abdel Razek AAK. Imaging of connective tissue diseases of the head and neck. NeuroRadiol J 2016; 29(3):222–30.

58. Myasoedova E, Crowson CS, Turesson C, et al. Incidence of extraarticular rheumatoid arthritis in Olmsted County, Minnesota, in 1995-2007 versus 1985-1994: a population-based study. J Rheumatol 2011;38(6):983–9.

59. Kunchok A, Aksamit AJ, Davis JM, et al. Association Between Tumor Necrosis Factor Inhibitor Exposure and Inflammatory Central Nervous System Events. JAMA Neurol 2020;77(8):937–46.

60. Ozkul A, Yılmaz A, Akyol A, et al. Cerebral vasculitis as a major manifestation of rheumatoid arthritis. Acta Clin Belg 2015;70(5):359–63.

61. Beck DO, Corbett JJ. Seizures due to central nervous system rheumatoid meningovasculitis. Neurology 1983;33(8):1058–61.

62. Brown AJ, Staugaitis SM. Central Nervous System Vasculitis Complicating Rheumatoid Arthritis in a Patient on a TNF Inhibitor: a Causal Association? Case Report and Systematic Review. J Vasc 2016;2(1).

63. Kurne A, Karabudak R, Karadag O, et al. An unusual central nervous system involvement in rheumatoid arthritis: combination of pachymeningitis and cerebral vasculitis. Rheumatol Int 2009;29(11):1349–53.

64. Makol A, Crowson CS, Wetter DA, et al. Vasculitis associated with rheumatoid arthritis: a case-control study. Rheumatology 2014;53(5):890–9.

65. Wiseman SJ, Ralston SH, Wardlaw JM. Cerebrovascular Disease in Rheumatic Diseases: A Systematic Review and Meta-Analysis. Stroke 2016;47(4): 943–50.

66. Nozaki K, Scott TF, Sohn M, et al. Isolated neurosarcoidosis: case series in 2 sarcoidosis centers. Neurol 2012;18(6):373–7.

67. Bradshaw MJ, Pawate S, Koth LL, et al. Neurosarcoidosis: Pathophysiology, Diagnosis, and Treatment. Neurol Neuroimmunol Neuroinflamm 2021; 8(6):e1084.

68. Ungprasert P, Matteson EL, Crowson CS. Increased Risk of Multimorbidity in Patients With Sarcoidosis: A Population-Based Cohort Study 1976 to 2013. Mayo Clin Proc 2017;92(12):1791–9.

69. Bathla G, Watal P, Gupta S, et al. Cerebrovascular manifestations in neurosarcoidosis: how common are they and does perivascular enhancement matter? Clin Radiol 2018;73(10):907.e15.

70. Saygin D, Jones S, Sundaram P, et al. Differentiation between neurosarcoidosis and primary central nervous system vasculitis based on demographic, cerebrospinal and imaging features. Clin Exp Rheumatol 2020;124(2):135–8.

71. Ferro JM, Oliveira Santos M. Neurology of inflammatory bowel disease. J Neurol Sci 2021;424:117426.

72. Gekka M, Sugiyama T, Nomura M, et al. Histologically confirmed case of cerebral vasculitis associated with Crohn's disease–a case report. BMC Neurol 2015;15:169.

73. Sy A, Khalidi N, Dehghan N, et al. Vasculitis in patients with inflammatory bowel diseases: A study of 32 patients and systematic review of the literature. Semin Arthritis Rheum 2016;45(4):475–82.

74. Salvarani C, Brown RD, Christianson TJH, et al. Primary central nervous system vasculitis associated with lymphoma. Neurology 2018;90(10):e847–55.

75. Singhal AB, Silverman SB, Romero JM, et al. Case 6-2023: a 68-year-old man with recurrent strokes. N Engl J Med 2023;388:747–57. Cabot RC, Rosenberg ES, Dudzinski DM, et al., eds.

76. Taccone FS, Salmon I, Marechal R, et al. Paraneoplastic vasculitis of central nervous system presenting as recurrent cryptogenic stroke. Int J Clin Oncol 2007;12(2):155–9.

Neuroimaging of Infectious Vasculopathy

Renato Hoffmann Nunes, MD[a,*,1], Diogo Goulart Corrêa, MD, PhD[b,c,1],
Felipe Torres Pacheco, MD, PhD[a,d,1], Ana Paula Alves Fonseca, MD[a,1],
Luiz Celso Hygino da Cruz Jr, MD, PhD[b,1], Antônio José da Rocha, MD, PhD[a,d,1]

KEYWORDS

- Vasculitis • Stroke • Tuberculosis • Syphilis • COVID • MRI • Intracranial vessel wall imaging

KEY POINTS

- Several infectious agents cause cerebral vasculopathy, including bacteria, viruses, fungi, and parasites.
- Infectious cerebral vasculopathy can be secondary to systemic or intracranial infections, leading to ischemic stroke, transient ischemic attack, intracranial hemorrhages, and aneurysm formation.
- Infectious vasculopathy involves inflammation of the blood vessels, hematological disorder due to a hypercoagulable state, and/or cardiovascular dysfunction.
- Intracranial vessel wall MRI is a technique tailored to evaluate vessel walls and their pathologies that can demonstrate vascular changes before stenosis occurs.

INTRODUCTION

Vasculopathy is a term used to describe any alteration affecting blood vessels, including those caused by degenerative, metabolic, inflammatory, embolic, coagulative, and other diseases.[1,2] Infectious agents can affect blood vessels in several ways, including direct vessel wall invasion and indirect mechanisms, through an immunological response.[3] Vasculitis is a form of vasculopathy defined by inflammation of the blood vessel wall.[2] Sustained inflammation mediated by the infectious agent or inflammatory response can lead to vasculitis, with intimal thickening, vessel occlusion, and consequent ischemic stroke.[4] Additionally, vessel wall fragmentation, intimal hyperplasia, medial fibrosis with muscle and elastic tissue loss, secondary to infection, can lead to aneurysm formation and hemorrhages.[5] Thrombosis, thrombophlebitis, and venous ischemia can occur when the venous system is involved.[6] Several infectious agents are potential causes of cerebrovascular diseases, including ischemic stroke, transient ischemic attack, intracranial hemorrhages, and aneurysm formation with or without rupture, due to vasculopathy.[7]

Vasculopathy can be caused by systemic infections, such as sepsis and infectious endocarditis with septic emboli, as well as by primary intracranial infections, such as meningitis.[8] In general, the diagnosis of infectious vasculopathy and its cause is challenging and requires a high degree of suspicion. Usually, a final diagnosis is reached using a combination of epidemiological and clinical data, neuroimaging features, blood work, and cerebrospinal fluid (CSF) analysis. The determination of the etiological agent is important because many of them are amenable to treatment and can have

[a] Division of Neuroradiology, DASA - Diagnósticos da América SA, Rua João Cachoeira, 743, Itaim Bibi, 04535-012, Sao Paulo, Sao Paulo, Brazil; [b] Department of Radiology, Clínica de Diagnóstico por Imagem (CDPI)/DASA, Avenida das Américas, 4666, Barra da Tijuca, 2640-102, Rio de Janeiro, Rio de Janeiro, Brazil; [c] Department of Radiology, Federal Fluminense University, Avenida Marquês de Paraná, 303, 24033-900, Niterói, Rio de Janeiro, Brazil; [d] Division of Neuroradiology, Santa Casa de Sao Paulo School of Medical Sciences, Rua Dr. Cesário Mota Júnior, 112, Vila Buarque, 01221-020, Sao Paulo, Sao Paulo, Brazil
[1] These authors contributed equally to this article.
* Corresponding author. Division of Neuroradiology, DASA – Department of Radiology, Rua João Cachoeira, 743 - Itaim Bibi, São Paulo, Sao Paulo 04535-012, Brazil.
E-mail address: renatohn@hotmail.com
Twitter: @renatohn (R.H.N.); @ofelipe_pacheco (F.T.P.)

Neuroimag Clin N Am 34 (2024) 93–111
https://doi.org/10.1016/j.nic.2023.07.006

a dismal prognosis if left untreated.[7,9] In this article, we will review the pathophysiology and the main imaging and clinical features that can lead to suspicion of infectious vasculopathy.

PATHOPHYSIOLOGY

The pathophysiological mechanisms of infectious vasculopathy involve the following: (1) inflammation of the blood vessels due to direct invasion of the infectious agent through the endoluminal vascular space or the vasa vasorum, direct extension from adjacent foci of infection, or an immune-mediated process in which the systemic activation of autoreactive B and T cells leads to vascular injury[4]; (2) a hypercoagulable state that in combination with endothelial dysfunction leads to the activation of inflammatory and procoagulant cascades[4,10]; and (3) cardiovascular disorder leading to distant embolism and systemic hypotension, or a combination of these factors (Fig. 1).[10]

Additionally, persistent inflammatory activity, even years after a resolved infection, has been demonstrated to increase the risk of stroke.[11]

WHEN TO SUSPECT OF AN INFECTIOUS VASCULOPATHY

The clinical manifestations of infectious vasculopathy in the central nervous system (CNS) overlap with those of noninfectious vascular diseases, making diagnosis challenging. The most common manifestations are nonspecific, including headache, seizures, and focal neurological signs.[4] Furthermore, infectious vasculopathy predicts a poor prognosis, often associated with poor neurological outcomes and even death.[9] Neuroimaging is essential to detecting vascular complications, identifying certain patterns, guiding treatment, and evaluating treatment efficacy.[4]

Lumbar puncture and CSF analysis are essential in the evaluation of a patient suspected to have

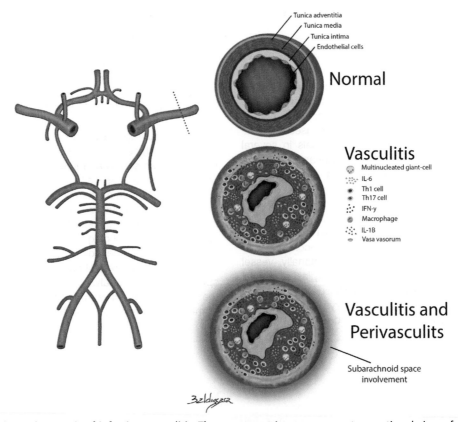

Fig. 1. The pathogenesis of infectious vasculitis. The uppermost image represents a sectional view of a normal artery, which shows the following main layers: tunica adventitia, tunica media, intima, and endothelial cells. Just below, thickening of all arterial layers is observed, with consequent reduction of the arterial lumen, highlighting the recruitment of local inflammatory cells, with secretion of inflammatory cytokines. Finally, in the bottom image, involvement of the subarachnoid space adjacent to the vessel is also observed, configuring perivasculitis, a recognizable pattern in some infectious vasculitis, such as syphilis and tuberculosis. (*Courtesy of* B Moreira, Rio de Janeiro, Brazil.)

infectious vasculopathy in the CNS. However, CSF analysis is not indicated in the clinical evaluation of a typical patient presenting with stroke. Associated clinical symptoms that can indicate infectious vasculopathy and lead to a lumbar puncture are fever, cutaneous lesions, neck stiffness, and a known earlier history of infection. Gradual onset of focal neurological deficits should also lead to a CSF analysis. For immunocompromised patients with a stroke, the suspicion for an infectious cause is higher, and a CSF analysis should be performed. Neuroimaging can demonstrate patterns suggestive of an infectious disease. Meningeal contrast enhancement and/or multifocal infarctions should raise suspicion for inflammatory (infectious or not) pathologic conditions.[8]

EXTRACRANIAL AND SYSTEMIC INFECTIOUS

There is an association between systemic infections and stroke. It is hypothesized that stimulation of the inflammatory response, through an immune-mediated process, is the pathophysiological mechanism of infection-induced stroke.[8] Excessive production of reactive oxygen species, such as superoxide and hypochlorous acid, proinflammatory cytokines and chemokines, elastases and matrix metalloproteinases, β2-integrins, and adhesion molecules, leads to a cerebral inflammatory response that may induce or exacerbate brain ischemia.[12] Although the pathogenetic linkage between infection and stroke is not completely understood, bacterial and viral infections can lead to cerebrovascular disease,[13] especially until 1 week to 1 month after the infection,[14,15] and in young and middle-aged patients[16] with no other vascular risk factors for strokes.[17] The most common associated infections are pulmonary and urinary tract infections.[14,16] However, sinusitis, enteritis, otitis media, and externa have also been associated with stroke.[17]

Sepsis

Patients with sepsis of any origin also present an increased risk for both ischemic and hemorrhagic stroke, even 1 year after the infection.[18] The pathophysiology involves systemic inflammation, hemodynamic dysfunction, and coagulopathy caused by sepsis.[19] The activation of the systemic inflammatory response and hemostatic system due to sepsis leads to hemodynamic collapse and coagulopathy, increasing the risks of thrombosis, embolisms, and hemorrhages.[20,21] Furthermore, patients with sepsis are prone to develop disseminated intravascular coagulation due to abnormal platelet-leukocyte aggregates involving activation of the clotting cascade, which leads to hypercoagulability

with thrombus formation, increasing the risk of stroke, as well as platelet and coagulation factor consumption, which in turn increase the risk of hemorrhages (Fig. 2).[22]

Sepsis and its complications, such as hypoxia or the need for extracorporeal membrane oxygenation, can be associated with microbleeds secondary to pyogenic vasculitis, subacute microvascular inflammatory processes, or endothelial dysfunction and microemboli.[23,24] These microbleeds are not usually manifested in conventional MRI sequences and can only be seen in susceptibility-weighted imaging (SWI) as multiple foci of low signal intensity (Fig. 3).[24]

Infective Endocarditis

Infective endocarditis is inflammation of the endocardium caused by bacteria. The most common causes are gram-positive streptococci, staphylococci, and enterococci, with *Staphylococcus aureus* responsible for approximately 30% of cases.[25] Less virulent coagulase-negative staphylococci, such as *Staphylococcus epidermidis*, can cause infective endocarditis from indwelling vascular devices or recently implanted prosthetic valves.[26]

Hemorrhagic and ischemic stroke, due to embolic events, are known complications of infective endocarditis. Strokes can be multiple and bilateral.[27] Risk factors for infectious endocarditis-induced strokes are older age, atrial fibrillation, multiple valvular involvements, mitral valve involvement, large vegetation size, earlier infective endocarditis with previous embolism, immunosuppression, delayed initiation of antibiotics, and *S aureus* or *Candida* as causative agents.[27]

The risk of stroke is higher at presentation of infective endocarditis and declines 1 to 2 weeks after antibiotic initiation.[8] Cerebrovascular complications occur in approximately one-fourth of patients with infective endocarditis.[28] Although the role of systematic brain MRI in patients with infective endocarditis is uncertain,[28,29] it may reveal brain abnormalities in up to 80% of cases, including cerebral embolism in approximately 50%, which is mostly asymptomatic.[30] Other brain MRI features of infective endocarditis are macrohemorrhages, microbleeds, subarachnoid hemorrhages, brain abscesses, and meningeal contrast-enhancement.[29]

Arterial wall lesions, secondary to septic emboli, lead to abnormal dilatations (mycotic aneurysms), which can be multiple and typically occur at distal branches of the cerebral arteries, mainly the middle cerebral artery (Fig. 4). These aneurysms can

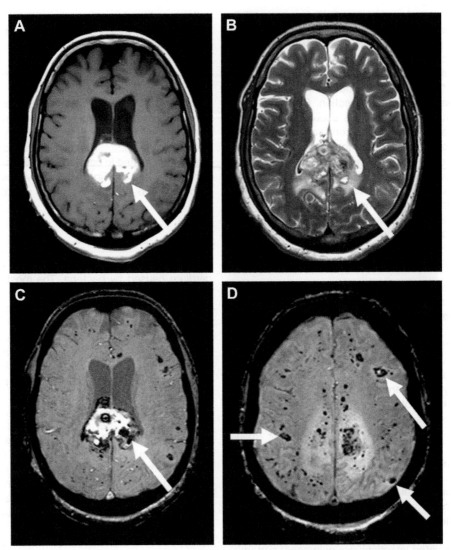

Fig. 2. A 40-year-old woman with a history of abortion and sepsis associated with disseminated intravascular coagulation. Brain MRI demonstrates an intraparenchymal hematoma in the splenium of the corpus callosum, with a hyperintense signal on T1-weighted imaging (*arrow* in *A*) and a heterogeneous signal on T2-weighted imaging (*arrow* in *B*). SWI also demonstrated a hematoma in the corpus callosum (*arrow* in *C*), as well as multiple microbleeds (*arrows* in *D*), due to sepsis-induced vasculopathy.

be fusiform, saccular, or complex in shape. Rapid changes in morphology can occur during follow-up.[30] Rupture of mycotic aneurysms is associated with a poor prognosis.[31]

INTRACRANIAL INFECTIOUS
Bacterial

Although the prevalence of stroke complicating bacterial meningitis varies depending on the agent,[8] vascular complications occur in up to 20% to 25% of patients with acute bacterial meningitis.[32,33] In patients with acute bacterial

meningitis, immunosuppression, associated otitis, and sinusitis are considered risk factors for cerebrovascular diseases.[32]

Cerebral infectious vasculopathy secondary to bacterial meningitis typically occurs early, during the first days to weeks following symptoms onset.[3] Any bacteria, including the most common causes of meningitis, such as *Streptococcus pneumoniae*, *Neisseria meningitidis* (Fig. 5), and *Haemophilus influenzae*, in the subarachnoid space can cause an inflammatory reaction that leads to strokes.[34]

Stroke is the result of the inflammatory response produced to eliminate the infectious agent.

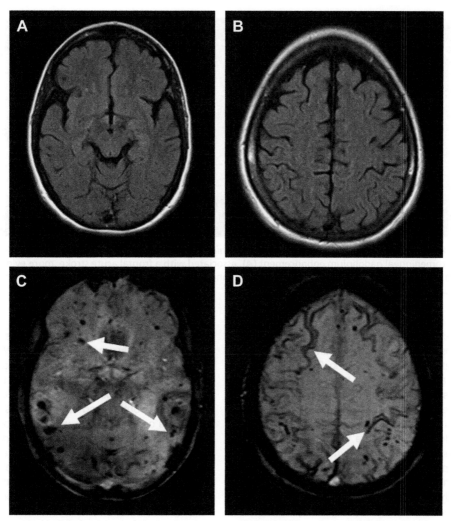

Fig. 3. A 40-year-old woman with urinary sepsis presented with seizures. Brain MRI showed a normal FLAIR (*A* and *B*) but SWI revealed multiple microbleeds (*arrows* in *C*) and subarachnoid hemorrhages (*arrows* in *D*) due to sepsis-induced vasculopathy, which was not seen on the other sequences.

Leukocytes are triggered to react to the infection due to the blood–brain barrier damage that occurs. Then, released cytokines cause additional damage to the blood–brain barrier, neuronal death, and the recruitment of prothrombotic factors, with the activation of the coagulation cascade, through the complement system. Finally, this inflammatory response causes vasculopathy and hypercoagulation of the cerebral blood vessels, leading to stroke.[35] Therefore, vasospasm and vasculitis are not the sole causes of cerebrovascular complications of bacterial meningitis.[36] Furthermore, brain ischemia can be caused by systemic inflammatory responses to meningitis, septic shock, acute respiratory distress syndrome, and/or disseminated intravascular coagulation.[37] Both small and large arteries can be affected, as well as cortical veins and dural sinuses (Fig. 6).[38]

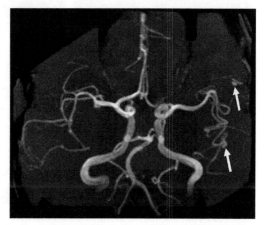

Fig. 4. A 45-year-old woman with a history of infective endocarditis after a dental manipulation. Brain MRA indicates 2 mycotic aneurysms in the distal branches of the left middle cerebral artery (*arrows*).

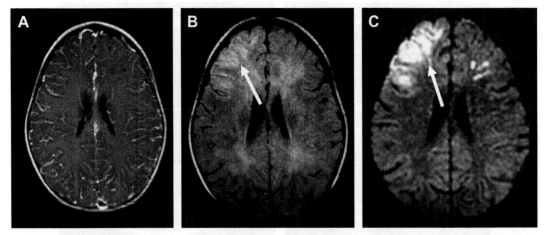

Fig. 5. An 8-month-old girl with meningitis due to *N meningitidis* complicated with seizures. Brain MRI indicates diffuse leptomeningeal gadolinium enhancement (*A*), associated with a frontal acute stroke, more evident on the right, with a hyperintense signal on FLAIR (*arrow* in *B*) and restricted diffusion (*arrow* in *C*), secondary to infectious vasculitis.

Tuberculosis

Tuberculosis remains a public health issue. Although the most affected organ is the lung, CNS involvement occurs in approximately 2% to 5% of patients with tuberculosis and in up to 15% of those with acquired immunodeficiency syndrome-related tuberculosis.[39] Meningitis is the most common form of neurotuberculosis. However, there are various forms of CNS involvement, such as parenchymal, meningeal, calvarial, spinal, or a combination of them.[40] Tuberculous meningitis is caused by the rupture of subependymal and meningeal tuberculomas in the subarachnoid space or hematogenic spread of the bacilli.[41]

Tuberculous meningitis typically affects the basal cisterns, especially around the circle of Willis. Neuroimaging, notably brain MRI, will demonstrate leptomeningeal contrast enhancement in the basal cisterns (especially the perimesencephalic, interpeduncular, prepontine, and suprasellar cisterns and around the cerebellar folia), with or without cranial nerve enhancement associated with hydrocephalus.[42] Hydrocephalus can be communicating, due to obstruction of CSF flow in basal cisterns by inflammatory exudate, or noncommunicating, secondary to obstruction caused by a tuberculoma. Some patients with tuberculous meningitis may present with only hydrocephalus on neuroimaging,

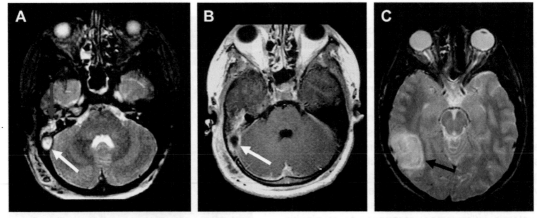

Fig. 6. A 30-year-old man with right acute otitis media complicated with transverse sinus thrombosis and venous stroke. Brain MRI shows an inflammatory fluid signal in the right middle ear cavity and mastoid cells, with a hyperintense signal on T2-weighted imaging (*red arrow* in *A*) and gadolinium enhancement (*red arrow* in *B*), associated with a lack of flow voids in the homolateral transverse sinus (*white arrow* in *A*) due to thrombosis (*white arrow* in *B*). Additionally, note the parenchymal edema due to a venous stroke (*arrow* in *C*).

without detectable leptomeningeal enhancement.[43] Postcontrast-fluid attenuated inversion recovery (FLAIR) is more sensitive than postcontrast T1-weighted imaging to detect leptomeningeal enhancement.[41]

Vasculitis is a known complication of tuberculous meningitis, which can occur as consequence of direct vascular invasion or immunologic injury, mostly involving the origins of the lenticulostriate and thalamoperforating arteries adjacent to the basal meninges. Angiographic studies, including magnetic resonance angiography (MRA) and computed tomography angiography (CTA), may demonstrate narrowing, beaded appearance, or occlusion of the basal cerebral arteries, associated with multiple basal ganglia small infarcts and basal cisterns leptomeningeal enhancement, on conventional MRI (Fig. 7).[42]

Syphilis

Syphilis is an infectious disease caused by the spirochete *Treponema pallidum* subspecies pallidum. Typically, it presents in 3 stages. The primary stage is characterized by a painless genital ulcer, called chancre, representing the site of invasion, associated with painless regional lymphadenopathy. The secondary stage is typically characterized by a nonpruritic cutaneous rash in the trunk, hands and/or feet, fever, and disseminated lymphadenopathy. The tertiary stage is characterized by a severe and self-destructive immune response to a persistent low level of spirochetemia, with lesions in the brain, nerves, spinal cord, eyes, heart, vessels, liver, bones, and joints. Neurosyphilis is not restricted to a late phase of the disease as *T pallidum* can enter the CNS at any time during the infection, even in the early stages.[44]

Meningovascular syphilis is a form of syphilitic meningitis with secondary vasculopathy and cerebral infarcts that is more common in immunosuppressed patients. Typically, this manifestation of meningovascular syphilis occurs with subacute symptoms, 5 to 10 years after the primary infection and is characterized by headache, dizziness, insomnia, and liability weeks to months before the cerebrovascular event.[44,45] It can occur with endarteritis obliterans of medium and large

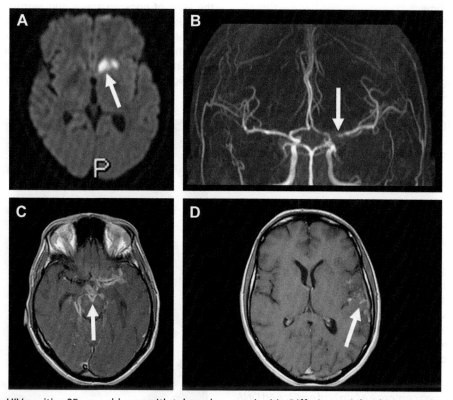

Fig. 7. An HIV-positive 35-year-old man with tuberculous meningitis. Diffusion-weighted imaging demonstrated acute ischemic stroke in the left basal ganglia (*arrow* in *A*). MRA showed narrowing and irregularity of flow in the left middle cerebral artery (*arrow* in *B*). Postcontrast T1-weighted imaging revealed leptomeningeal enhancement along the interpeduncular cistern (*white arrow* in *C*) and left temporal lobe (*arrow* in *D*). Additionally, note the vessel wall enhancement along the M1 segment of the left middle cerebral artery due to vasculitis (red *arrow* in *C*).

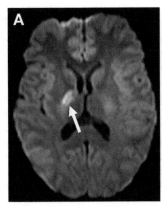
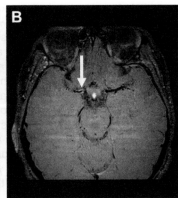
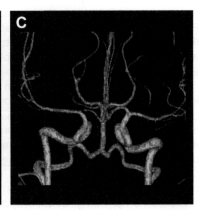

Fig. 8. A 37-year-old man with meningovascular syphilis. Venereal disease research laboratory and fluorescent treponemal antibody absorption tests of the CSF were positive. Brain MRI revealed ischemic stroke in the right basal ganglia on diffusion-weighted imaging (*arrow* in *A*). Intracranial vessel wall imaging showed concentric gadolinium enhancement in the right middle cerebral artery (*arrow* in *B*). MRA findings were normal (*C*).

arteries (Heubner arteritis) and/or small vessels (Nissl-Alzheimer arteritis). The most affected vessels are the middle cerebral arteries and their branches, especially the lenticulostriate arteries. However, multiple territories may be involved at the same time.[44]

Brain MRI can demonstrate infarcts of small and medium vessels, which may be associated with hemorrhage.[44,45] In general, a stroke involving the lenticulostriate and basilar arteries territories in a young patient with no cardiovascular risk factor, complicated or not by cognitive decline or psychiatric symptoms, should raise the suspicion of syphilis (Fig. 8).[46] Tuberculous meningitis is an important differential diagnosis, especially in human immunodeficiency virus (HIV)-positive patients.

Viral

Several viruses are causes of vasculopathy and are implicated in cerebrovascular diseases, including ischemic and hemorrhagic strokes. Varicella-zoster virus (VZV), cytomegalovirus, herpes simplex virus (HSV) 1 and 2, Epstein–Barr virus, HIV, human T-lymphotropic virus-1, hepatitis B and C viruses, parvovirus B19, West Nile virus, dengue, enterovirus, coxsackievirus, and severe acute respiratory syndrome coronavirus-2 (SARS-CoV-2) are causes of CNS vasculopathy.[47]

Herpesviridae
Herpesviruses compose a family of enveloped DNA viruses whose infection results in lifelong latency. This family includes HSV-1, HSV-2, HSV-6, VZV, Epstein–Barr virus, and cytomegalovirus.[48]

Most cases of herpes encephalitis in adults are caused by reactivation of HSV-1. The virus usually

stays in a latent state in the trigeminal ganglion. When reactivated due to any immunosuppression, the virus extends in a retrograde manner to infect the leptomeninges and brain due to its neurotropism. In general, patients present with a decline in the level of consciousness and seizures, with or without fever. Neuroimaging demonstrates a characteristic predilection for the limbic system, especially the temporal and inferior frontal lobes, insular and cingulate gyri, with hyperintense lesions on T2-weighted imaging and FLAIR, which may

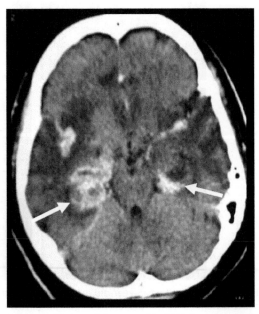

Fig. 9. A 45-year-old man with HSV 1 encephalitis. Brain CT demonstrated hypodense lesions in both temporal lobes and insular cortices, complicated by hemorrhages (*arrows*).

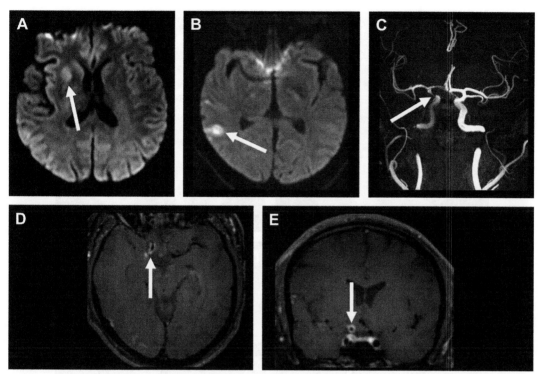

Fig. 10. Brain vasculitis due to HSV 2 infection. Brain MRI indicated multifocal acute ischemic strokes in the right basal ganglia (*arrow* in *A*) and right temporal lobe (*arrow* in *B*), with restricted diffusion. MRA showed stenosis of the right internal carotid artery (*arrow* in *C*). Intracranial vessel wall imaging after intravenous contrast injection revealed concentric arterial wall thickening and enhancement of the right internal carotid and proximal right middle cerebral arteries, compatible with inflammatory vasculopathy, in the axial and coronal planes (*arrows* in *D* and *E*).

demonstrate areas of restricted diffusion due to cytotoxic edema, as well as leptomeningeal and cortical contrast-enhancement. The disease rarely affects the hippocampus in isolation. It can be unilateral, especially in its early stage but it is generally bilateral and asymmetric.[49] Although there is no evidence to suggest that HSV-1 plays a role in ischemic stroke,[50] advanced disease presents with necrosis and parenchymal hemorrhages (Fig. 9).[8] However, HSV-2 infection can cause large-vessel vasculitis, leading to multifocal ischemia, independent of age, sex, and immunological status (Fig. 10).[51]

VZV is the most common herpesvirus that causes strokes.[52] VZV stays in a latent state in cranial nerves, including the trigeminal ganglion, dorsal roots, and autonomic nervous system ganglia. It can affect the brain parenchyma, spinal cord, and arteries via transaxonal migration after reactivation.[3] There is a 1.5-fold increase in stroke risk in the first month following a recent VZV infection, which may persist for several years, especially after ophthalmic Zoster and in young patients. However, cutaneous rash does not always precede stroke, making diagnosis difficult.[53] Furthermore,

polymerase chain reaction (PCR) is often negative in CSF. Thus, the diagnostic test of choice to identify the cause of vasculopathy is immunoassay detection of anti-VZV immunoglobulin G (IgG) antibody in the CSF.[54] The pathophysiology involves granulomatous angiitis that leads to vessel stenosis and occlusion.[53] It can involve small and large vessels. The most affected territories are the basal ganglia, internal capsules, and cerebral cortex, which are supplied by the middle cerebral artery (Fig. 11).[8]

Severe acute respiratory syndrome coronavirus-2

Coronavirus disease 2019 (COVID-19) rapidly spread across the world and became a global pandemic in 2020. Although the most common symptoms are secondary to respiratory system injury, extrapulmonary manifestations are also common, especially in severe cases. Approximately one-third of hospitalized patients with COVID-19 have neurological symptoms, such as dizziness, headache, impaired consciousness, ataxia, seizures, cranial nerve dysfunction, and cerebrovascular disease.[55,56] Neurological alterations

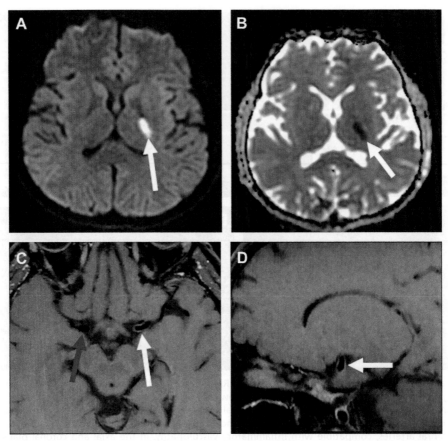

Fig. 11. Brain vasculitis secondary to varicella zoster virus. Brain MRI demonstrated acute ischemic stroke in the left basal ganglia, with restricted diffusion, a hyperintense signal on diffusion-weighted imaging (*arrow* in *A*), and a hypointense signal on the apparent diffusion coefficient map (*arrow* in *B*). Intracranial vessel wall imaging demonstrated subtle concentric vessel wall gadolinium enhancement in the left middle cerebral artery in the axial (*white arrow* in *C*) and sagittal planes (*white arrow* in *D*), with a normal right middle cerebral artery (red *arrow* in *C*). Polymerase chain reaction for VZV was positive in the CSF.

can be secondary to direct viral invasion, immune-mediated injury, or severe hypoxia secondary to acute respiratory failure.[56,57]

A recent review demonstrated that ischemic stroke occurs in 1.3% to 4.7% of patients with COVID-19, independent of disease severity (Fig. 12). The increased predisposition of these patients to develop ischemic stroke is multifactorial. The infection leads to a procoagulant state, with high D-dimer levels, hyperferritinemia, and an increased risk of ischemic events. The systemic inflammatory reaction to SARS-CoV-2 results in decreased levels of circulating lymphocytes, as well as a shift of the immune defense system toward natural killer cells, macrophages, and neutrophils, with elevated levels of proinflammatory cytokines and chemokines, which contribute to ischemia. Additionally, SARS-CoV-2 binds to angiotensin-converting enzyme-2 (ACE2) receptors, leading to endothelial damage and increased subintimal inflammation, followed by thrombosis.

The virus can increase the expression and activity of ACE2, unbalancing the renin-angiotensin system and leading to atherosclerosis. Finally, since cardiac arrhythmia and acute myocarditis are part of the clinical manifestations of COVID-19, cardioembolism can be the cause of ischemic stroke in patients with COVID-19.[58,59]

Intracranial hemorrhages are usually reported in patients with severe COVID-19. The common multifocal nature of the reported brain hemorrhages in patients with COVID-19 suggests some form of underlying vasculopathy (Fig. 13). Endothelial dysfunction, coagulopathy, and renal dysfunction associated with the disease, as well as therapeutic anticoagulation in critically ill patients, also cause intracranial hemorrhages.[58,59]

Human immunodeficiency virus

HIV-associated vasculopathy refers to any abnormality of the intracranial or extracranial cerebral blood vessels that results directly or indirectly

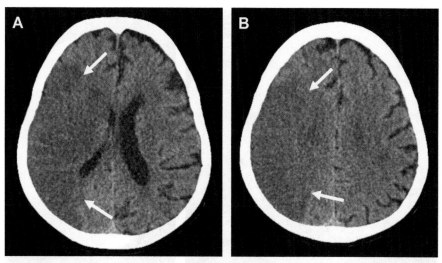

Fig. 12. An 80-year-old woman with COVID-19 with ischemic stroke. Brain CT demonstrated a hypodense lesion due to acute ischemic stroke, affecting the right middle cerebral artery territory (*arrows* in *A* and *B*).

from HIV infection, excluding vessel involvement in opportunistic infections or neoplasms.[60] Typically, HIV-associated vasculopathy is characterized by extracranial and/or intracranial fusiform aneurysmal dilatations (Fig. 14) and vascular stenosis/occlusion, which may cause hemorrhages and ischemia.[61,62] The pathogenesis of HIV-associated vasculopathy is related to endothelial dysfunction, which occurs secondary to exposure to circulating viruses, HIV proteins, and viral-induced proinflammatory cytokines. These factors damage the endothelium and then increase its permeability, leading to leukocyte invasion of the vessel wall and chronic inflammation that cause vascular stenosis and aneurysm formation.[63] HIV-positive patients may present white matter abnormalities secondary to small vessel ischemic disease or cerebrovascular insufficiency and Moya Moya-like phenomenon.[64] HIV-positive children due to congenital or perinatal transmission

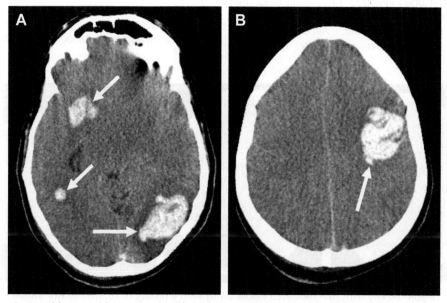

Fig. 13. A 49-year-old man with COVID-19 with multiple brain hematomas. Brain CT demonstrated multifocal lobar hyperdense lesions, with mass effect, due to cerebral hematomas (*arrows* in *A* and *B*).

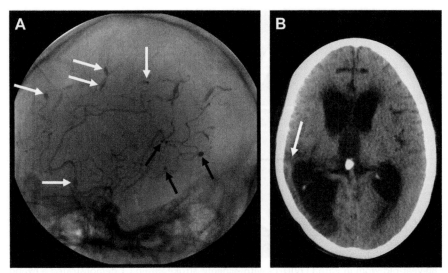

Fig. 14. HIV-associated vasculopathy in a 45-year-old man. Lateral view of the internal carotid artery distribution from the initial cerebral DSA demonstrated fusiform aneurysms on branches of the anterior cerebral artery (*white arrows* in A), as well as saccular aneurysms on branches of the middle cerebral artery (*black arrows* in A). The patient also had right parieto-occipital encephalomalacia (*arrow* in B).

may also have vasculopathy, with cerebral aneurysms being the most common manifestation (Fig. 15).[65]

Fungal

Fungal infections cause several different types of CNS lesions, including meningitis, encephalitis, hydrocephalus, abscess, expansive mass lesions, and ischemic and hemorrhagic strokes.[66] Fungal penetration across the blood–brain barrier is essential for brain infection. Circulating fungi are arrested in the brain microvasculature and then cross the blood–brain barrier.[67] Although cerebrovascular complications secondary to fungal

infections are rare, they occur more commonly because of angioinvasive molds, such as *Aspergillus* and *Mucor* spp, than yeasts, such as *Candida* and *Cryptococcus*.[66]

In immunocompromised patients, most CNS fungal infections, including *Aspergillus* and *Mucor* spp, are usually caused by hematogenous spread from a pulmonary infection (Figs. 16 and 17) or direct invasion through the paranasal sinus (Fig. 18). The fungi cause infectious vasculopathy due to direct invasion, vasculitis and/or thrombosis, causing acute infarction or hemorrhage.[67]

Molds, such as *Aspergillus* and *Mucor* spp (Fig. 19), invade large blood vessels, leading to

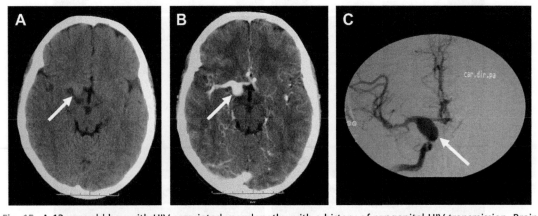

Fig. 15. A 12-year-old boy with HIV-associated vasculopathy with a history of congenital HIV transmission. Brain CT demonstrated a fusiform aneurysm in the right internal carotid/middle cerebral artery (*arrows* in A and B). Cerebral DSA confirmed the aneurysm (*arrow* in C).

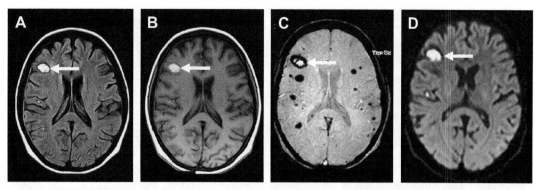

Fig. 16. A 35-year-old woman with acute myeloid leukemia with disseminated aspergillosis. Brain MRI revealed multiple hemorrhagic lesions. The largest lesion presented a hyperintense signal on FLAIR (*arrow* in *A*) and T1 (*arrow* in *B*), with a hypointense peripheral halo on SWI (*arrow* in *C*) and restricted diffusion (*arrow* in *D*). Note that SWI is more sensitive than the other sequences to detect minor hemorrhagic lesions.

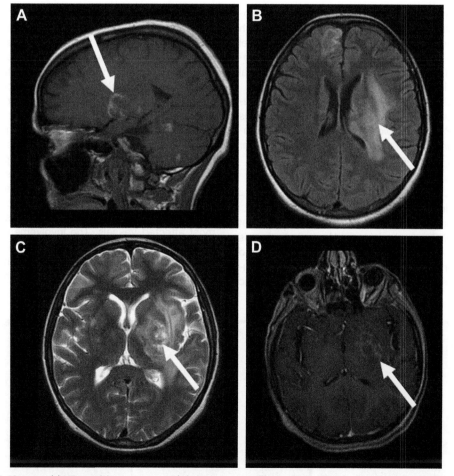

Fig. 17. A 42-year-old HIV-positive woman with invasive aspergillosis. Brain MRI demonstrated an infiltrative heterogeneous lesion, with a hyperintense component on T1-weighted imaging due to hemorrhage (*arrow* in *A*), heterogeneous signal on FLAIR (*arrow* in *B*) and T2-weighted imaging (*arrow* in *C*), and peripheral irregular gadolinium enhancement (*arrow* in *D*). Additionally, note the other hemorrhagic lesions in the cerebellum on sagittal T1-weighted imaging (*A*). Initially, toxoplasmosis was considered but biopsy of the lesion revealed angioinvasive aspergillosis.

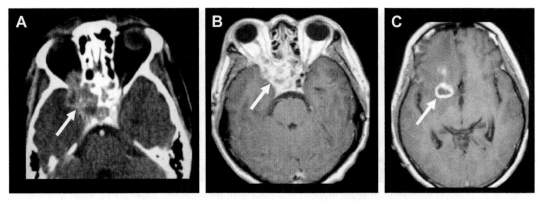

Fig. 18. A 58-year-old immunosuppressed woman with chronic sinusitis due to aspergillosis with brain invasion. Brain CT showed inflammatory sinusal disease with contrast enhancement associated with right orbital and intracranial invasion (*arrow* in *A*). Brain MRI also demonstrated the inflammatory sinusal disease, with contrast enhancement, associated with right orbital and intracranial invasion (*arrow* in *B*), as well as a peripheral enhancing lesion in the right basal ganglia due to invasive fungal disease (*arrow* in *C*).

mycotic aneurysm formation and vascular necrosis, causing hemorrhagic strokes. Yeasts, such as *Cryptococcus* and *Candida*, cause small vessel vasculitis that invades the capillaries and subarachnoid space, causing vasospasm and subpial ischemic lesions.[8,53,67]

Dimorphic fungi, such as *Histoplasma capsulatum*, *Blastomyces dermatitidis*, *Coccidioides immitis*, *Paracoccidioides brasiliensis*, and *Sporothrix schenckii*, are rare causes of cerebrovascular diseases, with a few cases reported.[8]

Parasitic

Parasitic infections can also cause vasculopathy.[8] Cysticercosis is the most important parasite that causes CNS vascular injury.[13] Neurocysticercosis can be classified into parenchymal and subarachnoid-cisternal cysticercosis. The parenchymal lesions cause seizures and focal neurologic deficits, whereas the subarachnoid-cisternal lesions cause arachnoiditis and vasculitis.[68] The presence of encysted larvae of *Taenia saginata* (*Cysticercus bovis*) in the subarachnoid space leads to inflammatory leptomeningeal thickening and consequent occlusions of small perforator vessels, resulting in lacunar infarcts. The involved vessels show advanced endarteritic changes with luminal narrowing, adventitial fibrosis, and chronic panarteritis.[69] Vasculitis of large vessels presents with segmental narrowing, beaded appearance, or vascular obstruction. Arteritis occurs in up to 53% of patients with subarachnoid-cisternal neurocysticercosis, including asymptomatic patients. Middle and posterior cerebral arteries are the most affected vessels. The involvement of more than one vessel is also possible (**Fig. 20**).[70]

Schistosomiasis can also cause cerebrovascular diseases. Schistosoma eggs can reach the

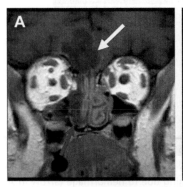
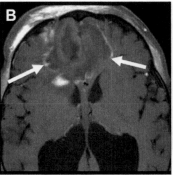
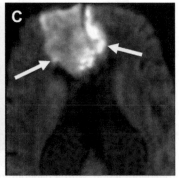

Fig. 19. A 72-year-old woman with poorly controlled diabetes mellitus with rhino-cerebral mucormycosis. Brain MRI demonstrated sinonasal inflammatory content (red *arrow* in *A*) associated with intracranial anterior fossa invasion (*white arrow* in *A*), determining an acute infarct in the frontobasal region, with peripheral gadolinium enhancement (*arrows* in *B*) and restricted diffusion (*arrows* in *C*).

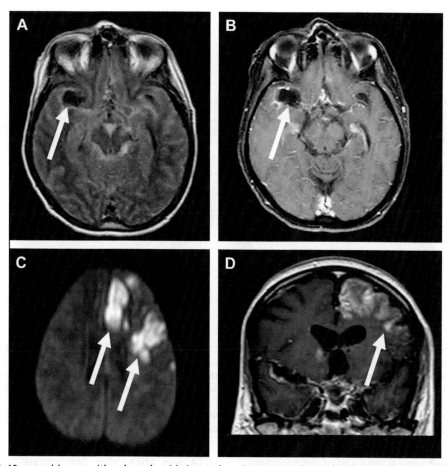

Fig. 20. A 40-year-old man with subarachnoid-cisternal cysticercosis and vasculitis. Brain MRI demonstrated leptomeningeal gadolinium enhancement on postcontrast FLAIR (red *arrow* in *A*) associated with a cystic lesion in the right Sylvian fissure (*white arrow* in *A* and *B*) and a smaller lesion in the left Sylvian fissure seen on FLAIR (*A*) and postgadolinium T1-weighted imaging (*B* and *D*). Note that postcontrast FLAIR demonstrated leptomeningeal enhancement better than postcontrast T1-weighted imaging. Diffusion-weighted imaging demonstrated restricted diffusion in the left frontal lobe (*arrows* in *C*), which was associated with cortical enhancement (*arrow* in *D*).

CNS through retrograde flow via the valveless venous plexus of Batson, which joins the deep iliac veins and inferior vena cava with the veins of the spinal cord and brain. Other routes include pulmonary and portalpulmonary arteriovenous shunts. In addition, adult worms can penetrate the cerebral veins and place their eggs directly at an ectopic site, including the CNS. Intracranial hemorrhages occur because of granulomatous meningitis around the Schistosoma eggs during the chronic stage of the infection.[71] In the acute stage of the infection, eosinophil-mediated cerebral vasculitis can cause distal ischemic strokes due to hypereosinophilic syndrome.[63]

Cerebral malaria caused by *Plasmodium falciparum* can present with multiple microbleeds in the brain as consequence of small venule and capillary endothelial wall injury, leading to occlusion of these vessels by infected erythrocytes.[72]

ROLE OF INTRACRANIAL HIGH-RESOLUTION VESSEL WALL IMAGING

Intracranial high-resolution vessel wall magnetic resonance imaging (VWI) is a technique tailored for the evaluation of vessel walls and their pathologies, providing diagnostic data beyond luminal changes.[73] This technique allows the intracranial vessel wall to be imaged with a detectable signal, whereas the signals from neighboring blood and CSF are suppressed.[74] Typically, vasculitis of any origin will present as concentric vessel-wall thickening with gadolinium enhancement (see **Fig. 10**), which may be associated with adjacent

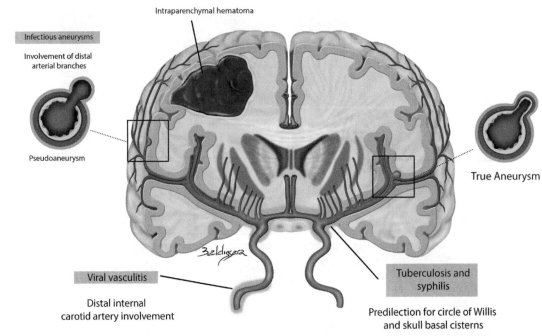

Fig. 21. The main involvement and complications of infectious vasculitis. Vessels highlighted in yellow indicate the most common sites involved: distal internal carotid artery for viral etiology; arterial polygon and intracranial cisterns for tuberculosis and syphilis; and distal arterial branches for embolic causes. In addition, there is an association of infectious aneurysms with distal arterial involvement and pseudoaneurysms. As a comparison, note the typical involvement of a true aneurysm (with all arterial layers) at the bifurcation of the M1 segment. In addition, there is a frontal intraparenchymal hematoma, which represents a common complication of angiocentric infections, particularly of fungal cause. (*Courtesy of* B Moreira, Rio de Janeiro, Brazil.)

brain parenchyma edema and/or enhancement.[75] In infectious vasculopathies, intracranial VWI is able to detect vessel wall abnormalities before stenosis occurs (see **Fig. 8**).[76] The addition of this sequence in the evaluation of a patient with suspected cerebral vasculitis helps in the differentiation of vasculitis from other vasculopathies, such as intracranial arterial dissection, intracranial atherosclerosis, reversible cerebral vasoconstriction syndrome, and Moya-Moya syndrome/disease,[74] as well as in the disease activity evaluation and guiding the best site for biopsy.[77]

SUMMARY

Vasculopathy is an important consequence of several intracranial and systemic infections, whose recognition is important because many of these diseases are amenable to treatment and have a poor prognosis if left untreated. Ischemic and/or hemorrhagic stroke, transient ischemic attack, aneurysm formation, and cerebral microbleeds are consequences of infectious vasculopathy. Neuroimaging, especially MRI, can be of utmost utility in demonstrating these complications. Lumen-based imaging modalities, such as

CTA and MRA, also demonstrate features of vasculitis. Finally, high-resolution intracranial VWI can directly evaluate the vessel wall and reveal signs of vasculitis (**Fig. 21**).

CLINICS CARE POINTS

- Cerebrovascular diseases associated with fever, cutaneous lesions, neck stiffness, gradual onset of focal neurological deficits, immunosuppression, and a known earlier history of infection should lead to suspicion of infectious vasculopathy.

- Although CSF analysis is not recommended for a typical patient with isolated stroke, it is essential in a patient with suspected brain infectious vasculopathy.

- Neuroimaging may demonstrate typical patterns of lesions of certain infectious causes of vasculopathy in the brain, such as tuberculosis, Herpes virus infection, or aspergillosis.

- Intracranial VWI should be added to the brain MRI protocol when there is a suspected brain infectious vasculopathy.

FUNDING

No funding was received for this study from funding agencies in the public, commercial, or not-for-profit sectors.

CONFLICT OF INTEREST

The authors declare that they have no conflict of interest.

REFERENCES

1. Berlit P. The spectrum of vasculopathies in the differential diagnosis of vasculitis. Semin Neurol 1994; 14(4):370–9.
2. Lie JT. Classification and histopathologic spectrum of central nervous system vasculitis. Neurol Clin 1997;15(4):805–19.
3. Younger DS, Coyle PK. Central Nervous System Vasculitis due to Infection. Neurol Clin 2019;37(2):441–63.
4. Shen G, Shen X, Pu W, et al. Imaging of cerebrovascular complications of infection. Quant Imaging Med Surg 2018;8(10):1039–51.
5. Clough RE, Taylor PR. Endovascular treatment of mycotic aortic aneurysms (review). Acta Chir Belg 2009;109(2):149–54.
6. Khatri IA, Wasay M. Septic cerebral venous sinus thrombosis. J Neurol Sci 2016;362:221–7.
7. Shulman JG, Cervantes-Arslanian AM. Infectious etiologies of stroke. Semin Neurol 2019;39(4):482–94.
8. Fugate JE, Lyons JL, Thakur KT, et al. Infectious causes of stroke. Lancet Infect Dis 2014;14(9):869–80.
9. Chow FC, Marra CM, Cho TA. Cerebrovascular disease in central nervous system infections. Semin Neurol 2011;31(3):286–306.
10. Takeoka M, Takahashi T. Infectious and inflammatory disorders of the circulatory system and stroke in childhood. Curr Opin Neurol 2002;15(2):159–64.
11. Ihara M, Yamamoto Y. Emerging evidence for pathogenesis of sporadic cerebral small vessel disease. Stroke 2016;47(2):554–60.
12. Jin R, Yang G, Li G. Inflammatory mechanisms in ischemic stroke: role of inflammatory cells. J Leukoc Biol 2010;87(5):779–89.
13. Grau AJ, Buggle F, Becher H, et al. Recent bacterial and viral infection is a risk factor for cerebrovascular ischemia: clinical and biochemical studies. Neurology 1998;50(1):196–203.
14. Bova IY, Bornstein NM, Korczyn AD. Acute infection as a risk factor for ischemic stroke. Stroke 1996; 27(12):2204–6.
15. Paganini-Hill A, Lozano E, Fischberg G, et al. Infection and risk of ischemic stroke: differences among stroke subtypes. Stroke 2003;34(2):452–7.
16. Clayton TC, Thompson M, Meade TW. Recent respiratory infection and risk of cardiovascular disease: case-control study through a general practice database. Eur Heart J 2008;29(1):96–103.
17. Syrjänen J, Valtonen VV, Iivanainen M, et al. Preceding infection as an important risk factor for ischaemic brain infarction in young and middle aged patients. Br Med J 1988;296(6630):1156–60.
18. Boehme AK, Ranawat P, Luna J, et al. Risk of acute stroke after hospitalization for sepsis: a case-crossover study. Stroke 2017;48(3):574–80.
19. Kellum JA, Kong L, Fink MP, et al. Understanding the inflammatory cytokine response in pneumonia and sepsis: results of the Genetic and Inflammatory Markers of Sepsis (GenIMS) Study. Arch Intern Med 2007;167(15):1655–63.
20. Lupu F, Keshari RS, Lambris JD, et al. Crosstalk between the coagulation and complement systems in sepsis. Thromb Res 2014;133(Suppl 1):S28–31.
21. Levi M, Schultz M, van der Poll T. Sepsis and thrombosis. Semin Thromb Hemost 2013;39(5):559–66.
22. Polito A, Eischwald F, Maho AL, et al. Pattern of brain injury in the acute setting of human septic shock. Crit Care 2013;17(5):R204.
23. Haller S, Vernooij MW, Kuijer JPA, et al. Cerebral microbleeds: imaging and clinical significance. Radiology 2018;287(1):11–28.
24. Corrêa DG, Cruz Júnior LC, Bahia PR, et al. Intracerebral microbleeds in sepsis: susceptibility-weighted MR imaging findings. Arq Neuropsiquiatr 2012;70(11):903–4.
25. Barnett R. Infective endocarditis. Lancet 2016; 388(10050):1148.
26. Hill EE, Herijgers P, Claus P, et al. Infective endocarditis: changing epidemiology and predictors of 6-month mortality: a prospective cohort study. Eur Heart J 2007;28(2):196–203.
27. Mishra AK, Sahu KK, Baddam V, et al. Stroke and infective endocarditis. QJM 2020;113(7):515–6.
28. Sotero FD, Rosário M, Fonseca AC, et al. Neurological complications of infective endocarditis. Curr Neurol Neurosci Rep 2019;19(5):23.
29. Champey J, Pavese P, Bouvaist H, et al. Value of brain MRI in infective endocarditis: a narrative literature review. Eur J Clin Microbiol Infect Dis 2016; 35(2):159–68.
30. Elsebaie N, Abdelzaher A, Gamaleldin O. Atypical intracranial aneurysms: spectrum of imaging findings in computed tomography and magnetic resonance imaging. Clin Imaging 2022;83:1–10.
31. Peters PJ, Harrison T, Lennox JL. A dangerous dilemma: management of infectious intracranial aneurysms complicating endocarditis. Lancet Infect Dis 2006;6(11):742–8.
32. Schut ES, Lucas MJ, Brouwer MC, et al. Cerebral infarction in adults with bacterial meningitis. Neurocrit Care 2012;16(3):421–7.

33. Klein M, Koedel U, Pfefferkorn T, et al. Arterial cerebrovascular complications in 94 adults with acute bacterial meningitis. Crit Care 2011;15(6):R281.

34. Chen M. Stroke as a complication of medical disease. Semin Neurol 2009;29(2):154–62.

35. Siegel JL. Acute bacterial meningitis and stroke. Neurol Neurochir Pol 2019;53(4):242–50.

36. Weisfelt M, Determann RM, de Gans J, et al. Procoagulant and fibrinolytic activity in cerebrospinal fluid from adults with bacterial meningitis. J Infect 2007; 54(6):545–50.

37. Pfister HW, Feiden W, Einhäupl KM. Spectrum of complications during bacterial meningitis in adults. Results of a prospective clinical study. Arch Neurol 1993;50(6):575–81.

38. Pfister HW, Borasio GD, Dirnagl U, et al. Cerebrovascular complications of bacterial meningitis in adults. Neurology 1992;42(8):1497–504.

39. Burrill J, Williams CJ, Bain G, et al. Tuberculosis: a radiologic review. Radiographics 2007;27(5): 1255–73.

40. Skoura E, Zumla A, Bomanji J. Imaging in tuberculosis. Int J Infect Dis 2015;32:87–93.

41. Salvador GLO, Basso ACN, Barbieri PP, et al. Central nervous system and spinal cord tuberculosis: Revisiting an important disease. Clin Imaging 2021;69:158–68.

42. Baloji A, Ghasi RG. MRI in intracranial tuberculosis: Have we seen it all? Clin Imaging 2020;68:263–77.

43. Katrak SM. Central nervous system tuberculosis. J Neurol Sci 2021;421:117278.

44. Corrêa DG, de Souza SR, Freddi TAL, et al. Imaging features of neurosyphilis. J Neuroradiol 2023;50(2): 241–52.

45. Akgoz A, Mukundan S, Lee TC. Imaging of rickettsial, spirochetal, and parasitic infections. Neuroimaging Clin N Am 2012;22(4):633–57.

46. Bhai S, Lyons JL. Neurosyphilis update: atypical is the new typical. Curr Infect Dis Rep 2015;17(5):481.

47. Vyas S, Choudhary N, Modi M, et al. High-resolution intracranial vessel wall imaging in cerebral viral infections evaluations. Neuroradiology 2022;64(5): 915–24.

48. Baskin HJ, Hedlund G. Neuroimaging of herpesvirus infections in children. Pediatr Radiol 2007;37(10): 949–63.

49. Soares BP, Provenzale JM. Imaging of Herpesvirus Infections of the CNS. AJR Am J Roentgenol 2016; 206(1):39–48.

50. Alexandri NM, Tavernarakis A, Potagas C, et al. Accident vasculaire ischémique cérébral et méningoencéphalite à herpès simplex 1. Rev Neurol (Paris) 2004;160(5 Pt 1):579–81.

51. Hauer L, Pikija S, Schulte EC, et al. Cerebrovascular manifestations of herpes simplex virus infection of the central nervous system: a systematic review. J Neuroinflammation 2019;16(1):19.

52. Amlie-Lefond C, Gilden D. Varicella zoster virus: a common cause of stroke in children and adults. J Stroke Cerebrovasc Dis 2016;25(7):1561–9.

53. Jillella DV, Wisco DR. Infectious causes of stroke. Curr Opin Infect Dis 2019;32(3):285–92.

54. Nagel MA, Forghani B, Mahalingam R, et al. The value of detecting anti-VZV IgG antibody in CSF to diagnose VZV vasculopathy. Neurology 2007; 68(13):1069–73.

55. Mao L, Jin H, Wang M, et al. Neurologic manifestations of hospitalized patients with coronavirus disease 2019 in Wuhan, China. JAMA Neurol 2020; 77(6):683–90.

56. Corrêa DG, Hygino da Cruz LC Jr, Lopes FCR, et al. Magnetic resonance imaging features of COVID-19-related cranial nerve lesions. J Neurovirol 2021; 27(1):171–7.

57. Corrêa DG, da Cruz LCH Jr. Critical illness-associated brain microhemorrhages in a child with multisystem inflammatory syndrome secondary to coronavirus disease 2019. Pediatr Neonatol 2021; 62(3):329–30.

58. Alves VPV, Altoé A, Veloso V, et al. Computed tomography features of cerebrovascular complications in intensive care unit patients with severe COVID-19. Radiol Bras 2021;54(5):283–8.

59. Maury A, Lyoubi A, Peiffer-Smadja N, et al. Neurological manifestations associated with SARS-CoV-2 and other coronaviruses: a narrative review for clinicians. Rev Neurol (Paris) 2021;177(1–2):51–64.

60. Benjamin LA, Bryer A, Emsley HC, et al. HIV infection and stroke: current perspectives and future directions. Lancet Neurol 2012;11(10):878–90.

61. Bulsara KR, Raja A, Owen J. HIV and cerebral aneurysms. Neurosurg Rev 2005;28(2):92–5.

62. Tipping B, de Villiers L, Candy S, et al. Stroke caused by human immunodeficiency virus-associated intracranial large-vessel aneurysmal vasculopathy. Arch Neurol 2006;63(11):1640–2.

63. Jauréguiberry S, Ansart S, Perez L, et al. Acute neuroschistosomiasis: two cases associated with cerebral vasculitis. Am J Trop Med Hyg 2007;76(5): 964–6.

64. Schneider CL, Mohajeri-Moghaddam S, Mbewe EG, et al. Cerebrovascular disease in children perinatally infected with human immunodeficiency virus in Zambia. Pediatr Neurol 2020;112:14–21.

65. Schieffelin JS, Williams PL, Djokic D, et al. Central nervous system vasculopathy in HIV-infected children enrolled in the pediatric AIDS clinical trials group 219/ 219C study. J Pediatric Infect Dis Soc 2013;2(1):50–6.

66. Panackal AA, Williamson PR. Fungal infections of the central nervous system. Continuum 2015;21(6 Neuroinfectious Disease):1662–78.

67. Góralska K, Blaszkowska J, Dzikowiec M. Neuroinfections caused by fungi. Infection 2018;46(4): 443–59.

68. Kim JS, Caplan LR. Non-atherosclerotic intracranial arterial diseases. Front Neurol Neurosci 2016;40: 179–203.

69. Cantú C, Barinagarrementeria F. Cerebrovascular complications of neurocysticercosis. Clinical and neuroimaging spectrum. Arch Neurol 1996;53(3): 233–9.

70. Barinagarrementeria F, Cantú C. Frequency of cerebral arteritis in subarachnoid cysticercosis: an angiographic study. Stroke 1998;29(1):123–5.

71. Preidler KW, Riepl T, Szolar D, et al. Cerebral schistosomiasis: MR and CT appearance. AJNR Am J Neuroradiol 1996;17(8):1598–600.

72. Nickerson JP, Tong KA, Raghavan R. Imaging cerebral malaria with a susceptibility-weighted MR sequence. AJNR Am J Neuroradiol 2009;30(6): e85–6.

73. Lindenholz A, van der Kolk AG, Zwanenburg JJM, et al. The use and pitfalls of intracranial vessel wall imaging: how we do it. Radiology 2018;286(1): 12–28. https://doi.org/10.1148/radiol.2017162096.

74. Mandell DM, Mossa-Basha M, Qiao Y, et al. Intracranial vessel wall MRI: principles and expert consensus recommendations of the american society of neuroradiology. AJNR Am J Neuroradiol 2017;38(2):218–29.

75. Mattay RR, Saucedo JF, Lehman VT, et al. Current clinical applications of intracranial vessel wall MR imaging. Semin Ultrasound CT MR 2021;42(5): 463–73.

76. Corrêa DG, Pacheco FT, da Cruz LCH Jr, et al. Intracranial vessel wall magnetic resonance imaging features of infectious vasculitis. Clin Imaging 2023;98: 26–35.

77. Fushimi Y, Yoshida K, Okawa M, et al. Vessel wall MR imaging in neuroradiology. Radiol Med 2022; 127(9):1032–45.

Imaging of Drug-Related Vasculopathy

Paulo Puac-Polanco, MD, MSc[a], Àlex Rovira, MD[b], Lubdha M. Shah, MD[c],
Richard H. Wiggins, MD[d], Francisco Rivas Rodriguez, MD[e], Carlos Torres, MD, FRCPC, FCAR[a],*

KEYWORDS

- CNS • Vasculitis • Vasculopathy • Drug-related • Cocaine-induced • Levamisole • RCVS • PRES

KEY POINTS

- Cocaine-induced CNS vasculitis is produced by additives/contaminants added to cocaine, mainly levamisole.
- Cocaine-induced midline destructive lesion should be considered in any structural lesion of the sinonasal complex in the context of a positive toxicologic screening or confirmed cocaine-snorting habit.
- Marijuana is the most prevalent triggering factor in reversible vasoconstriction syndrome secondary to substance abuse.
- The risk of CNS vasculopathy associated with sympathomimetic or immunosuppressant drug therapy increases in patients with impaired renal and hepatic function.

INTRODUCTION

Illicit drugs and medications represent an important etiologic factor in patients with vasculopathy. This type of vascular injury has been recognized as a separate entity under the 2012 revised Chapel Hill Consensus Conference Nomenclature of Vasculitides.[1] Drug-associated antineutrophil cytoplasmic antibodies (ANCA) vasculitis has been described with cocaine, antithyroid drugs, and hydralazine. Other drugs may have direct toxicity on the vascular endothelium (immunosuppressants and oncologic medications) or affect the integrity of the vessels through their sympathomimetic mechanism (marijuana, amphetamines, sympathomimetic drugs). This article reviews the pathomechanism, clinical presentation, and imaging findings of vasculopathy related to recreational drug abuse and prescribed medications.

IMAGING TECHNIQUE AND PROTOCOL

Magnetic resonance (MR) imaging is the modality of choice for the evaluation of patients with suspected central nervous system (CNS) vasculopathy. Recommended sequences include diffusion-weighted imaging (DWI), susceptibility-weighted imaging (SWI), T2-weighted images (WI), fluid-attenuated inversion recovery (FLAIR), and T1WI-post intravenous contrast administration. MR time of flight (TOF) or MR angiography (MRA) is recommended to visualize the vessels' lumen to detect stenosis, occlusion, or aneurysms. CT, combined with CT-angiography (CTA), is an alternative to MR imaging when this is contraindicated or unavailable.

Vascular lumen imaging has been the cornerstone in evaluating intracranial and extracranial vascular diseases. Imaging modalities such as

[a] Department of Radiology, Radiation Oncology and Medical Physics, Box 232, General Campus Room 1466e, 501 Smyth Road, Ottawa, Ontario K1H 8L6, Canada; [b] Neuroradiology Section, Department of Radiology, Hospital Vall d'Hebron Passeig Vall d'Hebron 119-129 08035 Barcelona, Spain; [c] Division of Neuroradiology, University of Utah, 50 Medical Drive North, Salt Lake City, UT 84132, USA; [d] Department of Radiology and Imaging Sciences, University of Utah School of Medicine, University of Utah Health Sciences Center, 50 Medical Drive North, Salt Lake City, UT 84132, USA; [e] Radiology, Division of Neuroradiology, University of Michigan, 1500 East Medical Center Drive, B2A205 Ann Arbor, MI 48109-5302, USA
* Corresponding author. Department of Radiology, Radiation Oncology and Medical Physics, Box 232, General Campus Room 1466e, 501 Smyth Road, Ottawa, Ontario K1H 8L6, Canada.
E-mail address: catorres@toh.ca

Neuroimag Clin N Am 34 (2024) 113–128
https://doi.org/10.1016/j.nic.2023.07.003

CTA, digital subtraction angiography (DSA), and MRA rely on the opacification of the vascular lumen following intra-arterial (DSA) or intravenous (CTA, MRA) contrast administration. Alternatively, the development and dissemination of MR pulse sequences with high spatial resolution, multiplanar 2D or 3D acquisition, multiple tissue weightings, and suppression of signal in luminal blood and CSF have allowed the use of specific MR sequences to evaluate the vascular wall of the circle of Willis and second-third order intracranial arterial vessels.[2] As a result, the direct visualization of the vessel wall on vessel wall MR imaging (VW-MR) is a valuable adjunct to conventional imaging to differentiate among causes of intracranial arterial narrowing such as atherosclerosis, vasculitis, reversible cerebral vasoconstriction syndrome (RCVS), and arterial dissection.

ILLICIT DRUG-ASSOCIATED VASCULOPATHY
Central Nervous System Complications Associated with Cocaine Abuse

Cocaine is the most common illegal stimulant drug worldwide. It is highly addictive and has a high lipid solubility, which accounts for its rapid diffusion across cell membranes. This substance blocks catecholamine absorption, resulting in the vasoconstriction of blood vessels, elevation of blood pressure, tachycardia, and increased cardiac output.[3,4] Most commonly, cocaine is sniffed as cocaine hydrochloride, although it can also be smoked (the alkaloidal form known as crack) or injected.[4,5] Drug effects include a brief but intense euphoria, enhanced energy, and alertness.

Cocaine abuse has been associated with various neurologic complications, mainly ischemic and hemorrhagic strokes, induced directly or indirectly by additive substances in contaminated samples. For unknown reasons, the drug's hydrochloride form is linked to significantly greater rates of hemorrhagic strokes than its alkaloidal form, which causes an equal frequency of ischemic and hemorrhagic events.[6]

Around 40% to 50% of patients with hemorrhagic strokes (intraparenchymal and subarachnoid) have concurrent pathology, such as cerebral arteriovenous malformations or aneurysms (Fig. 1), which rupture as a result of cocaine's sympathetic effects.[4,7,8] In cases where it is impossible to document concomitant vascular pathology, intraparenchymal bleeding is most commonly located in the basal ganglia and thalami.[9]

The causes of ischemic stroke are diverse and include drug-induced thrombosis caused by increased platelet aggregation, vasospasm, cardioembolism, accelerated atherosclerosis, and cerebral vasculitis.[5,10,11] Brain infarcts are primarily located in the subcortical white matter (watershed infarctions), in the middle cerebral artery territory (see Fig. 1), and in the mesencephalon. The latter is more frequently involved when cocaine is combined with amphetamines.[9]

Cocaine-induced CNS vasculitis, which seems to be produced by additives/contaminants added to cocaine, mainly levamisole, is usually associated with intranasal drug administration.[12] In addition to brain infarcts found in cross-sectional imaging studies, focal constrictions of the main arteries might be identified in angiographic studies. In contrast, VW-MR imaging identifies concentric enhancement of the vessel wall, a feature that distinguishes this condition from isolated drug-induced vasospasm.[9]

Rarely, cocaine produces a toxic encephalopathy from direct effects after intravenous or nasal administration. Brain MR imaging shows diffuse high-signal intensity lesions on T2-WI involving the subcortical and deep white matter, the corpus callosum, and the deep gray matter (pallidum) associated with diffusion restriction (Fig. 2).[13] Cocaine-induced blood pressure imbalance can even cause reversible cerebral vasoconstriction syndrome (RCVS) and posterior reversible encephalopathy syndrome (PRES) (Fig. 3).[8,14] Finally, transitory spinal cord ischemia or infarction has been described in cocaine users, and it should be considered in the differential diagnosis of acute nontraumatic myelopathy.[15]

Levamisole-induced Multifocal Inflammatory Leukoencephalopathy

Levamisole is an anthelmintic agent with significant immunomodulatory properties, commonly used as an additive to cocaine[16] as it enhances and extends its stimulating effects. Chronic exposure to levamisole may cause serious side effects, including skin necrosis, agranulocytosis, cutaneous and CNS vasculitis, and a potentially lethal MIL.

The physiopathology of levamisole-induced MIL likely depends to a large extent on an immunologic mechanism, given that biopsy specimens show lymphocytic infiltrates, the condition responds to immunosuppressive therapy, and it typically has a latent period of at least 2 weeks after cocaine use.[17]

Imaging findings in MIL include multiple inflammatory-demyelinating-like lesions, predominantly involving the frontal and parietal subcortical and periventricular white matter (Fig. 4), the basal ganglia, and the brainstem.[18] The lesions show

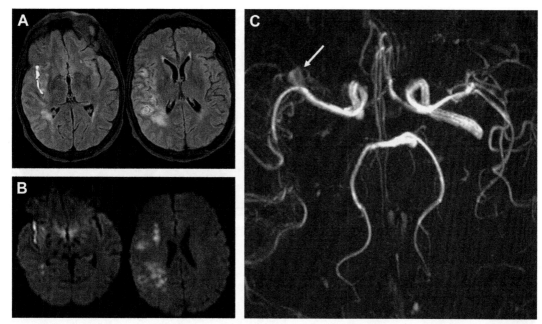

Fig. 1. Acute infarctions associated with subarachnoid hemorrhage in a patient with a history of cocaine abuse. Axial FLAIR (*A*) and diffusion-weighted (*B*) images show acute infarcts in the right MCA territory and subarachnoid hemorrhage within the right Sylvian fissure. MRA shows a small saccular aneurysm at the right MCA bifurcation (*arrow* in C).

variable degrees of surrounding vasogenic edema and peripheral restricted diffusion, with mild or no mass effect. Ring enhancement can be detected in up to one-third of cases.[18] Single or multifocal tumefactive and Balo-like demyelinating lesions, with the typical concentric rings on T2-WI, associated with peripheral diffusion restriction and contrast enhancement, are unusual findings (Fig. 5).[19,20]

The diagnosis of levamisole-induced MIL based on MRI findings is complex, and it should always be considered in the context of the patient's clinical setting (chronic cocaine use) or following positive results of toxicologic screening tests. Differential diagnosis includes inflammatory-demyelinating disorders such as multiple sclerosis (MS) or acute disseminated encephalomyelitis (ADEM). Patients with levamisole-induced MIL are commonly treated with steroids and have a good clinical outcome.[20]

Cocaine-induced Midline Destructive Lesions

The recurrent vasoconstrictive effect in the nasal mucosa induced by chronic intranasal cocaine use has the potential to produce the so-called CIMDL. This repetitive vasoconstriction causes progressive damage leading to ischemia and subsequent necrosis of the mucosa lining and underlying structures.[21,22] Additional pathomechanisms include chemical irritation, mechanical trauma from high-velocity inhalation, the toxic effect of adulterants mixed with cocaine (amphetamines or caffeine), secondary bacterial infection, antineutrophil cytoplasmic antibodies formation, immunosuppression, and osteoblast inhibition.[22–24]

Patients with CIDML present self-limiting epistaxis, rhinorrhea, and scabs, sometimes associated with olfactory dysfunction (hyposmia or anosmia), likely induced by direct damage to the neuroepithelium by cocaine or its adulterants or by the potential obstruction of the olfactory cleft by inflammation and mucosal edema.[25,26]

The typical features of CIDML are usually detected on CT. Common imaging findings include the opacification of the paranasal sinuses and mucoperiosteal thickening of the nasal cavity and paranasal cavities. Progressive involvement of the sinonasal region with eventual erosion and destruction of the mucosa and bony structures is typical. The starting point of CIDML seems to be the nasal septum, which may spread across the inferior third of the sinonasal complex, including the nasal floor and the inferolateral nasal wall (inferior turbinate and maxilla) (Fig. 6). From this point, the disease may extend superiorly toward the middle third of the sinonasal complex (middle

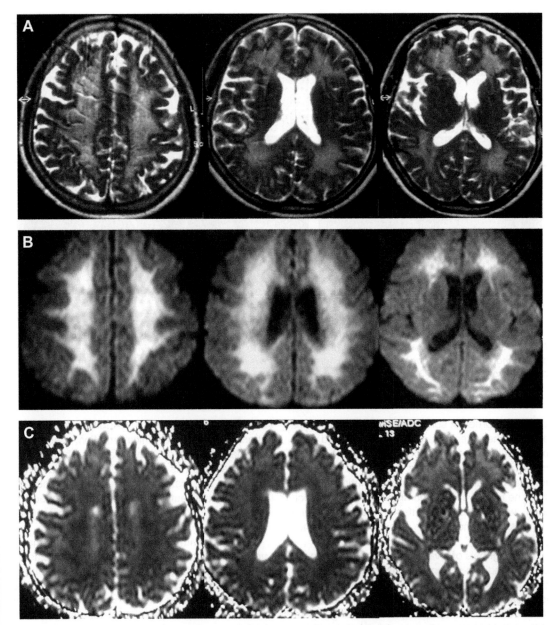

Fig. 2. Cocaine-induced encephalopathy. MR imaging shows diffuse symmetric and confluent T2WI hyperintense lesions (*A*) involving the subcortical and deep white matter of both hemispheres, associated with high signal intensity on diffusion-weighted images (*B*) and mild low signal on the ADC maps (*C*), indicating partial restricted diffusion.

turbinate and ethmoid) (**Fig. 7**). Finally, there could be the involvement of the neurocranium (anterior skull base, lamina papyracea, and orbit).[27,28]

CIMDL should be considered, according to Seyer and colleagues[21] when two of the following three findings are present: nasal septal perforation, palatal perforation, or lateral nasal wall destruction. An alternative and more simplistic diagnostic criteria of CIMDL include demonstrating any structural lesion of the sinonasal complex in the context of a positive toxicologic screening or confirmed cocaine-snorting habit.[29] A classification based on this distribution pattern has also been proposed (**Table 1**) (**Fig. 8**).[28]

Differential considerations of midline destructive lesions include granulomatosis with polyangiitis (GPA), Churg-Strauss Syndrome (CSS), T-cell lymphoma, and trauma. Although a positive antineutrophil cytoplasmic antibodies (ANCA) test would support the diagnosis of GPA, positive ANCA

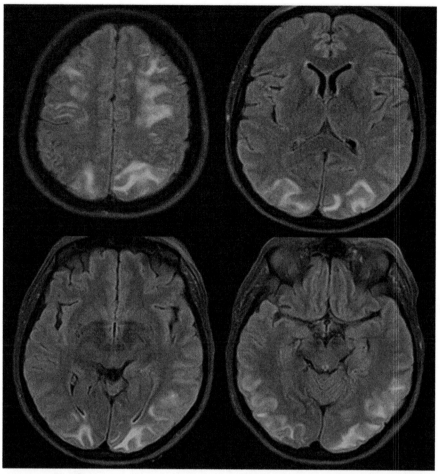

Fig. 3. PRES in a middle-aged cocaine abuser female. Axial FLAIR images show bilateral asymmetric subcortical white matter signal abnormality consistent with vasogenic edema in the parieto-occipital regions and frontal lobes.

test results have also been found in an unexpectedly large proportion of patients with CIMDL,[27,30] which makes the discrimination between the 2 challenging in the absence of documented cocaine addiction. Ultimately, the absence of systemic manifestations and the lack of response to treatment for GPA will lead to the confirmation of CIMDL in a cocaine user. On imaging, early destruction of the nasal septum, nasal floor, and inferolateral nasal wall supports CIMDL, given that these structures are more likely preserved in other diseases, such as GPA.[29] Given patients' noncompliant lifestyle, CIDML management is complex. Regular debridement of necrotic tissues and crusts and local and systemic antibiotic medication are all part of the conservative treatment. Surgical reconstruction of bone and cartilaginous lesions and correction of mucosal and cutaneous defects can be performed in complex cases.[31] However, surgical treatment should be withheld until there is evidence of lesion stability for at least 12 months, along with the confirmation of cocaine abuse discontinuation.

Marijuana-related Reversible Cerebral Vasoconstriction Syndrome

RCVS often affects young adults. Patients present with severe thunderclap headaches, which may or may not be associated with neurologic deficits. Intracranial arterial segmental vasoconstriction may result in multifocal luminal narrowing with a beading appearance on imaging studies (Fig. 9). These findings are expected to resolve within 12 weeks from onset.[32] While most patients follow a benign course, some may experience permanent neurologic deficits or death from intracranial hemorrhage or ischemic stroke.[33]

While RCVS occurs spontaneously in about 40% of cases, 60% of RCVS cases may be

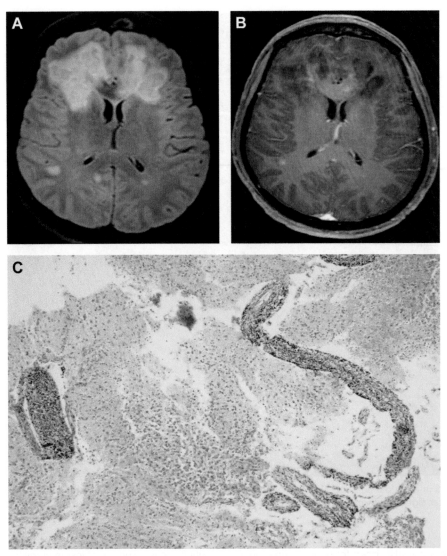

Fig. 4. Levamisole-induced MIL. Young male with a history of daily cocaine abuse who presented with progressive confusion, behavioral change, and visual hallucinations. Axial FLAIR (*A*) and contrast-enhanced T1-weighted (*B*) images show confluent white matter lesions mainly affecting the frontal lobes, with minimal mass effect and mild contrast enhancement. Brain biopsy shows perivascular lymphocytic infiltration (CD3+ and CD4+) (hematoxylin-eosin, original magnification X10) (*C*). (*From* Pessini LM, Kremer S, Auger C, et al. Tumefactive inflammatory leukoencephalopathy in cocaine users: Report of three cases. Mult Scler Relat Disord. 2020;38:101496.)

associated with vasoactive substances, pregnancy, uncontrolled hypertension, head trauma, and neurosurgical procedures.[34] Use of vasoactive substances, including marijuana, selective serotonin reuptake inhibitors, exercise stimulants, energy drinks, alcohol, triptans, methamphetamines, or sympathomimetic drugs, is the most frequently documented cause of RCVS. Among these substances, marijuana is the most prevalent triggering factor, reported in up to 30% of secondary RCVS cases.[35]

Intracranial VW-MR imaging is a valuable adjunct to conventional imaging to distinguish between RCVS and its relevant differential diagnosis of vasculitis. On MR imaging, these two entities may show multiple, likely bilateral, parenchymal infarctions of different ages and in different vascular territories (Fig. 10). CTA, MRA, or DSA demonstrate focal or multifocal segmental narrowing of small and medium size arterial vessels (Fig. 11). Differentiation between RCVS and vasculitis has clinical relevance; RCVS is treated with observation or

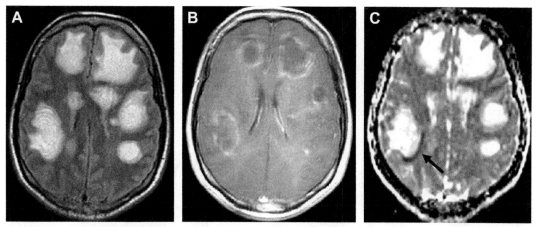

Fig. 5. Levamisole-induced MIL with Baló-like lesions. A middle-aged male with a history of chronic cocaine abuse presented with confusion, disorientation, speech, and behavioral impairment. Axial FLAIR (A) and contrast-enhanced T1-weighted (B) images show several pseudo tumoral lesions affecting the subcortical frontoparietal white matter of both cerebral hemispheres, with incomplete ring-enhancement and peripheral diffusion restriction on the ADC map (arrow in C). A concentric ring pattern (onion bulb appearance) is noted on the FLAIR image (A). Postmortem hair samples showed significant concentrations of cocaine and levamisole. (From Pessini LM, Kremer S, Auger C, et al. Tumefactive inflammatory leukoencephalopathy in cocaine users: Report of three cases. Mult Scler Relat Disord. 2020;38:101496.)

calcium channel blockers, whereas vasculitis is treated with steroids and immunosuppressive drugs. VW-MR imaging may help differentiate these entities; while both disorders may result in arterial wall thickening, the vessel wall in RCVS typically does not enhance, in contrast to the characteristic intense concentric vessel wall enhancement in vasculitis.[36] The relative paucity of arterial wall enhancement is concordant with limited histopathologic data in RCVS, which has shown a lack of arterial wall inflammation.

Heroin Toxicity

Heroin is a semi-synthetic opioid made from chemically processed morphine. It can be sniffed,

inhaled, or injected. Heroin may cause acute or chronic effects on the brain, including neurovascular disorders, leukoencephalopathy, and atrophy.[37] Ischemia is the most commonly encountered acute neurovascular complication, typically seen following intravenous injection. Proposed pathomechanisms include vasospasm as a direct effect of heroin in vascular smooth muscle receptors, vasculitis from immune-mediated responses, or embolic events from impure additives.[9]

Symmetric spongiform degeneration occurs in the setting of heroin-induced leukoencephalopathy affecting the cerebral and cerebellar white matter and the corticospinal and solitary tracts.[38] This is exclusively seen after drug inhalation ("chasing the dragon"), and the clinical manifestations

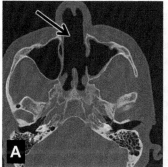
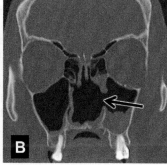
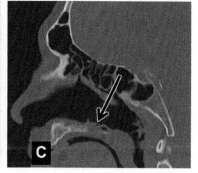

Fig. 6. 59-year-old man with a significant history of cocaine abuse and cocaine-induced midline destructive lesions (CIMDL). Noncontrast bone algorithm CT images through the nasal vault demonstrate a widely perforated nasal septum (arrow, A). Coronal image shows the absence of middle and inferior turbinates (arrow, B). Sagittal reconstruction to the left of midline shows the osseous destruction of the posterior hard palate (arrow, C), which is also seen on the coronal B image.

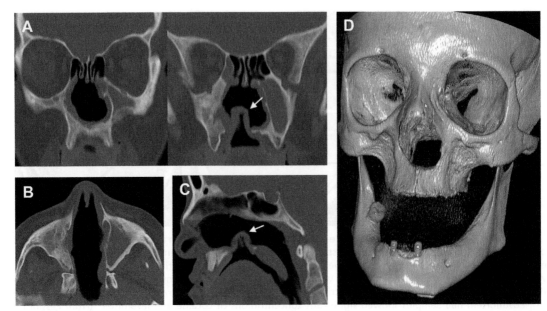

Fig. 7. CIMDL in a patient with a history of chronic intranasal cocaine abuse. Coronal (*A*), axial (*B*), and sagittal (*C*) bone window views of a CT scan of the facial bones show absence of the nasal septum, of the bilateral inferior, middle, and superior turbinates, of the medial walls of the maxillary sinuses, as well as palatal perforation with herniation of oral cavity mucosa into the nasal cavity (*arrows* in *A* and *C*). Volume-rendered 3D image (*D*) was acquired to help plan the surgical repair of the sinonasal cavity.

develop days to months after consumption.[37] On MR imaging, this is seen as symmetric T2WI and FLAIR hyperintensity in the cerebellum and posterior limbs of the internal capsules, sparing the anterior limbs (Fig. 12). Sparing of the subcortical white matter is typical.[39] These findings are presumed to reflect mitochondrial toxicity as MR spectroscopy typically shows reduced N-acetyl aspartate and increased lactate in the affected areas.[40]

MEDICATION-ASSOCIATED CENTRAL NERVOUS SYSTEM VASCULOPATHY
Sympathomimetic Drugs

Sympathomimetic agents are used to augment the endogenous catecholamines of the sympathetic CNS for therapeutic purposes. Sympathomimetic drugs, such as pseudoephedrine, can cause intracranial vasculopathy. Pseudoephedrine relieves cold, flu, sinusitis, asthma, and bronchitis symptoms. Cerebral angiography studies in patients with stroke, associated with over-the-counter sympathomimetic medications, have shown "vasculitis-like" abnormalities, including widespread segmental narrowing and beading, usually in both the carotid and vertebrobasilar territories.[41] Sympathomimetic drug use has been identified as a risk factor for intracranial hemorrhage[42,43] and occasionally for ischemic stroke (Fig. 13).[44] The risk of complication increases in patients with impaired renal and hepatic function. Proposed mechanisms by which these drugs cause cerebrovascular complications include the development of hypertensive crisis[45] due to direct vasoconstrictive action and the result of angiitis.[46,47]

Table 1
Classification Proposal for lesion location and grading of cocaine-induced midline destructive lesions

Localization	Grade	Frequency
Nasal septum	1	99%
Grade 1 + inferolateral region (inferior turbinate and medial wall of maxillary sinus)	2a	59%
Grade 1 + palate	2b	30%
Grade 2 + ethmoid bone, middle turbinate, and superior turbinate	3	23%
Grade 3 + neurocranium (lamina papyracea, orbit or anterior skull base)	4	8%

Modified from Nitro L, Pipolo C, Fadda GL, et al. Distribution of cocaine-induced midline destructive lesions: systematic review and classification. Eur Arch Otorhinolaryngol. 2022;279(7):3257-3267.

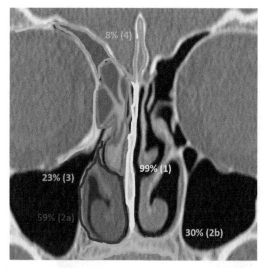

Fig. 8. Prevalence of CIMDL according to location. Coronal CT scan from a healthy subject is used as an anatomic reference. Yellow: grade 1 (nasal septum); red: grade 2a (inferior turbinate and medial wall of maxillary sinus); green: grade 2b (palate); blue: grade 3 (ethmoid bone, middle turbinate, and superior turbinate); orange, grade 4 (lamina papyracea, orbit or skull base). (*Modified from* Nitro L, Pipolo C, Fadda GL, et al. Distribution of cocaine-induced midline destructive lesions: systematic review and classification. Eur Arch Oto-Rhino-Laryngology. 2022;279(7):3257-3267.)

Antithyroid Drugs

Methimazole (MMI) and propylthiouracil (PTU) have long been used to treat hyperthyroidism secondary to Grave's disease (GD). ANCA-associated vasculitis is a rare and potentially life-threatening complication associated with these drugs. The median time between drug initiation and disease onset is 42 months, with PTU reported to have a higher incidence of vasculitis than MMI.[48] The pathogenesis is not well understood. Still, it has been postulated that MMI and PTU influence the production of myeloperoxidase (MPO)-ANCA, leading to vascular injury.[48] MPO-ANCA-associated vasculitis affects a single organ in 44% of patients, two organs in 34%, and more than two in 22%. In approximately 2% of cases, CNS vasculitis can occur, and it is seen in patients with more than two-organ involvement.[48] Typical manifestations include multiple lower cranial nerve deficits, cerebral hemorrhage, or hypertrophic pachymeningitis.

Prognosis is, however, favorable if the condition is detected early, if antithyroid drugs are discontinued, and if patients are treated with corticosteroids or immunosuppressants.[48,49]

Oncologic Drugs

Methotrexate (MTX) is an anti-metabolite agent that inhibits the enzyme dihydrofolate reductase (DHFR), which catalyzes the conversion of dihydrofolate into tetrahydrofolate, the active form of folic acid. Tetrahydrofolate is necessary for the synthesis of nucleotides of both DNA and RNA.[50] The incidence of MTX neurotoxicity ranges from 3% to 8%.[51,52] Acute MTX neurotoxicity, most often seen 10 to 11 days after intrathecal MTX administration,[51,52] usually results in stroke-like symptoms, such as aphasia, weakness, sensory deficits, ataxia, and seizures. Symptoms typically resolve within 24 to 36 hours. The inhibition of tetrahydrofolate by MTX also appears to affect the synthesis of macromolecules, such as myelin. Therefore, the presence of MTX-induced leukoencephalopathy is considered to be secondary to the impairment of myelin turnover. DHFR inhibition also leads to increased levels of homocysteine, which is toxic to vascular endothelium and may cause direct vascular damage. This is the proposed mechanism behind mineralizing angiopathy (**Fig. 14**) and vascular occlusion.[53]

On MR imaging, acute MTX-related leukoencephalopathy often demonstrates restricted diffusion in the deep periventricular white matter without corresponding FLAIR signal abnormality. Interestingly, in the subacute stage, high T2WI/FLAIR signal abnormality appears in a delayed fashion in the same regions of DWI signal change, a finding that is seen in 15% to 75% of patients (**Fig. 15**). These imaging findings, however, do not consistently correlate with neurologic deficits.[51] DWI abnormalities in acute MTX neurotoxicity indicate cerebral dysfunction but not necessarily overt structural injury to the cerebrum.[54] Most patients have a benign course with no long-term sequelae and can usually resume MTX therapy.[52]

Immunosuppressive Drugs

Immunosuppressive drugs (eg, cyclosporine, tacrolimus) are common precipitants of PRES. Although the pathophysiology remains unclear, these drugs are believed to have a direct toxic effect on vascular endothelial cells with secondary damage to the blood-brain barrier.[55] Hypertension and renal failure are risk factors for developing neurologic symptoms in patients treated with immunosuppressants.[55] Patients present with headache, mental confusion, vomiting, visual disturbances, or seizures. On imaging, subcortical vasogenic edema is typically seen in the parieto-occipital regions on CT or MR imaging, often with the additional involvement of the posterior

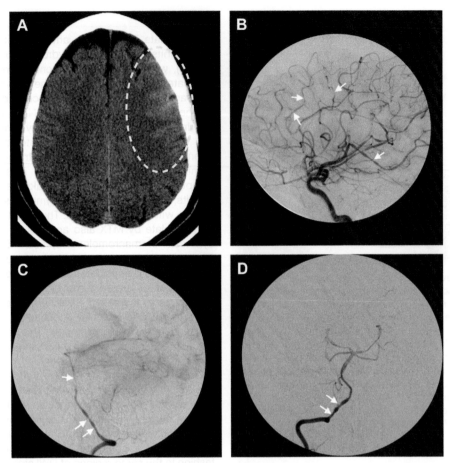

Fig. 9. Marijuana-induced RCVS. 27-year-old male patient with post-coital headache and marijuana consumption. Non-contrast CT head shows acute subarachnoid hemorrhage in the left frontal region (*dashed circle* in *A*). DSA shows multifocal narrowing of ipsilateral distal ACA and MCA branches (*arrows* in *B*). There is also multifocal narrowing of the basilar artery (*arrows* in *C and D*) and both proximal posterior cerebral arteries, giving a "beaded appearance" of the vessels.

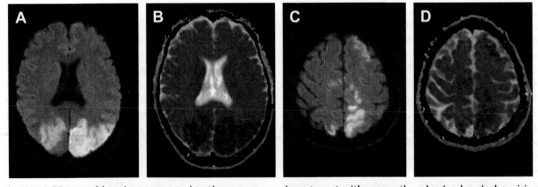

Fig. 10. A 38-year-old patient presented to the emergency department with severe thunderclap headache, vision loss, and mental status changes. The patient disclosed daily exposure to smoked marijuana and caffeinated energy drinks. DWI MR imaging (*A-D*) at admission demonstrates multifocal acute and subacute infarcts involving the bilateral occipital and parietal lobes, as well as the frontal lobes, the latter left more than right.

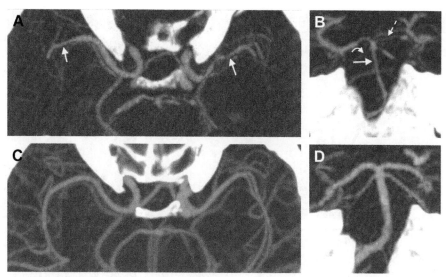

Fig. 11. Same patient from Fig. 10. Thick 10 mm axial (*A*) and coronal (*B*) MIP reconstructions of CTA COW at admission demonstrate moderate to severe multifocal short and long segment luminal narrowing, representing vasospasm, involving the left supraclinoid ICA, the bilateral MCAs, left worse than right (*arrows* in *A*), the basilar artery (*arrow* in *B*), the right superior cerebellar artery (*curved arrow* in *B*) and left PCA (*dashed arrow* in *B*). 12 weeks follow up CTA (*C* and *D*) demonstrate complete resolution of vasospasm.

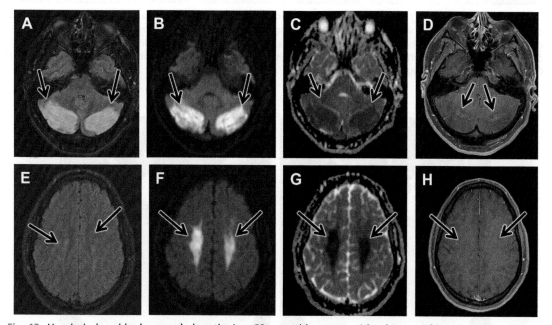

Fig. 12. Heroin-induced leukoencephalopathy in a 23-year-old woman with a history of heroin abuse, Adderall overdose, and hypnotic toxidrome. Top row (*A-D*): the posterior fossa demonstrates abnormally increased FLAIR signal intensity bilaterally within the cerebellar hemispheres (*arrows, A*), with bright diffusion signal intensity (*arrows, B*) and low signal intensity on ADC (*arrows, C*). There is linear enhancement of small folia on axial T1-post contrast fat-saturated image (*arrows, D*). Lower row (*E-H*) demonstrates subtle increased FLAIR signal within the bilateral centrum semiovale (*arrows, E*) but significant restricted diffusion (*arrows in F and G*). There are small foci of enhancement on postcontrast T1WI (*arrows in H*).

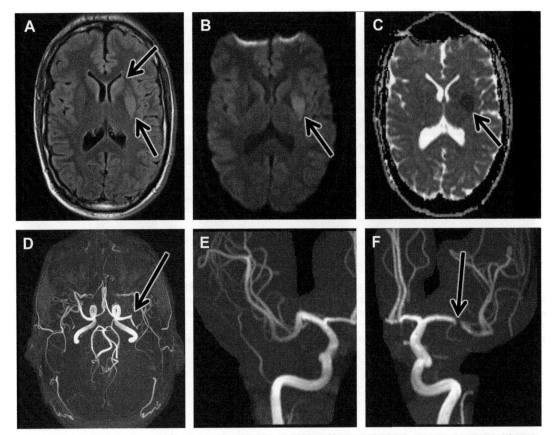

Fig. 13. Acute infarct in a 27-year-old woman with a history of methamphetamine abuse presenting with severe dysarthria and right-sided weakness. Axial FLAIR image demonstrates bright signal intensity within the left caudate head and putamen (*arrows in A*). DWI shows corresponding restricted diffusion (*arrows in B and C*) consistent with an acute infarct. MRA shows focal occlusion of the distal left M1 segment (*arrows in D and F*). Contralateral normal M1 segment for comparison (*E*).

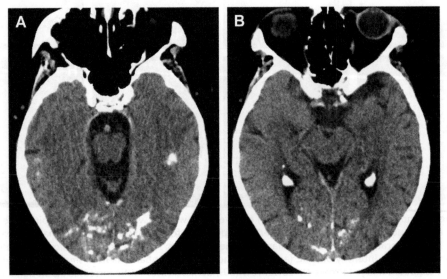

Fig. 14. Mineralizing microangiopathy. CT brain images (*A and B*) show multiple parenchymal calcifications in both occipital and temporal lobes in a patient with remote history of MTX treatment.

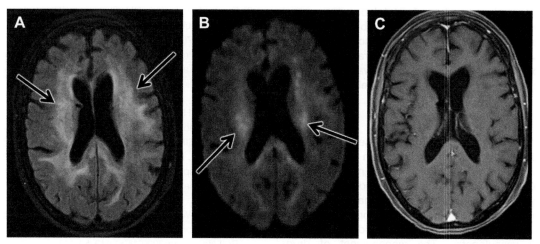

Fig. 15. MTX-related leukoencephalopathy. 69-year-old woman with a history of chronic lymphocytic leukemia recently started on methotrexate therapy who presented with falls, confusion, and weakness. Axial FLAIR image shows diffuse high signal intensity of the deep white matter (*arrows* in *A*), associated with patchy restricted diffusion (*arrows* in *B*). There is no enhancement on axial T1 post-contrast fat-saturated image (*C*).

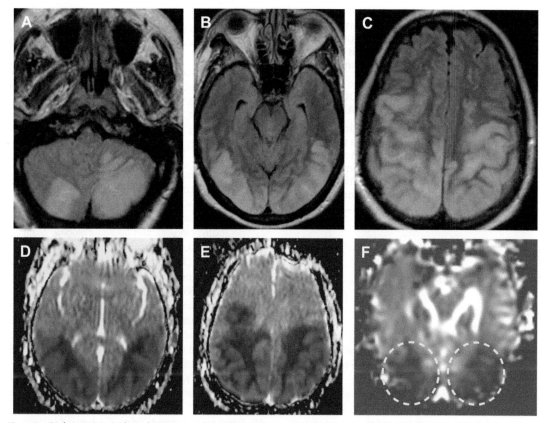

Fig. 16. Cyclosporine-induced PRES. Axial FLAIR (*A–C*) images demonstrate diffuse bilateral slightly asymmetric subcortical edema in the cerebellum, occipitotemporal and frontoparietal regions associated with restricted diffusion on ADC map (*D–E*) and low perfusion on dynamic susceptibility contrast perfusion (*dashed circles* in *F*).

temporal, parietal, or frontal lobes (**Fig. 16**).[56] Additional structures such as the brainstem, cerebellum, and basal ganglia can also be affected.[56] Most patients usually have a full gradual resolution of symptoms after drug withdrawal, and imaging abnormalities resolve within 2 weeks.

SUMMARY

Vasculopathy secondary to the use of recreational drugs or certain medications can lead to significant complications in the central nervous system (CNS) and sinonasal cavity, including intracranial hemorrhage and stroke. MR imaging, VW-MR, and CT/CTA are valuable tools for the evaluation of patients with suspected drug-induced vasculitis or vasculopathy. The management of drug-associated vasculopathy relies on drug withdrawal and supportive therapy to avoid secondary toxic effects. Most patients have a benign course with no long-term sequelae.

CLINICS CARE POINTS

- Approximately half of patients with hemorrhagic strokes due to cocaine abuse have a concomitant pathology such as cerebral vascular malformations or aneurysms.

- The pattern of involvement of the sinonasal complex helps differentiate CIMDL from its primary differential diagnosis, GPA.

- Over-the-counter sympathomimetics medications to relieve cold, flu, or asthma symptoms have been identified as a risk factor for CNS vasculopathy, intracranial hemorrhage, or ischemic strokes, especially in patients with impaired renal and hepatic function.

DISCLOSURE

The authors have nothing to disclose.

REFERENCES

1. Jennette J.C., Falk R.J., Bacon P.A., et al., 2012 revised International Chapel Hill Consensus Conference Nomenclature of Vasculitides. Arthritis Rheum. 2013;65(1):1-11.

2. Mandell DM, Mossa-Basha M, Qiao Y, et al. Intracranial vessel wall MRI: Principles and expert consensus recommendations of the American society of neuroradiology. Am J Neuroradiol 2017; 38(2):218–29.

3. Fessler RD, Esshaki CM, Stankewitz RC, et al. The neurovascular complications of cocaine. Surg Neurol 1997;47(4):339–45.

4. Brown E, Prager J, Lee HY, et al. CNS complications of cocaine abuse: Prevalence, pathophysiology, and neuroradiology. Am J Roentgenol 1992;159(1):137–47.

5. Toossi S, Hess CP, Hills NK, et al. Neurovascular Complications of Cocaine Use at a Tertiary Stroke Center. J Stroke Cerebrovasc Dis 2010;19(4):273–8.

6. Levine SR, Brust JCM, Futrell N, et al. Cerebrovascular Complications of the Use of the Crack Form of Alkaloidal Cocaine. N Engl J Med 1990;323(11):699–704.

7. McEvoy AW, Kitchen ND, Thomas DGT. Intracerebral haemorrhage and drug abuse in young adults. Br J Neurosurg 2000;14(5):449–54.

8. Tamrazi B, Almast J. Your brain on drugs: Imaging of drug-related changes in the central nervous system. Radiographics 2012;32(3):701–19.

9. Geibprasert S, Gallucci M, Krings T. Addictive illegal drugs: Structural neuroimaging. Am J Neuroradiol 2010;31(5):803–8.

10. Koch S, Sacco RL. Cocaine-associated stroke: Some new insights? Nat Clin Pract Neurol 2008;4(11):579.

11. Erwin MB, Hoyle JR, Smith CH, et al. Cocaine and accelerated atherosclerosis: Insights from intravascular ultrasound [4]. Int J Cardiol 2004;93(2–3):301–3.

12. Daras M, Tuchman AJ, Marks S. Central nervous system infarction related to cocaine abuse. Stroke 1991;22(10):1320–5.

13. De Roock S, Hantson P, Laterre PF, et al. Extensive pallidal and white matter injury following cocaine overdose [3]. Intensive Care Med 2007;33(11):2030–1.

14. Hagan IG, Burney K. Radiology of recreational drug abuse. Radiographics 2007;27(4):919–40.

15. Di Lazzaro V, Restuccia D, Oliviero A, et al. Ischaemic myelopathy associated with cocaine: Clinical, neurophysiological, and neuroradiological features. J Neurol Neurosurg Psychiatry 1997;63(4):531–3.

16. Chang A, Osterloh J, Thomas J. Levamisole: A dangerous new cocaine adulterant. Clin Pharmacol Ther 2010;88(3):408–11.

17. Wu VC, Huang JW, Lien HC, et al. Levamisole-induced multifocal inflammatory leukoencephalopathy: Clinical characteristics, outcome, and impact of treatment in 31 patients. Medicine (Baltim) 2006; 85(4):203–13.

18. Xu N, Zhou W, Li S, et al. Clinical and MRI characteristics of levamisole-induced leukoencephalopathy in 16 patients. J Neuroimaging 2009;19(4):326–31.

19. Sagduyu Kocaman A, Yalinay Dikmen P, Karaarslan E. Cocaine-induced multifocal leukoencephalopathy mimicking Balo's concentric sclerosis: A 2-year

follow-up with serial imaging of a single patient. Mult Scler Relat Disord 2018;19:96–8.

20. Pessini LM, Kremer S, Auger C, et al. Tumefactive inflammatory leukoencephalopathy in cocaine users: Report of three cases. Mult Scler Relat Disord 2020; 38. https://doi.org/10.1016/j.msard.2019.101496.

21. Seyer BA, Grist W, Muller S. Aggressive destructive midfacial lesion from cocaine abuse. Oral Surg Oral Med Oral Pathol Oral Radiol Endod 2002;94(4): 465–70.

22. Rubin K. The manifestation of cocaine-induced midline destructive lesion in bone tissue and its identification in human skeletal remains. Forensic Sci Int 2013;231(1–3):408.e11.

23. Kuriloff DB, Kimmelman CP. Osteocartilaginous necrosis of the sinonasal tract following cocaine abuse. Laryngoscope 1989;99(9):918–24.

24. Deutsch HL, Millard DR. A New Cocaine Abuse Complex: Involvement of Nose, Septum, Palate, and Pharynx. Arch Otolaryngol Neck Surg 1989; 115(2):235–7.

25. Gordon AS, Moran DT, Jafek BW, et al. The Effect of Chronic Cocaine Abuse on Human Olfaction. Arch Otolaryngol Neck Surg 1990;116(12):1415–8.

26. Armengot M, Garćia-Lliberós A, Gómez MJ, et al. Sinonasal Involvement in Systemic Vasculitides and Cocaine-Induced Midline Destructive Lesions: Diagnostic Controversies. Allergy Rhinol 2013;4(2). https://doi.org/10.2500/ar.2013.4.0051.

27. Trimarchi M, Nicolai P, Lombardi D, et al. Sinonasal osteocartilaginous necrosis in cocaine abusers: Experience in 25 patients. Am J Rhinol 2003;17(1):33–43.

28. Nitro L, Pipolo C, Fadda GL, et al. Distribution of cocaine-induced midline destructive lesions: systematic review and classification. Eur Arch Oto-Rhino-Laryngology. 2022;279(7):3257–67.

29. Trimarchi M, Gregorini G, Facchetti F, et al. Cocaine-induced midline destructive lesions: Clinical, radiographic, histopathologic, and serologic features and their differentiation from Wegener granulomatosis. Medicine (Baltim) 2001;80(6):391–404.

30. Di Cosola M, Ambrosino M, Limongelli L, et al. Cocaine-induced midline destructive lesions (CIMDL): A real challenge in diagnosis. Int J Environ Res Public Health 2021;18(15). https://doi.org/10.3390/ijerph18157831.

31. Colletti G, Autelitano L, Chiapasco M, et al. Comprehensive surgical management of cocaine-induced midline destructive lesions. J Oral Maxillofac Surg 2014;72(7):1395.e1–10.

32. Ducros A. Reversible cerebral vasoconstriction syndrome. Lancet Neurol 2012;11(10):906–17.

33. Katz BS, Fugate JE, Ameriso SF, et al. Clinical worsening in reversible cerebral vasoconstriction syndrome. JAMA Neurol 2014;71(1):68–73.

34. Calabrese LH, Dodick DW, Schwedt TJ, et al. Narrative review: Reversible cerebral vasoconstriction syndromes. Ann Intern Med 2007;146(1):34–44.

35. Jensen J, Leonard J, Salottolo K, et al. The Epidemiology of Reversible Cerebral Vasoconstriction Syndrome in Patients at a Colorado Comprehensive Stroke Center. J Vasc Interv Neurol 2018; 10(1):32–8.

36. Hajj-Ali RA, Furlan A, Abou-Chebel A, et al. Benign angiopathy of the central nervous system: Cohort of 16 patients with clinical course and long-term followup. Arthritis Care Res 2002;47(6):662–9.

37. Büttner A, Mall G, Penning R, et al. The neuropathology of heroin abuse. Forensic Sci Int 2000;113: 435–42.

38. Wolters EC, Stam FC, Lousberg RJ, et al. Leucoencephalopathy after inhaling "heroin" pyrolysate. Lancet 1982;320(8310):1233–7.

39. Keogh CF, Andrews GT, Spacey SD, et al. Neuroimaging features of heroin inhalation toxicity: "Chasing the dragon.". Am J Roentgenol 2003; 180(3):847–50.

40. Kriegstein AR, Shungu DC, Millar WS, et al. Leukoencephalopathy and raised brain lactate from heroin vapor inhalation ('chasing the dragon'). Neurology 1999;53(8):1765–73.

41. Cantu C, Arauz A, Murillo-Bonilla LM, et al. Stroke associated with sympathomimetics contained in over-the-counter cough and cold drugs. Stroke 2003;34(7):1667–72.

42. Maertens P, Lum G, Powell Williams J, et al. Intracranial hemorrhage and cerebral angiopathic changes in a suicidal phenylpropanolamine poisoning. South Med J 1987;80(12):1584–6.

43. Kernan WN, Viscoli CM, Brass LM, et al. Phenylpropanolamine and the Risk of Hemorrhagic Stroke. N Engl J Med 2000;343(25):1826–32.

44. Johnson DA, Etter HS, Reeves DM. STROKE AND PHENYLPROPANOLAMINE USE. Lancet 1983; 322(8356):970.

45. Lake CR, Gallant S, Masson E, et al. Adverse drug effects attributed to phenylpropanolamine: A review of 142 case reports. Am J Med 1990;89(2):195–208.

46. Fallis RJ, Fisher M. Cerebral vasculitis and hemorrhage associated with phenylpropanolamine. Neurology 1985;35(3):405–7.

47. Forman HP, Levin S, Stewart B, et al. Cerebral vasculitis and hemorrhage in an adolescent taking diet pills containing phenylpropanolamine: Case report and review of literature. Pediatrics 1989;83(5):737–41.

48. Noh JY, Yasuda S, Sato S, et al. Clinical characteristics of myeloperoxidase antineutrophil cytoplasmic antibody-associated vasculitis caused by antithyroid drugs. J Clin Endocrinol Metab 2009;94(8): 2806–11.

49. Alidoost M, Cheng J, Alpert DR. Propylthiouracil-induced anti-neutrophil cytoplasmic antibody vasculitis presenting with red eye followed by pulmonary hemorrhage: Diagnostic and management considerations. Am J Case Rep 2020;21:1–5.

50. Koźmiński P, Halik PK, Chesori R, et al. Overview of dual-acting drug methotrexate in different neurological diseases, autoimmune pathologies and cancers. Int J Mol Sci 2020;21(10).

51. Mahoney DH, Shuster JJ, Nitschke R, et al. Acute neurotoxicity in children with B-precursor acute lymphoid leukemia: An association with intermediate-dose intravenous methotrexate and intrathecal triple therapy - A Pediatric Oncology Group study. J Clin Oncol 1998; 16(5):1712–22.

52. Rubnitz JE, Relling MV, Harrison PL, et al. Transient encephalopathy following high-dose methotrexate treatment in childhood acute lymphoblastic leukemia. Leukemia 1998;12(8):1176–81.

53. Shuper A, Stark B, Kornreich L, et al. Methotrexate treatment protocols and the central nervous system: Significant cure with significant neurotoxicity. J Child Neurol 2000;15(9):573–80.

54. Rollins N, Winick N, Bash R, et al. Acute methotrexate neurotoxicity: Findings on diffusion-weighted imaging and correlation with clinical outcome. Am J Neuroradiol 2004;25(10):1688–95.

55. Hinchey J, Chaves C, Appignani B, et al. A reversible posterior leukoencephalopathy syndrome. N Engl J Med 1996;334(8):494–500.

56. Schwartz RB, Bravo SM, Klufas RA, et al. Cyclosporine neurotoxicity and its relationship to hypertensive encephalopathy: CT and MR findings in 16 cases. Am J Roentgenol 1995;165(3):627–31.

Imaging of Reversible Cerebral Vasoconstriction Syndrome and Posterior Reversible Encephalopathy Syndrome

Bilal Battal, MD*, Mauricio Castillo, MD

KEYWORDS

- Neuroimaging • Posterior reversible encephalopathy syndrome (PRES)
- Reversible cerebral vasoconstriction syndrome (RCVS) • Magnetic resonance imaging (MRI)
- Vasculitis • Vessel wall imaging • Seizure • Brain

KEY POINTS

- Exact pathogenesis remains unclear for both PRESS and RCVS, but primarily proposed mechanisms focus on blood flow dysregulation due to abnormal cerebrovascular tone and endothelial dysfunction.
- PRES is mainly characterized by encephalopathy and seizures with hallmark imaging findings of vasogenic edema in a symmetric mainly subcortical white matter pattern centered at the watershed areas.
- RCVS is characterized by reversible segmental arterial vasoconstriction, causing severe thunderclap headache and neurologic complications, including ischemic infarcts and hemorrhage, that may occur during the course of the disease.
- PRES and RCVS have common triggers and share some clinical and imaging features.
- Imaging plays an important role in confirming the diagnosis and guiding management and has a pivotal role in determining the temporal progression, detecting complications, and predicting prognosis.

INTRODUCTION

Posterior reversible encephalopathy syndrome (PRES) and reversible cerebral vasoconstriction syndrome (RCVS) have progressively been recognized mainly due to the wider use of brain magnetic resonance imaging (MRI) and increasing clinical awareness. PRES and RCVS are descriptive terms, each with similar imaging findings, clinical manifestations, and even common pathophysiological causal factors. PRES is characterized by a combination of clinical features and neuroimaging findings in the presence of various risk factors but it may occur in healthy subjects.[1,2] Key clinical and imaging findings include impaired consciousness, seizures, headache, focal neurologic deficits, and vasogenic edema involving bilateral parietal and occipital cortical/subcortical regions.[1–4] RCVS represents a group of conditions that show identical clinical, imaging, and prognostic features regardless of their associated conditions. RCVS is characterized by reversible segmental constriction of cerebral arteries causing severe thunderclap headache which is usually

Division of Neuroradiology, Department of Radiology, University of North Carolina School of Medicine, Chapel Hill, NC 27599, USA
* Corresponding author. Division of Neuroradiology, Department of Radiology, The University of North Carolina at Chapel Hill, 101 Manning Drive, CB 7510, 2000 Old Clinic, Chapel Hill, NC 27599.
E-mail addresses: bilbat_23@yahoo.com; bilal_battal@med.unc.edu

Neuroimag Clin N Am 34 (2024) 129–147
https://doi.org/10.1016/j.nic.2023.07.004
1052-5149/24/© 2023 Elsevier Inc. All rights reserved.

reversible, but neurologic complications, including ischemic infarcts, and hemorrhage, may occur during the course of the disease.

Although there is debate about the pathophysiology of PRES and RCVS, whether they are completely separate or a continuum of a pathologic spectrum, the underlying pathophysiology in both is mainly related to the reversible dysregulation of the cerebral vasculature. PRES and RCVS may occur simultaneously in cases of hypertension, preeclampsia or eclampsia, autoimmune diseases, intracranial hypotension, and use of vasoactive or cytotoxic drugs.[3–6] Overlapping of imaging findings can occur between these entities as well: typical PRES findings can be observed in 8% to 38% of patients with RCVS and some patients with PRES may demonstrate reversible segmental vasoconstriction of intracranial arteries.[7–11]

Imaging plays an important role in confirming the diagnosis and providing appropriate clinical management guidelines for PRES and RCVS. It also has a pivotal role in determining the temporal progression of these pathologies, detecting complications, and predicting prognosis. In this review, we aim to describe PRES and RCVS, discuss their possible pathophysiological mechanisms, and present imaging methods that are useful in the diagnosis, management, and follow-up of patients.

POSTERIOR REVERSIBLE ENCEPHALOPATHY SYNDROME
Terminology and pathophysiology

PRES is a clinicoradiologic entity defined as posterior leukoencephalopathy syndrome, hyperperfusion encephalopathy, and brain capillary leak syndrome. However, these descriptions do not definitely explain the pathophysiological and clinical features of the disease because brain injury not always reversible, involvement is not necessarily confined to the white matter or the posterior regions of the brain, and the syndrome can cause irreversible brain damage.[1–4]

The exact pathogenesis remains unclear for both PRESS and RCVS. Several pathophysiological mechanisms have been proposed primarily focusing a blood flow dysregulation due to abnormal cerebrovascular tone and endothelial dysfunction, but other mechanisms, such as immune system dysregulation, may also play a role.[1] Some authors hypothesized that PRES and RCVS are a continuum of reversible disorders of cerebral vascular function with different expressions.[4,7] However, the pathologic mechanism differs as PRES involves failure of autoregulation with increased blood flow through arterioles opposite to RCVS that involves excessive vasospasm

with resultant inadequate blood flow through arterioles (Table 1).[1–4,7]

Regarding the failure of blood flow autoregulation and hypertension theories, hyperperfusion is thought to play a critical role. Normally, brain tissue is protected from the harmful effects of hypertension by the vasoconstriction of arterioles with blood flow autoregulation. In the case of extremely high blood pressure, failure of autoregulation may lead to fluid exudation and tissue edema.[12] Patients with baseline hypotension or highly labile blood pressure are more susceptible to developing PRES, whereas chronic hypertensive patients can tolerate extremely high blood pressures without developing PRES.[13] The posterior brain regions are particularly susceptible to failure of autoregulation and hyperperfusion due to relatively less sympathetic innervation.[12] Endothelial dysfunction may also be responsible for the exudation of fluid and tissue edema, particularly in patients with preeclampsia and undergoing treatment with cytotoxic chemotherapy.[14] Another mechanism is focal vasoconstriction and cerebral ischemia that can be seen in some patients with PRES, in which, dysfunctional attempts at autoregulation may further cause reactive focal vasoconstriction and resultant focal hypoperfusion and infarction.[13] In this situation, a combined syndrome involving both PRES and RCVS can occur. However, all these mechanisms do not explain all PRES cases, and in some clinical settings, hypercalcemia, hypomagnesemia, hypoalbuminemia, uremia, sepsis, and other metabolic disturbances and fluid overload may cause PRES possibly due to disturbance of the vascular endothelium function.[2,15]

Clinical findings

Although PRES may affect all age groups, increased prevalence has been reported among young or middle-aged adults with a female predominance.[16–18] PRES was initially thought to affect patients with hypertension, but there are various associated conditions and risk factors, including abrupt elevations of blood pressure, impaired renal function, preeclampsia/eclampsia, autoimmune diseases, infection, sepsis, malignancy, transplantation, and chemotherapeutic agents. However, the disease may be seen in normotensive patients and may even be idiopathic (see Table 1).[19]

Headache, visual symptoms, seizures, and confusion may occur in PRES and RCVS. However, encephalopathy and seizures are distinct and frequent symptoms in PRES, whereas recurrent thunderclap headaches are the leading symptom in RCVS. Although more than 90% of patients

Table 1
Pathophysiologic, clinic, and radiologic features of PRES and RCVS.

	PRES	RCVS
Proposed pathophysiologic mechanism		
	Failure of cerebral vascular autoregulation and endothelial dysfunction with excess blood flow through the arterioles	Diffuse multifocal vasospasm of cerebral arteries due to autonomic over-activity, endothelial dysfunction, and oxidative stress with inadequate blood flow through the arterioles
Associated clinical risk factors/triggers		
	Hypertension, pre-eclampsia/ eclampsia, immunosuppression, malignancy, post-transplant, renal failure, dialysis, autoimmune disorders, infection, sepsis, shock, metabolic disorders, chemotherapeutic medications, tumor lysis syndrome, erythropoietin, IVIG, idiopathic	Pregnancy and postpartum states, exposure to vasoactive/ recreational drugs and blood products, erythropoietin, IVIG, head trauma, head and neck surgery, carotid dissection, unruptured aneurysm, tumors (pheochromocytoma, paraganglioma), migraines, environmental exposure, idiopathic
Clinical features		
Headache	Dull headache (moderate-severe)	Thunderclap headache
Encephalopathy	Common	Uncommon
Seizure	Common	Uncommon
Visual disturbances	Common	Uncommon
Focal neurologic deficit	Uncommon	Common with complicated infarction and hemorrhage
CSF analysis	Normal/near normal	Normal/near normal
Radiological features		
Vasoconstriction	Uncommon	Common, multifocal, string-of-beads
Lesion distribution	Generally symmetric	Generally asymmetric
Edema	Common; parietooccipital pattern, holohemispherical pattern, superior frontal sulcus pattern	Uncommon; PRES-like pattern
Ischemic lesions	Uncommon	Common in a symmetric watershed distribution
Hemorrhage	Punctate type common, ICH/SAH uncommon	Lobar intraparenchymal/convexity SAH common
Contrast enhancement	Common, superficial leptomeningeal and cortical gyral pattern	Uncommon

Abbreviations: CSF, cerebrospinal fluid; ICH, intra-cerebral hemorrhage; IVIG, intravenous immunoglobulin; PRES, posterior reversible encephalopathy syndrome; RCVS, reversible cerebral vasoconstriction syndrome; SAH, subarachnoid hemorrhage.

demonstrate typical clinical and neuroradiological imaging findings, the clinical presentation may be significantly variable and related to the underlying precipitating factors and comorbidities.[20] Seizure is a major presenting manifestation that may occur in different types and recur, though a small number of patients with mild disease may be seizure-free. Hypertension is a frequent precipitating factor. Constant, non-localized, moderate to severe headache is typical, and analgesic response is poor. Other symptoms include encephalopathy varying in degree from somnolence to coma, visual disturbances including aura, diplopia, blurred vision, visual hallucinations and visual field deficits due to cortical blindness, and focal neurologic deficits such as hemiparesis, aphasia/dysarthria, or ataxia depending on the involved brain regions (see Table 1).[1–3,14–16]

PRES was initially described as a benign monophasic reversible entity with favorable prognosis, but during the last 2 decades, mortality has been observed in 19% of patients, and varying degree long-term functional impairments including epilepsy and motor deficits have been reported in 44% of patients.[21–23] In rare occurrences, recurrences have also been reported.[24]

Imaging findings

Brain imaging is a main pillar along with clinical findings in confirming the diagnosis of PRES. Hallmark imaging finding is vasogenic edema that typically tends to occur in a bilateral symmetric pattern within the cortex and subcortical white matter centered at the watershed areas. Distribution is usually not confined to a single vascular territory and commonly involves the posterior parieto-occipital regions.[12,25] Beyond the classic parieto-occipital pattern, several atypical/rare patterns have been documented including holo-hemispherical watershed pattern, and superior frontal sulcus pattern, and central pattern (Fig. 1).[17,26,27] Occasionally, extensive edema of central brain structures may result in brainstem compression and hydrocephalus.[28]

PRES has been classified into different grades as mild, moderate, and severe.[25] Cortical or subcortical scattered white matter edema without apparent hemorrhage, mass effect, or herniation and minimal involvement one of the cerebellum, brain stem, or basal ganglia is defined as mild PRES. In moderate PRES, there is confluent edema extending from cortex to deep white matter without the involvement of the ventricular margins, mild mass effect without herniation or midline shift, presence of parenchymal hemorrhage or mild involvement of at least 2 other regions (cerebellum, brainstem, or basal ganglia). In severe PRES, there is confluent vasogenic edema that extends from the cortex to the ventricular margins, midline shift, or herniation due to extensive edema, parenchymal hemorrhage, or involvement of all three regions of cerebellum, brainstem, and basal ganglia (Fig. 2).[25]

Despite vasogenic edema can be visualized on non-contrast computed tomography (CT) as patchy hypodensities in severe cases, which may be non-specific and difficult to differentiate from other pathologies, and mild cases may even demonstrate normal CT appearance. Brain MRI, especially the T2-weighted and fluid-attenuated inversion recovery (FLAIR) sequences are useful in the evaluation of its distribution and determination of white/gray matter involvement of vasogenic/cytotoxic edema.[17] FLAIR sequences improve sensitivity and detect subtle peripheral and cortical lesions which are understood to be more common than once thought.[29] Diffusion-weighted imaging (DWI) combined with apparent diffusion coefficient (ADC) maps help differentiate cytotoxic from vasogenic edema and aid in differentiating PRES from ischemic lesions (Fig. 3).[30,31] However, in severe and complicated cases, diffusion restriction may also be detected in PRES.

Knowledge of the different presentations of PRES is important, as atypical imaging findings should not dissuade a diagnosis of PRES in the correct clinical context.[32] Atypical findings including asymmetric involvement of the cerebral hemispheres (rarely unilateral), restricted diffusion suggesting cytotoxic edema (seen in 30% of patients), intracerebral hemorrhage seen in 10% to 30% of cases, and contrast enhancement may also occur (Fig. 4).[25,33,34] Junewar and colleagues[35] demonstrated a higher incidence of cytotoxic edema in patients with PRES with eclampsia which may be related to reactive vasoconstriction. Previous findings are inconclusive regarding the relationship between cytotoxic edema and clinical prognosis of PRES, but the presence of restricted diffusion may be associated with incomplete recovery.[36] A study by Covarrubias and colleagues[31] showed that diffusion restriction may be the earliest sign of irreversible lesions though other studies report no significant correlation between diffusion restriction and mortality. Moreover, complete resolution of diffusion restriction during follow-up without abnormal imaging sequelae has also been reported.[37]

PRES related hemorrhage usually occurs in areas of cerebral edema and is primarily seen in patients after allogenic bone marrow transplantation and coagulopathy and can represent as a minute focal hemorrhages (<5 mm), sulcal SAH, or focal hematomas (Fig. 5). Susceptibility-weighted imaging (SWI) is more sensitive in detecting micro hemorrhages that have been observed in PRES but its correlation with severity of edema and its clinical relevance is still unknown.[25,33,34,38,39] Either, hyper perfusion induced by loss of cerebral autoregulation or damage of blood-brain barrier (BBB) caused by endothelial cell injury can lead to increase of capillary permeability and exudation of plasma and erythrocytes into the subarachnoid

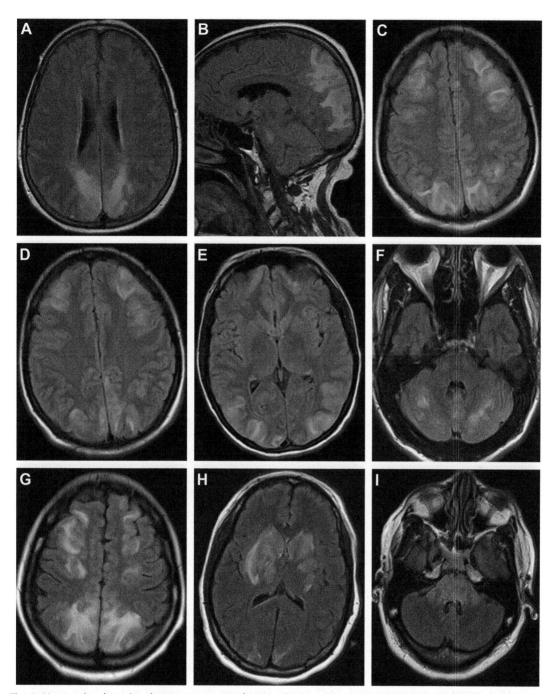

Fig. 1. Vasogenic edema involvement patterns of PRES. *Classic parieto-occipital pattern,* (*A*) axial and (*B*) sagittal FLAIR images demonstrate cortical and subcortical white matter vasogenic edema confined in bilateral parieto-occipital lobes. *Holo-hemispherical watershed pattern,* (*C-F*) FLAIR images show vasogenic edema predominantly involves ACA, MCA, and PCA watershed zones and cerebellum. *Superior frontal sulcus pattern,* (*G*) FLAIR image reveals vasogenic edema predominantly involving ACA/MCA watershed zone at the depth of superior frontal sulcus. *Central pattern,* (*H*) and (*I*) FLAIR images show vasogenic edema preferentially located in the deep white matter, basal ganglia, thalami, and brainstem.

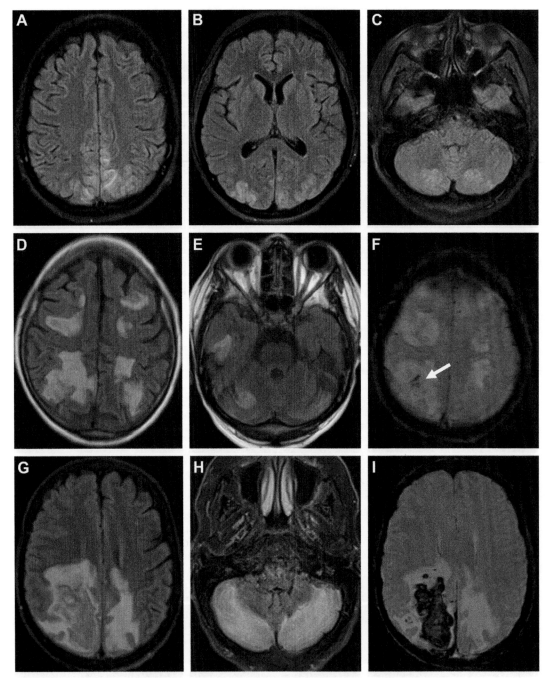

Fig. 2. Mild, moderate, and severe PRES. (*A-C*) Axial FLAIR images show cerebral and cerebellar cortical and subcortical white matter edema without apparent hemorrhage, mass effect or basal ganglia and brainstem involvement consistent with mild PRES. (*D*) and (*E*) FLAIR and (*F*) SWI images demonstrate confluent cortical and subcortical edema extending cortex to the deep white matter as well as cerebellar involvement and micro hemorrhagic foci (*white arrow*) in the right parietal parenchyma consistent with moderate PRES. (*G*) and (*H*) FLAIR and (*I*) SWI images show extensive confluent vasogenic edema extending cortex to the ventricular margin, significant cerebellar involvement and large parietal parenchymal hemorrhage consistent with severe PRES.

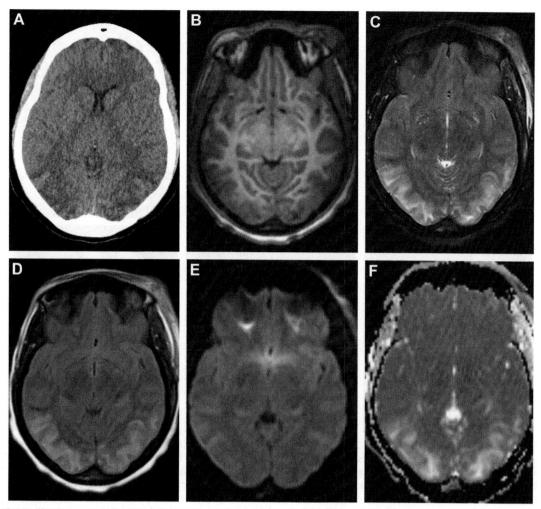

Fig. 3. Classic imaging findings of PRES in a 22-year-old female with chronic renal failure. (*A*) CT image with brain parenchyma window settings shows patch hypodensity in bilateral occipital regions suggestive of edema. (*B*) T1, (*C*) T2 and (*D*) FLAIR images demonstrate cortical and subcortical white matter T1 hypointense, T2 and FLAIR hyperintense signal abnormality in occipital regions bilaterally. (*E*) DWI and (*F*) ADC map images demonstrate facilitated diffusion in affected occipital regions consistent with vasogenic edema.

space and brain parenchyma resulting in SAH and punctate hemorrhages.

Contrast enhancement on T1-weighted imaging, most commonly involving leptomeningeal and cortical regions, is seen in approximately 40% of patients without correlation with age, imaging severity, or outcome (Fig. 6).[40]

In vascular imaging, including conventional cerebral angiography and CT/MR angiography, moderate to severe vessel irregularities suggestive of focal or diffuse vasoconstriction, vasodilation, or a "string-of-beads" appearance is seen in more than 80% of patients.[41] These findings may be confused with other diagnoses, such as vasospasm or vasculitis but on follow-up there is the reversal of spasm in the majority and residual spasm in few patients.[42,43] Perfusion imaging

studies have demonstrated decreased cerebral blood flow, particularly more than a day after the onset of symptoms, but in certain cases, hyperperfusion may be observed in the early disease course (Fig. 7).[42]

Differential diagnosis

Differentiating atypical features of PRES such as central PRES and hemorrhagic PRES from other disorders including toxic leukoencephalopathy, meningoencephalitis, central/extra pontine myelinolysis, lupus cerebritis, malignancy, hypoxicischemic encephalopathy, progressive multifocal leukoencephalopathy, and postictal state requires a thorough review of risk factors, additional testing and follow up imaging.[44,45] Frequent differential

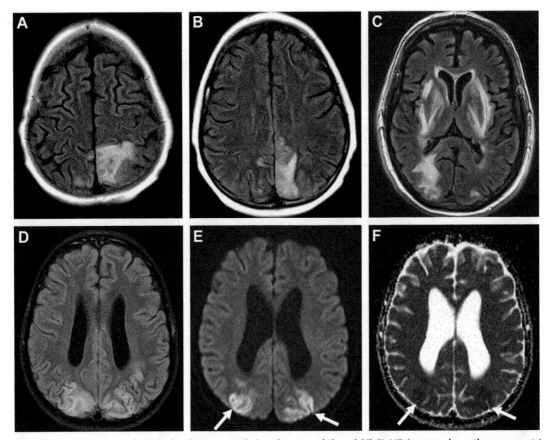

Fig. 4. Atypical findings of PRES. *(A-C) Asymmetric involvement.* (*A*) and (*B*) FLAIR images show the asymmetric involvement of parieto-occipital lobes with subtle edema on the right and large confluent edema on the left. (*C*) FLAIR image of a different patient demonstrates asymmetric right occipital white matter edema and associated bilateral basal ganglia and internal/external capsular involvement. *(D-F) Diffusion restriction/cytotoxic edema.* (*D*) FLAIR image shows bilateral parieto-occipital high signal involving the cortex and subcortical white matter in a patient with Fanconi anemia. (*E*) DWI and (*F*) ADC map show bilateral cortical restricted diffusion (*arrows*) consistent with complicated PRES with cytotoxic edema/ischemia.

considerations and their distinctive clinical and radiologic features are presented in Table 2.

REVERSIBLE CEREBRAL VASOCONSTRICTION SYNDROME
Terminology and pathophysiology

RCVS is another increasingly recognized vasculopathy representing a group of conditions associated with various triggering factors. The main pathophysiologic characteristic of RCVS is the segmental constriction of cerebral arteries that is always monophasic and usually resolves spontaneously within 3 months. This disease has also been previously called migrainous vasospasm/migraine angiitis, thunderclap headache-associated vasospasm, postpartum cerebral angiopathy, and drug-induced cerebral arteritis.

The primary problem seems to be a diffuse, multifocal vasospasm of intracranial arteries with resultant *inadequate* blood flow through arterioles possibly secondary to a transitory spontaneous or triggered autonomic over-activity, endothelial dysfunction, and oxidative stress.[46] The pathogenesis of the acute and severe headache (thunderclap) in RCVS may result from a positive feed-forward cycle involving increasing pain, increasing sympathetic tone, and increasing vasospasm due to the innervation of arteries via sensory afferents from the trigeminal nerve.[46] There are multiple risk factors associated with RCVS, but more than 50% of cases are associated with vasoactive adrenergic or serotonergic drugs, especially in the postpartum period, likely due to endothelial vasoconstriction triggered by directly vasoactive substances and sudden decreases in the concentration of estrogen and progesterone suggesting a hormonal contribution.[4,47,48] Ducros and colleagues[7] proposed that vasoconstriction begins in the distal small arteries and progresses centrally over time, eventually affecting

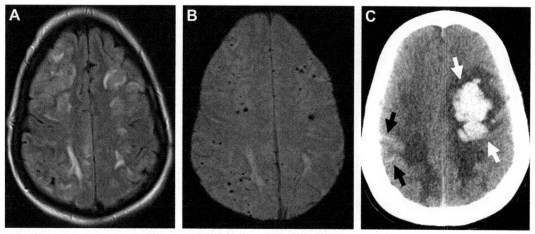

Fig. 5. PRES-related hemorrhages. (*A*) FLAIR and (*B*) SWI images show holo-hemispherical PRES with frontoparietal region edema and multiple foci of minute focal hemorrhages. (*C*) Axial CT image of different patient demonstrates significant parietal and posterior centrum semiovale edema in the settings of known PRES and associated right parietal sulcal subarachnoid hemorrhage (*black arrows*) and left frontal parenchymal acute hematoma (*white arrows*).

medium and large size arteries as well. Considering that thunderclap headache is probably the result of leptomeningeal trigeminal afferents in the distal small arteriole walls, vasoconstriction may rarely be detected by imaging in the early thunderclap headache period due to low sensitivity of angiographic studies, whereas vasoconstriction can be more frequently detected by angiography in later periods when the headache has resolved due to peripheral vasoconstriction that progresses centripetally to involve medium- and large-size arteries.[2]

Clinical findings

The incidence of RCVS is uncertain, but the recently increasing number of cases is probably due to elevated awareness and increased use of sensitive diagnostic imaging tools.[1,7,49] RCVS is more common in women than men (2:1) and occurs predominantly between ages of 20 to 60 years with a peak at around 42 years.[4]

The clinical setting of RCVS is different from that of PRES. Thunderclap headache, which is defined as high-intensity headache of abrupt onset reaching its peak intensity within less than 1 minute and lasting for more than 5 minutes, is the main symptom that 90% of patients experience and often remains its only manifestation. Less than 10% of patients present with subacute or less severe headaches. Thunderclap headache is usually bilateral in a posterior location that becomes diffuse pain and is frequently be associated with nausea, vomiting, photophobia, phonophobia, and visual changes. The patients typically report triggering factors such as exertion, emotion,

orgasm, swimming, bathing/showering, or Valsalva maneuvers (coughing, sneezing, defecation).[1,2,4–8] RCVS is usually self-limiting, resolution of symptoms happens within 3 weeks, and resolution of vasoconstriction should occur within 3 months. However, recurrences and complications including death may occur.[50,51] Although thunderclap headache in RCVS can be as short as a few minutes, cases lasting several days have been reported. The absence of headache at the onset of other symptoms is exceptional. Usually, headache improves within 1 to 3 hours, which helps differentiate it from SAH. A single attack of headache is possible, but usually, thunderclap headaches in RCVS tend to *recur* over a span of days to weeks and moderate headache frequently persists between exacerbations.[7,52,53] Co-existing *neck pain* should prompt investigation for cervical arterial dissection due to the co-existence of both pathologies in up to 12% of cases.[54]

More than 90% of patients with RCVS have a benign course. A rapidly progressive course of RCVS may lead to permanent disability or even in-hospital death in 5% to 10% of patients.[1] Approximately 75% of admitted patients develop parenchymal lesions and related additional symptoms including convexity SAH, intraparenchymal hemorrhage, subdural hemorrhage, watershed ischemic strokes, brain edema, PRES, focal neurologic deficits, and seizures.[55] Less than 5% of patients develop coma or die secondary to progressive arterial vasoconstriction causing massive brain edema, large ischemic strokes, and intraparenchymal hemorrhages. Factors, such as glucocorticoid and intra-arterial vasodilator therapies and infarction

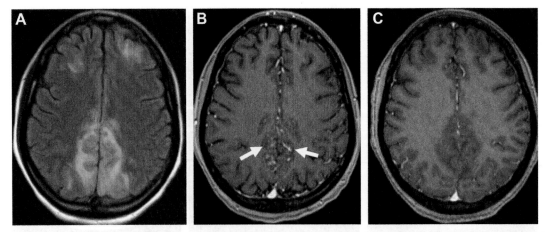

Fig. 6. A 19-year-old female with Lupus-associated PRES. (*A*) FLAIR image shows frontal and parieto-occipital ACA/MCA and ACA/PCA watershed distribution vasogenic edema of PRES. (*B*) Post-contrast T1 MR image shows cortical/leptomeningeal contrast enhancement in the region of PRES involving biparietal and posterior insular cortex (*white arrows*). (*C*) Post-treatment follow-up post-contrast T1 MR image obtained 1 week later demonstrates near complete resolution of abnormal contrast enhancement.

on baseline imaging are associated with poor outcomes.[1,56]

Imaging findings

Abnormal cerebral angiography findings are the primary diagnostic feature of RCVS. However, brain imaging of many patients in initial clinical presentation, including conventional angiography, may be normal, and maintaining a high degree of suspicion is essential for diagnosis.[57] MR/CT angiography or conventional angiography demonstrates cerebral vasoconstriction, generally widespread, bilateral,

and with proximal progression along the circle of Willis and its branches over time. Angiography shows the characteristic beaded arterial vasoconstriction that is seen as smooth, tapered narrowing involving large to medium-sized arteries followed by abnormally dilated segments of distal second- and third-order branches (Fig. 8). Chen and colleagues[9] reported that peak arterial vasoconstriction occurs in proximal arterial structures at approximately 16 days after symptom onset. Initial CT/MR angiography and catheter angiography can be normal due to the fact that vasoconstriction starts in distal small arteries. The vasoconstriction

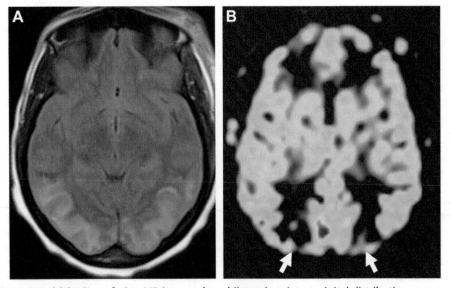

Fig. 7. (*A*) FLAIR and (*B*) ASL perfusion MR images show bilateral parieto-occipital distribution vasogenic edema consistent with PRES and associated decreased perfusion (*arrows*).

Table 2
Differential diagnoses for PRES

HIE	PRES
• Increased DWI signal with low ADC, subtle FLAIR signal in acute phase • Increased FLAIR signal and faded DW signal in subacute phase • Usually, involvement of deep gray matter	• Usually, vasogenic edema, T2 shine through, high ADC • Rarely, complicated cases may show diffusion restriction/infarct • Deep gray matter involvement is atypical

Stroke/Posterior border-zone infarcts	PRES
• In acute setting increased DW signal with low ADC values • Generally unilateral and history of ischemic insult	• Usually, vasogenic edema, T2 sine through, high ADC • Rarely, complicated cases may show diffusion restriction/infarct

Postictal state	PRES
• Hippocampal involvement and unilateral distribution • Cortical signal without subcortical involvement • Splenial involvement	• Usually posterior watershed zone involvement • Cortical and subcortical white matter involvement • Splenial involvement is atypical

Acute toxic leukoencephalopathy	PRES
• Acute neurologic deterioration with reversible vasogenic edema and restricted diffusion centered in the periventricular white matter • Lack of cortical involvement	• Usually, vasogenic edema, T2 shine through, high ADC, centered in cortical and subcortical regions

SMART syndrome	PRES
• Prominent gyriform cortical and leptomeningeal enhancement with mild mass effect and cortical thickening with or without diffusion restriction • Cortical laminar necrosis may be associated • Typically, unilateral and patients with cranial irradiation history	• Usually bilateral, symmetric, posterior involvement • Vasogenic edema, T2 shine through, high ADC, centered in cortical and subcortical regions

Malignancy/Gliomatosis cerebri	PRES
• Persistent abnormalities on follow-up scans commonly enlarging over time, asymmetrical distribution • Elevated choline/NAA peak	• Usually bilateral, symmetric, posterior involvement • Reversibility of the lesions

Paraneoplastic encephalitis	PRES
• Temporofrontal predominant involvement with hippocampal and basal ganglia involvement • Inflammatory CSF, positive antineuronal antibodie	• Usually bilateral, symmetric, posterior involvement • Normal CSF analysis

Progressive multifocal leukoencephalopathy (PML)	PRES
• Periventricular and subcortical involvement, sparing the cortex • Little or no mass effect or enhancement	• Usually bilateral, symmetric, posterior cortical and subcortical involvement

Abbreviations: ADC, apparent diffusion coefficient; CSF, cerebrospinal fluid; DWI, diffusion-weighted imaging; FLAIR, fluid attenuated inversion recovery; HIE, hypoxic-ischemic encephalopathy; NAA, N-acetyl aspartate; PML, progressive multifocal leukoencephalopathy; PRES, posterior reversible encephalopathy syndrome; SMART, stroke-like migraine attacks after radiation therapy.

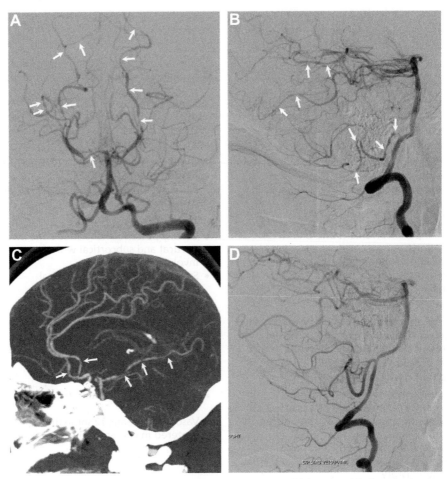

Fig. 8. Catheter angiography and CTA findings of RCVS in a 49-year-old female with thunderclap headache. (*A*) and (*B*) catheter angiography images of vertebrobasilar system with left vertebral artery injection show multiple severe beaded arterial vasoconstriction of intracranial arteries, most prominent in posterior cerebral and posterior inferior cerebellar arteries (*arrows*). (*C*) Sagittal Maximum-Intensity-Projection (MIP) CTA image demonstrates multisegment beaded vasoconstriction of bilateral anterior and posterior cerebral arteries (*arrows*). (*D*) Sagittal catheter angiography image of vertebrobasilar system shows near complete resolution of multisegment arterial stenosis following intra-arterial vasodilator administration.

progresses proximally with the resolution of distal vasoconstriction around the same time as headache resolution. In patients with a high degree of clinical suspicion for RCVS, follow-up non-invasive angiographic studies after 5 to 7 days are helpful in demonstrating classic multifocal vasoconstriction. Additional cervical CT/MR angiography may be useful for the detection of cervical arterial dissection which may occur with RCVS.

Catheter digital angiography is the gold standard diagnostic test due to its superior spatial resolution for small distal cerebral arteries, though it is invasive and less commonly used in clinical practice.[4,58] Additionally, DSA may provide information that aids in the diagnosis, including reversibility of vasoconstriction following intra-arterial administration of a vasodilator distinguishing it

from other entities such as primary angiitis of the central nervous system (PACNS), Moya Moya, or arteriosclerotic disease which show only partial or incomplete improvement (see **Fig. 8**).[59] Ducros and colleagues[7] reported that DSA was associated with a risk of provoking transient neurologic deficits in 9% of their cases. However, other studies did not find an increase in complication rates following catheter angiography for RCVS.[58,60] Since more than 90% of patients improve spontaneously and there is no proven therapy for RCVS, it may be safer to use repeat CT and MR angiography in routine clinical scenarios and to reserve DSA for complicated cases such as those with progressive clinical deterioration despite conservative management or an inability to exclude aneurysmal SAH (**Fig. 9**).

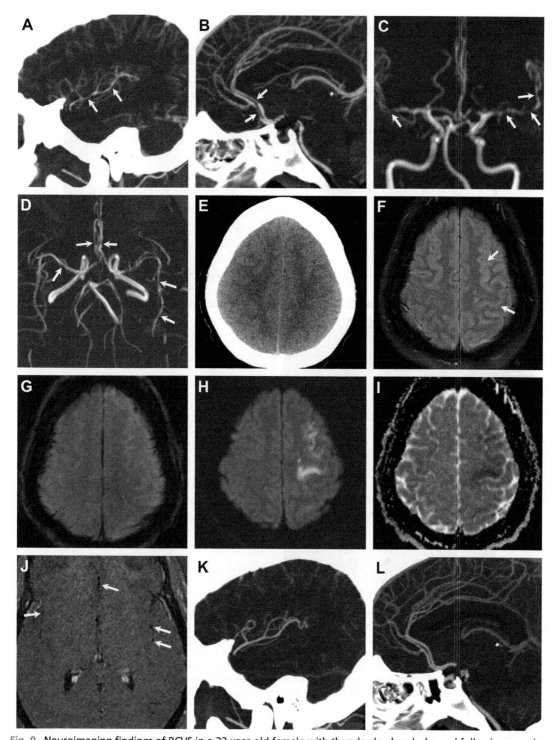

Fig. 9. Neuroimaging findings of RCVS in a 32-year-old female with thunderclap headache and following superimposed stroke. (*A*) and (*B*) MIP CTA and (*C*) and (*D*) MIP MRA images demonstrate multisegment beaded vasoconstriction/stenosis in the proximal and distal branches of ACA and MCA (*arrows*). (*E*) Initial unenhanced CT is unremarkable. (*F*) FLAIR and (*G*) SWI images demonstrate linear hyperintense signal along the left frontoparietal sulci without SWI signal dropout suggesting slow flow in leptomeningeal vessels (*arrows*). The patient had right-sided weakness 2 days later, and (*H*) DWI and (*I*) ADC map images showed left frontal cortical/subcortical patchy diffusion restriction consistent with superimposed infarct. (*J*) Axial vessel wall image shows mild narrowing of ACA and MCA branches without abnormal vessel wall enhancement (*arrows*). (*K*) and (*L*) 3 months later follow-up sagittal MIP CTA images show the complete resolution of multisegment intracranial arterial vasoconstrictions.

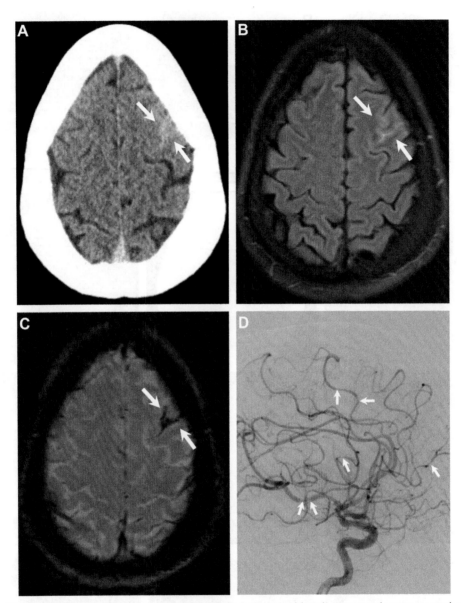

Fig. 10. Subarachnoid hemorrhage in a case with RCVS. A 47-year-old male presented acute onset thunderclap headache without resolution for 7 days. Initial unenhanced head CT was unremarkable (not seen). The patient was re-evaluated with unenhanced CT head (*A*) due to increased intensity of headache and associated seizure, which shows left frontal convexity sulcal subarachnoid hemorrhage (*arrows*). (*B*) FLAIR and (*C*) SWI images show abnormal linear FLAIR hyperintense signal and SWI signal dropout, keeping with sulcal subarachnoid hemorrhage (*arrows*). (*D*) Catheter angiography image of the left ICA injection demonstrates multisegment vasoconstriction in middle and distal branches of ACA and MCA (*arrows*).

CT and MRI are often initially normal in patients with RCVS but they may be used to evaluate alternative diagnoses, and to detect and follow up complications associated with the disease including lobar ICH, convexity SAH, subdural hemorrhage and ischemic infarction. An imaging correlate for angiographically occult peripheral arterial vasoconstriction is slow flow in leptomeningeal vessels is FLAIR hyperintense blood vessels along cerebral sulci. The presence of hyperintense blood vessels on FLAIR leads to a higher risk of ischemic stroke and PRES and correlates with more severe vasoconstriction as measured by transcranial Doppler (TCD).[61,62] This finding is also associated with other conditions including severe cerebral artery stenosis or

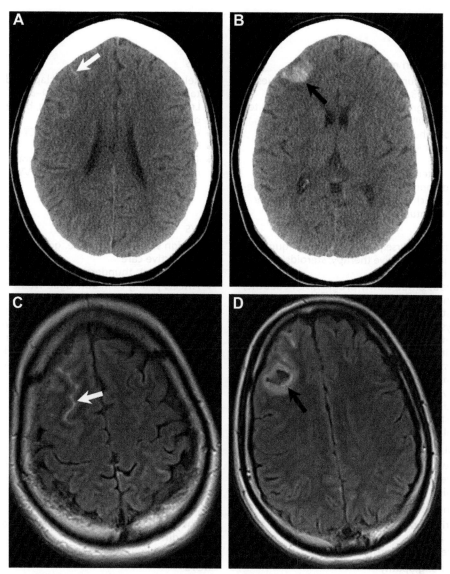

Fig. 11. RCVS complicated with subarachnoid and lobar intra-parenchymal hemorrhage. (*A*) and (*B*) unenhanced CT and (*C*) and (*D*) FLAIR images show right frontal sulcal subarachnoid hemorrhage (*white arrows*) and intra-parenchymal acute hematoma (*black arrows*).

occlusion and Moya Moya disease. Subarachnoid hemorrhage, which may be present in patients with RCVS and also demonstrates hyperintense signal along cerebral sulci on FLAIR should be included in the differential diagnosis. SWI may be helpful to identify SAH (see **Fig. 9**; **Fig. 10**).[58,61,62]

Non-cisternal convexity SAH is the most common complication of RCVS and affects one-third of patients. RCVS is the most common cause of convexity SAH in patients less than 60 year old (see **Fig. 10**). In a minority of patients with RCVS, both SAH and PRES findings may occur in the first week of clinical symptoms.[8,10] However, ischemic complications of RCVS typically occur in cortical subcortical regions in *bilateral and symmetric* distributions along anterior-posterior watershed zones generally at the end of the second week often after the resolution of headaches presumably reflecting a delay in the resolution of cerebral vasoconstriction. The earlier onset of SAH and PRES is hypothesized to reflect the sequela of smaller and more peripherally located artery vasoconstriction, whereas the later onset of positive angiographic studies and ischemic stroke is thought to reflect the sequela of larger and more centrally located artery vasoconstriction.[4,57]

Parenchymal hemorrhage tends to be seen in the first week after thunderclap headaches

Table 3
Differential diagnoses for RCVS.

Aneurysmal/peri mesencephalic SAH	RCVS
• Constant thunderclap headache continues more than 3 h • Acute progressive neurologic decline due to acute SAH/IVH and communicating hydrocephalus • Remarkable pathologic findings on initial NCCT • Basal cistern/circle of Willis centered SAH • VWI demonstrates aneurysmal wall enhancement which could represent inflammation/recent rupture	• Relapsing-remitting thunderclap headache attacks usually improves within 1–3 h • Less severe neurologic symptom, better clinical grade, younger patient age, • Usually, unremarkable initial NCCT • Superficial sulcal localized SAH • Transient luminal narrowing without or minimal vessel wall enhancement on VWI
PACNS	**RCVS**
• Fulminant course/poor prognosis, requires immunosuppressive therapy; steroids/cytotoxic agent • Insidious onset, slowly progressive headache, • Often seen in older men • Elevated protein and WBC count in CSF analysis • Multifocal varying age infarcts in initial MRI • Multifocal narrowing and irregularity of mid-to-distal cerebral arteries • Partial/incomplete improvement in cerebral artery narrowing following intra-arterial vasodilator therapy • Persistent luminal narrowing with circumferential vessel wall enhancement on VWI	• Benign self-limited course, good outcome, supportive care • Acute onset, thunderclap headache • Affects young to middle-aged women • Usually, normal CSF analysis • Unremarkable imaging findings in initial MRI • In complicated cases; infarcts, sulcal SAH, parenchymal hemorrhage, concomitant PRES • Complete improvement in cerebral artery narrowing following intra-arterial vasodilator therapy • Transient luminal narrowing without or minimal vessel wall enhancement on VWI
Cortical vein/DVS thrombosis	**RCVS**
• MRI with 3D contrast enhanced T1, SWI and MR venography show venous thrombosis • Requires anticoagulant therapy	• Sulcal SAH, parenchymal hemorrhage/infarct without venous thrombosis • Supportive care
Migraine headache and stroke	**RCVS**
• Severity and quality of headache similar to prior attacks • Single vascular territory infarct	• The severity and quality of headache are usually different • Multifocal/multi-territory infarcts
Amyloid angiopathy	**RCVS**
• Elderly patient • Without thunderclap or acute headache • Evidence of leukoaraiosis and microhemorrhages	• Young women • Typical thunderclap headache • Initial MRI is usually unremarkable

Abbreviations: 3D, three-dimensional; CSF, cerebrospinal fluid; IVH, intra-ventricular hemorrhage; MRI, magnetic resonance imaging; NCCT, non-contrast computed tomography; PACNS, primary angiitis of the central nervous system; PRES, posterior reversible encephalopathy syndrome; RCVS, reversible cerebral vasoconstriction syndrome; SAH, subarachnoid hemorrhage; SWI, susceptibility-weighted imaging; VWI, vessel wall imaging; WBC, white blood cell.

suggesting a mechanistic role for reperfusion injury. These bleeds are usually small and lobar but isolated deep ones may occur (Fig. 11).[10] Migraine history, older age, and female gender have been defined as factors leading to parenchymal hemorrhage in RCVS but over 90% of patients have similar lengths of hospital stays and good clinical outcomes.[7,56]

TCD has been used to diagnose and monitor the evolution of vasoconstriction in patients with RCVS by measuring mean and peak blood flow velocities in proximal cerebral arteries around the circle of Willis.[53,63]

Perfusion imaging in RCVS may show multifocal areas of hypoperfusion that often include cerebral watershed zones.[64,65] These areas of perfusion abnormalities may worsen acutely and, in some instances, progress to watershed infarctions.[65]

Vessel wall imaging (VWI) shows concentric wall thickening but none or minimal contrast enhancement in arteries.[66] Absence of contrast enhancement or a minimal contrast enhancement is concordant with histopathological absent inflammation in RCVS (see Fig. 9). Follow-up imaging shows the resolution of wall thickening and enhancement within a median interval of 3 months in all cases.[67] This is in contradistinction to cerebral vasculitis which shows multifocal circumferential enhancement associated with regions of stenosis and persistence of luminal narrowing on follow-up imaging.[66–68] Brain biopsies in RCVS show normal arterial histology with absent vessel wall inflammation as seen in vasculitis.[4]

Differential diagnosis

Presenting symptoms, sequelae, and imaging features of RCVS can significantly overlap with other pathologies including aneurysmal SAH, PACNS, migraine, cortical vein thrombosis, pituitary apoplexy, amyloid angiopathy, hypertensive hemorrhage, PRES, giant cell arteritis, arterial dissection, spontaneous intracranial hypotension, and meningitis. Furthermore, the treatment of these alternative diagnoses, including aneurysmal SAH and PACNS, varies considerably from that of RCVS making an accurate diagnosis critical to ensure appropriate patient care.[58,69] Frequent differential considerations and their distinctive clinical and imaging features are presented in Table 3.

SUMMARY

Pathophysiological mechanisms of PRES and RCVS are still not fully understood. Although distinct clinical and imaging features have been described, shared precipitating factors, clinical and imaging features frequently co-exist suggesting common pathophysiological mechanisms related to reversible dysregulation of cerebral vasculature, endothelial dysfunction, and breakdown of the blood-brain barrier. Although PRES and RCVS are usually fully reversible with early diagnosis and prompt treatment, some patients develop hemorrhage or ischemia often resulting in permanent disabilities. Radiologists need to be aware of the typical and atypical imaging manifestations of these syndromes to make an accurate diagnosis. Neuroimaging helps in early diagnosis avoiding unnecessary or dangerous treatments, improving outcomes, and may give new insights into understanding etiologies and pathophysiology as well.

CLINICS CARE POINTS

- Currently, the precise pathogenesis of PRES and RCVS remains uncertain; however, both conditions have common triggers and share certain clinical and imaging features.
- Initially described as favorable, the prognosis of PRES and RCVS can be affected by their potential to cause intracranial hemorrhage, ischemic strokes, varying degrees of long-term functional impairments, and even mortality.
- Early diagnosis and prompt treatment are crucial to prevent complications and permanent disabilities. Neuroimaging plays a vital role in confirming the diagnosis, guiding management, and is pivotal in determining the temporal progression, detecting complications, and predicting prognosis.

DISCLOSURE

The authors have nothing to disclose.

REFERENCES

1. Pilato F, Distefano M, Calandrelli R. Posterior Reversible Encephalopathy Syndrome and Reversible Cerebral Vasoconstriction Syndrome: Clinical and Radiological Considerations. Front Neurol 2020;11:34.
2. Levitt A, Zampolin R, Burns J, et al. Posterior Reversible Encephalopathy Syndrome and Reversible Cerebral Vasoconstriction Syndrome: Distinct Clinical Entities with Overlapping Pathophysiology. Radiol Clin North Am 2019;57:1133–46.
3. Hinchey J, Chaves C, Appignani B, et al. A reversible posterior leukoencephalopathy syndrome. N Engl J Med 1996;334:494–500.
4. Ducros A. Reversible cerebral vasoconstriction syndrome. Lancet Neurol 2012;11:906–17.
5. Feil K, Forbrig R, Thaler FS, et al. Reversible cerebral vasoconstriction syndrome and posterior reversible encephalopathy syndrome associated with intracranial hypotension. Neurocrit Care 2017;26:103–8.
6. Lee WJ, Yeon JY, Jo KI, et al. Reversible cerebral vasoconstriction syndrome and posterior reversible encephalopathy syndrome presenting with deep intracerebral hemorrhage in young women. J Cerebrovasc Endovasc Neurosurg 2015;17:239–45.
7. Ducros A, Boukobza M, Porcher R, et al. The clinical and radiological spectrum of reversible cerebral vasoconstriction syndrome. A prospective series of 67 patients. Brain 2007;130:3091–101.
8. Singhal AB, Hajj-Ali RA, Topcuoglu MA, et al. Reversible cerebral vasoconstriction syndromes: analysis of 139 cases. Arch Neurol 2011;68:1005–12.

9. Chen SP, Fuh JL, Wang SJ, et al. Magnetic resonance angiography in reversible cerebral vasoconstriction syndromes. Ann Neurol 2010;67:648–56.

10. Ducros A, Fiedler U, Porcher R, et al. Hemorrhagic manifestations of reversible cerebral vasoconstriction syndrome: frequency, features, and risk factors. Stroke 2010;41:2505–11.

11. Schwartz R, Mulkern R, Vajapeyam S, et al. Catheter angiography, MR angiography, and MR perfusion in posterior reversible encephalopathy syndrome. AJNR Am J Neuroradiol 2009;30:E19.

12. Fugate JE, Rabinstein AA. Posterior reversible encephalopathy syndrome: clinical and radiological manifestations, pathophysiology, and outstanding questions. Lancet Neurol 2015;14:914–25.

13. Tetsuka S, Ogawa T. Posterior reversible encephalopathy syndrome: A review with emphasis on neuroimaging characteristics. J Neurol Sci 2019;404:72–9.

14. Gewirtz AN, Gao V, Parauda SC, et al. Posterior Reversible Encephalopathy Syndrome. Curr Pain Headache Rep 2021;25:19.

15. Toledano M, Fugate JE. Posterior reversible encephalopathy in the intensive care unit. Handb Clin Neurol 2017;141:467–83.

16. Lee VH, Wijdicks EF, Manno EM, et al. Clinical spectrum of reversible posterior leukoencephalopathy syndrome. Arch Neurol 2008;65:205–10.

17. Bartynski WS, Boardman JF. Distinct imaging patterns and lesion distribution in posterior reversible encephalopathy syndrome. AJNR Am J Neuroradiol 2007;28:1320–7.

18. Fugate JE, Claassen DO, Cloft HJ, et al. Posterior reversible encephalopathy syndrome: associated clinical and radiologic findings. Mayo Clin Proc 2010;85:427–32.

19. Hinduja A. Posterior Reversible Encephalopathy Syndrome: Clinical Features and Outcome. Front Neurol 2020;11:71.

20. Gao B, Lyu C, Lerner A, et al. Controversy of posterior reversible encephalopathy syndrome: what have we learnt in the last 20 years? J Neurol Neurosurg Psychiatry 2018;89:14–20.

21. Jacquot C, Glastonbury CM, Tihan T. Is posterior reversible encephalopathy syndrome really reversible? Autopsy findings 4.5 years after radiographic resolution. NP 2015;34:26–33.

22. Legriel S, Schraub O, Azoulay E, et al. Determinants of recovery from severe posterior reversible encephalopathy syndrome. PLoS One 2012;7:e44534.

23. Alhilali LM, Reynolds AR, Fakhran S. A multi-disciplinary model of risk factors for fatal outcome in posterior reversible encephalopathy syndrome. J Neurol Sci 2014;347:59–65.

24. Sweany JM, Bartynski WS, Boardman JF. "Recurrent" posterior reversible encephalopathy syndrome: report of 3 cases–PRES can strike twice. J Comput Assist Tomogr 2007;31:148–56.

25. McKinney AM, Short J, Truwit CL, et al. Posterior reversible encephalopathy syndrome: incidence of atypical regions of involvement and imaging findings. AJR Am J Roentgenol 2007;189:904–12.

26. Liman TG, Siebert E, Endres M. Posterior reversible encephalopathy syndrome. Curr Opin Neurol 2019;32:25–35.

27. Fischer M, Schmutzhard E. Posterior reversible encephalopathy syndrome. J Neurol 2017;264:1608–16.

28. Keyserling HF, Provenzale JM. Atypical imaging findings in a near-fatal case of posterior reversible encephalopathy syndrome in a child. AJR Am J Roentgenol 2007;188:219–21.

29. Casey SO, Sampaio RC, Michel E, et al. Posterior reversible encephalopathy syndrome: utility of fluid-attenuated inversion recovery MR imaging in the detection of cortical and subcortical lesions. AJNR Am J Neuroradiol 2000;21:1199–206.

30. Provenzale JM, Petrella JR, Cruz LC Jr, et al. Quantitative assessment of diffusion abnormalities in posterior reversible encephalopathy syndrome. AJNR Am J Neuroradiol 2001;22:1455–61.

31. Covarrubias DJ, Luetmer PH, Campeau NG. Posterior reversible encephalopathy syndrome: prognostic utility of quantitative diffusion-weighted MR images. AJNR Am J Neuroradiol 2002;23:1038–48.

32. Stevens CJ, Heran MK. The many faces of posterior reversible encephalopathy syndrome. Br J Radiol 2012;85:1566–75.

33. Liman TG, Bohner G, Heuschmann PU, et al. The clinical and radiological spectrum of posterior reversible encephalopathy syndrome: the retrospective Berlin PRES study. J Neurol 2012;259:155–64.

34. Hefzy HM, Bartynski WS, Boardman JF, et al. Hemorrhage in posterior reversible encephalopathy syndrome: imaging and clinical features. AJNR Am J Neuroradiol 2009;30:1371–9.

35. Junewar V, Verma R, Sankhwar PL, et al. Neuroimaging features and predictors of outcome in eclamptic encephalopathy: a prospective observational study. AJNR Am J Neuroradiol 2014;35:1728–34.

36. Moon SN, Jeon SJ, Choi SS, et al. Can clinical and MRI findings predict the prognosis of variant and classical type of posterior reversible encephalopathy syndrome (PRES)? Acta Radiol 2013;54:1182–90.

37. Pande AR, Ando K, IshikurA R, et al. Clinicoradiological factors influencing the reversibility of posterior reversible encephalopathy syndrome: a multicenter study. Radiat Med 2006;24:659–68.

38. McKinney AM, Sarikaya B, Gustafson C, et al. Detection of microhemorrhage in posterior reversible encephalopathy syndrome using susceptibility-weighted imaging. AJNR Am J Neuroradiol 2012;33:896–903.

39. Chen Z, Zhang G, Lerner A, et al. Risk factors for poor outcome in posterior reversible encephalopathy syndrome: systematic review and meta-analysis. Quant Imaging Med Surg 2018;8:421–32.

40. Karia SJ, Rykken JB, McKinney ZJ, et al. Utility and significance of gadolinium-based contrast enhancement in posterior reversible encephalopathy syndrome. AJNR Am J Neuroradiol 2016;37:415–22.

41. Bartynski WS, Boardman JF. Catheter angiography, MR angiography, and MR perfusion in posterior reversible encephalopathy syndrome. AJNR Am J Neuroradiol 2008;29:447–55.

42. Bartynski WS. Posterior reversible encephalopathy syndrome. Part 1. Fundamental imaging and clinical features. AJNR Am J Neuroradiol 2008;29:1036–42.

43. Sengar AR, Gupta RK, Dhanuka AK, et al. MR imaging, MR angiography, and MR spectroscopy of the brain in eclampsia. AJNR Am J Neuroradiol 1997; 18:1485–90.

44. McKinney AM, Jagadeesan BD, Truwit CL. Central-variant posterior reversible encephalopathy syndrome: brainstem or basal ganglia involvement lacking cortical or subcortical cerebral edema. AJR Am J Roentgenol 2013;201:631–8.

45. Rykken JB, McKinney AM. Posterior reversible encephalopathy syndrome. Semin Ultrasound CT MR 2014;35:118–35.

46. Arrigan MT, Heran MKS, Shewchuk JR. Reversible cerebral vasoconstriction syndrome: an important and common cause of thunderclap and recurrent headaches. Clin Radiol 2018;73:417–27.

47. Freilinger T, Schmidt C, Duering M, et al. Reversible cerebral vasoconstriction syndrome associated with hormone therapy for intrauterine insemination. Cephalalgia 2010;30:1127–32.

48. Moussavi M, Korya D, Panezai S, et al. Reversible cerebral vasoconstriction syndrome in a 35-year-old woman following hysterectomy and bilateral salpingo-oophorectomy. J Neurointerv Surg 2012;4:e35.

49. Miller TR, Shivashankar R, Mossa-Basha M, et al. Reversible cerebral vasoconstriction syndrome, part 1: epidemiology, pathogenesis, and clinical course. AJNR Am J Neuroradiol 2015;36:1392–9.

50. Marshall N, Maclaurin WA, Koulouris G. MRA captures vasospasm in fatal migrainous infarction. Headache 2007;47:280–3.

51. Soltanolkotabi M, Ansari SA, Shaibani A, et al. Spontaneous post-partum cervical carotid artery dissection in a patient with reversible cerebral vasoconstriction syndrome. Interv Neuroradiol 2011;17:486–9.

52. Chen SP, Fuh JL, Lirng JF, et al. Recurrent primary thunderclap headache and benign CNS angiopathy: spectra of the same disorder? Neurology 2006;67:2164–9.

53. Chen SP, Fuh JL, Chang FC, et al. Transcranial color doppler study for reversible cerebral vasoconstriction syndromes. Ann Neurol 2008;63:751–7.

54. Mawet J, Boukobza M, Franc J, et al. Reversible cerebral vasoconstriction syndrome and cervical artery dissection in 20 patients. Neurology 2013;81:821–4.

55. Cappelen-Smith C, Calic Z, Cordato D. Reversible Cerebral Vasoconstriction Syndrome: Recognition and Treatment. Curr Treat Options Neurol 2017;19:21.

56. Singhal AB, Topcuoglu MA. Glucocorticoid-associated worsening in reversible cerebral vasoconstriction syndrome. Neurology 2017;88:228–36.

57. Chen SP, Wang SJ. Hyperintense vessels: an early MRI marker of reversible cerebral vasoconstriction syndrome? Cephalalgia 2014;34:1038–9.

58. Miller TR, Shivashankar R, Mossa-Basha M, et al. Reversible cerebral vasoconstriction syndrome, part 2: diagnostic work-up, imaging evaluation, and differential diagnosis. AJNR Am J Neuroradiol 2015;36:1580–8.

59. Linn J, Fesl G, Ottomeyer C, et al. Intraarterial application of nimodipine in reversible cerebral vasoconstriction syndrome: a diagnostic tool in select cases? Cephalalgia 2011;31:1074–81.

60. Katz BS, Fugate JE, Ameriso SF, et al. Clinical worsening in reversible cerebral vasoconstriction syndrome. JAMA Neurol 2014;71:68–73.

61. Chen SP, Fuh JL, Lirng JF, et al. Hyperintense vessels on FLAIR imaging in reversible cerebral vasoconstriction syndrome. Cephalalgia 2012;32:271–8.

62. Kameda T, Namekawa M, Shimazaki H, et al. Unique combination of hyperintense vessel sign on initial FLAIR and delayed vasoconstriction on MRA in reversible cerebral vasoconstriction syndrome: a case report. Cephalalgia 2014;34:1093–6.

63. Ducros A. L37: reversible cerebral vasoconstriction syndrome—distinction from CNS vasculitis. Presse Med 2013;42:602–4.

64. Komatsu T, Kimura T, Yagishita A, et al. A case of reversible cerebral vasoconstriction syndrome presenting with recurrent neurological deficits: evaluation using noninvasive arterial spin labeling MRI. Clin Neurol Neurosurg 2014;126:96–8.

65. Rosenbloom MH, Singhal AB. CT angiography and diffusion-perfusion MR imaging in a patient with ipsilateral reversible cerebral vasoconstriction after carotid endarterectomy. AJNR Am J Neuroradiol 2007;28:920–2.

66. Mandell DM, Matouk CC, Farb RI, et al. Vessel wall MRI to differentiate between reversible cerebral vasoconstriction syndrome and central nervous system vasculitis. Stroke 2012;43:860–2.

67. Obusez EC, Hui F, Hajj-Ali RA, et al. High-resolution MRI vessel wall imaging: Spatial and temporal patterns of reversible cerebral vasoconstriction syndrome and central nervous system vasculitis. Am J Neuroradiol 2014;35:1527–32.

68. Mossa-Basha M, Alexander M, Gaddikeri S, et al. Vessel wall imaging for intracranial vascular disease evaluation. J Neurointerv Surg 2016;8:1154–9.

69. Hajj-Ali RA, Furlan A, Abou-Chebel A, et al. Benign angiopathy of the central nervous system: cohort of 16 patients with clinical course and long-term followup. Arthritis Rheum 2002;47:662–9.

Imaging of Childhood Cerebral Vasculitis

Sheng-Che Hung, MD, PhD*, Carolina Guimaraes, MD

KEYWORDS

- Childhood cerebral vasculitis • Primary angiitis of CNS • Secondary vasculitis • Systemic vasculitis
- Inflammatory vasculopathy

KEY POINTS

- Evaluation of children with suspected cerebral vasculitis requires a stepwise approach and a multidisciplinary team of specialists including neurologists, neuroradiologists, rheumatologists, immunologists, infectious disease specialists, and hematologists.
- MR imaging is the preferred imaging modality for workup of children with suspected cerebral vasculitis.
- Timely identification of cerebral vasculitis and initiation of immunosuppressive therapy can improve outcomes.
- Childhood cerebral vasculitis can be divided into primary and secondary.
- Childhood primary angiitis of the central nervous system (cPACNS) can be further divide into three subtypes based on the size of the affected vessels and disease course: angiography-positive nonprogressive cPACNS, angiography-positive progressive cPACNS, and angiography-negative cPACNS.

INTRODUCTION

Childhood cerebral vasculitis (CCV) is a varied condition that affects blood vessels in children's brains resulting in inflammation and a range of neurologic symptoms such as headache, seizure, stroke, psychiatric manifestations, and encephalopathy. Recent studies have shown that CCV is a common cause of arterial ischemic stroke in children, but due to its rarity and heterogeneous clinical presentation, it remains a challenging diagnosis. The use of imaging techniques is crucial for detecting and managing CCV. Over the past decade, imaging for CCV has made significant advancements, with several modalities emerging as useful tools for diagnosis, monitoring, and follow-up. This review aims to provide a detailed overview of the current state of imaging for CCV, including its diagnostic algorithm, imaging techniques, and imaging spectrum of primary and secondary CCV in children.

CLASSIFICATION

The classification of CCV is ever evolving and can be approached from various angles. Predominantly affected vessel sizes are used to classify CCV as small, medium, or large vessel vasculitis.[1] Another approach involves categorizing vasculitides into granulomatous or non-granulomatous based on the histologic patterns of their inflammatory infiltrates.[2] In addition, CCV can be classified etiologically as primary or secondary.[3] Primary CCV, also known as childhood primary angiitis of the central nervous system (cPACNS) is divided into angiography-positive cPACNS (AP-cPACNS) and angiography-negative cPACNS (AN-cPACNS) based on the affected vessel sizes and catheter angiographic findings. AP-cPACNS is further classified based on the disease course into progressive and nonprogressive AP-cPACNS (angiography-positive progressive cPACNS [APP-cPACNS] and angiography-positive nonprogressive cPACNS

Department of Radiology, University of North Carolina, 2000 Old Clinic, CB# 7510, Chapel Hill, NC 27599, USA
* Corresponding author.
E-mail address: hsz829@gmail.com

Neuroimag Clin N Am 34 (2024) 149–166
https://doi.org/10.1016/j.nic.2023.07.005
1052-5149/24/Published by Elsevier Inc.

[APNP-cPACNS]) (Figs. 1 and 2).[4] Secondary CCV is linked to various systemic conditions such as infection, systemic vasculitis, systemic inflammatory diseases, drugs, radiation, malignancy, and genetic diseases (Table 1).[5]

DIAGNOSTIC ALGORITHM

Diagnosing CCV is challenging, as its symptoms overlap with other neurologic conditions. However, timely identification and initiation of immunosuppressive therapy can improve outcomes in cPACNS.[6] To achieve this, a multidisciplinary team of specialists is required, including neurologists, neuroradiologists, rheumatologists, immunologists, infectious disease specialists, and hematologists. The stepwise diagnostic algorithm for CNS vasculitis in children consists of four steps, including:

Step 1. History and Physical Examination: To evaluate preexisting underlying conditions including infections, malignancies, rheumatological diseases, other systemic diseases, family history, and treatment history.

Step 2. Laboratory: Comprehensive laboratory studies including hematology and acute phase reactants, basic biochemistry, infection survey, immunologic tests, and cerebrospinal fluid (CSF) analysis.[7]

Step 3. Neuroimaging: MR imaging with contrast, magnetic resonance angiography (MRA), and vessel wall imaging (VWI). In some cases, serial neuroimaging studies may be necessary to diagnose AN-cPACNS.

Step 4. Biopsy: Performed when necessary, to establish the diagnosis and exclude other inflammatory brain diseases, malignancies, or infections, especially in cases where AN-cPACNS is suspected.

METHODS OF IMAGING EVALUATION
MR Imaging

MR imaging is the preferred imaging method due to its ability to visualize parenchymal and most vascular changes. A comprehensive MR imaging protocol should include various sequences and techniques such as MRA and VWI (Table 2). Structural MR imaging can identify parenchymal changes such as edema, infarction, and hemorrhages, differentiate vasogenic, and cytotoxic edema and determine the age of ischemic and hemorrhagic changes. Time-of-flight MRA is the most commonly used MRA technique and can assess proximal arteries' luminal caliber changes, but it is less reliable in evaluating distal intracranial arteries.[8] VWI detects vessel inflammatory changes in CCV, including arterial wall thickening and contrast enhancement. It is crucial to consider the patient's clinical presentation, laboratory findings, and histopathology when interpreting MR imaging results.[9]

Ultrasound Doppler

Ultrasound Doppler can be used to evaluate the medium-sized to large-sized extracranial vessels and provides information on wall thickness, luminal narrowing, and blood flow abnormalities.

Computed Tomography

Computed tomography (CT) has limited utility in the evaluation of CCV due to several factors. Although non-contrast CT is better than MR imaging in ruling out acute hemorrhage and post-contrast CT can show parenchymal lesions and enhancement of parenchymal/leptomeninges, the accuracy of these findings is lower compared with MR imaging. CT angiography can assess medium to large-sized vessels for luminal narrowing or occlusion, but it is not reliable in evaluating distal intracranial arteries and has limited capability in assessing vessel walls compared with VWI. In addition, the use of CT should be avoided to decrease radiation exposure.[10]

Catheter Angiography

Catheter angiography is an invasive procedure that offers excellent imaging resolution in detecting medium-to-large sized vascular stenosis, occlusion, beaded appearance of vessels, and aneurysms. However, it is usually reserved for

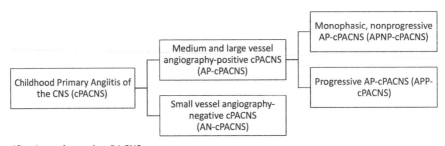

Fig. 1. Classification scheme in cPACNS.

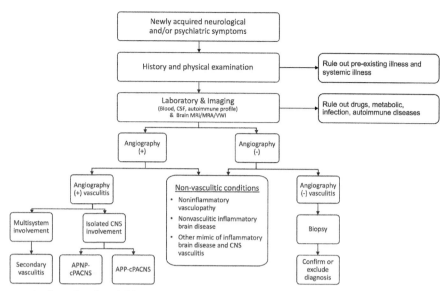

Fig. 2. Diagnostic algorithm for children with suspected cerebral vasculitis.

cases where other imaging modalities have failed to provide conclusive results due to its invasive nature and associated risks. Digital subtraction angiography (DSA) has superior resolution in assessing distal intracranial arteries compared with CTA and MRA, but its sensitivity and specificity in detecting small-vessel CCV are limited as some pathologic changes in small vessels are beyond its resolution. DSA depends on the contrast opacification of vessel lumens and cannot evaluate the vessel wall.

IMAGING FINDINGS IN CHILDHOOD CEREBRAL VASCULITIS

The imaging findings observed in CCV are dependent on the specific type of blood vessels involved. Medium-to-large sized vessel vasculitis often affects the carotid, vertebral arteries, and circle of Willis, with unifocal or multifocal infarcts being the most common parenchymal findings. Ischemic lesions localized in the deep or subcortical white and gray

Table 1
Causes of secondary childhood central nervous system vasculitis[5,14]

Infection	• Bacterial (TB, mycoplasma, GAS, GBS) • Viral (HBV, HCV, HIV, VZV, CMV, SARS-CoV-2) • Fungal (*Candida, Actinomycosis, Aspergillus*) • Spirochete (*Borrelia burgdorferi*, syphilis)
Systemic vasculitis	• Small vessel: IgA vasculitis/Henoch–Schönlein purpura, childhood-onset anti-neutrophil cytoplasmic antibody (ANCA)-associated vasculitides • Medium vessel: childhood-onset polyarteritis nodosa, Kawasaki disease • Large vessel: childhood-onset Takayasu arteritis • Variable: Behçet's disease
Rheumatic and inflammatory diseases	• Juvenile SLE, juvenile systemic sclerosis, juvenile dermatomyositis • Sjögren's syndrome • Inflammatory bowel disease • Hemophagocytic lymphohistiocytosis
Genetic diseases	• DADA2 • Aicardi–Goutières syndrome
Other	• Drug-induced vasculitis • Radiation-induced vasculitis • Malignancy-associated vasculitis • Graft vs host disease

Abbreviations: CMV, cytomegalovirus; GAS, group-A *Streptococcus*; GBS, group-B *Streptococcus*; HBV, hepatitis B virus; HCV, hepatitis C virus; HIV, human immunodeficiency virus; SARS-Cov-2, severe acute respiratory syndrome coronavirus 2; SLE, systemic lupus erythematosus; TB, *Mycobacterium* tuberculosis.

Table 2
Roles of MR imaging techniques in evaluation of childhood cerebral vasculitis

Sequences	Role	Pathologic Changes
Non-contrast T1W	Anatomic evaluation	Atrophy, encephalomalacia, subacute hemorrhage
Post-contrast T1W	Evaluate integrity of blood-brain barrier	Abnormal parenchymal and leptomeningeal enhancement
T2W/FLAIR	Tissue water content	Edema, gliosis, ischemia/infarction
Diffusion-weighted imaging (DWI)	Extracellular diffusion of water molecules	Distinguish acute vs chronic ischemic changes; cytotoxic edema vs vasogenic edema
Susceptibility-weighted imaging	Sensitive to compounds which distort the local magnetic field	Hemorrhages/blood products; calcium; acute thrombi
MR angiography (MRA)	Visualize intraluminal vessel flow	Luminal calibers change and tortuosity; aneurysm
Vessel wall imaging (VWI)	Evaluate arterial wall	Vessel wall thickening and intramural enhancement; distinguish vasculitis, dissection, and intracranial atherosclerotic disease

matter may result from the involvement of perforating arteries. Infarctions in both cortex and white matter can be found when larger arteries are occluded.[10] T2-weighted (T2W), FLuid Attenution Inversion Recovery (FLAIR), and diffusion-weighted imaging (DWI) sequences can aid in the differentiation of cytotoxic versus vasogenic edema and determine the age of infarction. MRA and VWI are useful in demonstrating stenosis and/or occlusion of affected blood vessels, vessel wall thickening and enhancement, and/or surrounding tissue changes. In cases of small-sized vessel vasculitis, multifocal nonspecific demyelination-like or inflammation-like parenchymal lesions with normal MRA and VWI are often present. Punctate or patchy areas of enhancement can be visible in the affected regions. Leptomeningeal enhancement is also common.[5]

CHILDREN PRIMARY ANGIITIS OF THE CNS

Primary angiitis of the CNS is a rare vascular disease that is increasingly recognized as a leading cause of arterial ischemic stroke in children.[11] However, the exact prevalence and incidence of cPACNS is unknown. The common presentations of cPACNS include neurologic deficits, stroke-like events, new-onset seizures, and psychiatric symptoms. Although the pathogenesis is often idiopathic, it may be associated with infectious (eg, human immunodeficiency virus, *Mycobacterium tuberculosis*, *Streptococcus*), post-infectious (post-varicella), and autoimmune and chronic inflammatory diseases.[12]

The diagnosis of cPACNS can be challenging and is often one of exclusion. The modified Calabrese Criteria for cPACNS require (1) an acquired and otherwise unexplained neurologic or psychological deficit, (2) classic angiographic or histopathological features of angiitis within the CNS, and (3) the absence of another systemic disorder to explain these features.[13] Based on the sizes of the affected vessels and the disease course, cPACNS can be classified into three subtypes: APNP-cPACNS and APP-cPACNS, which affect medium to large-sized vessels, and AN-cPACNS, which primarily affects small vessels (see Fig. 1). These subtypes can be distinguished based on characteristic clinical presentations, laboratory tests, and imaging features (Table 3).[12,14]

APNP-cPACNS is the most common subtype of cPACNS and has a limited, monophasic course of unilateral vessel wall inflammation. This subtype is characterized by inflammatory stenosis of the distal internal carotid artery and/or proximal circle of Willis and increased adherence of platelets to the vessel wall, leading to thrombus formation and artery-to-artery embolisms.[15,16] The most common clinical presentations include sudden-onset neurologic deficits and headaches. Typically, there are no systemic features of inflammation associated with this subtype.

Imaging findings for APNP-cPACNS include multifocal unilateral ischemic lesions in medium to large-vessel distributions, predominantly involving the basal ganglia of the lateral lenticulostriate artery territory.[15] MRA findings typically

Table 3
Childhood primary angiitis of central nervous system: Subtypes and their characteristics

	APNP-cPACNS	APP-cPACNS	AN-cPACNS
Sizes of affected vessels	Medium to large	Medium to large	Small
Affected vessels	Internal carotid artery, proximal circle of Willis; often unilateral focal or segmental	Internal carotid artery, proximal circle of Willis; unilateral or and bilateral	Arterioles, capillaries, venules
Gender	boys > girls	Boys > girls	Girls >> boys
Onset	Acute	Acute/subacute	Slowly progressive
Course	Monophasic, nonprogressive	Progressive	Progressive
Clinical presentations	Unilateral stroke, acute focal neurologic deficit, headache, encephalopathy	Focal and diffuse neurologic deficits, headache, encephalopathy, seizures, confusion, lethargy, impaired memory	Seizures, focal and diffuse neurologic deficits, and psychiatric symptoms
Inflammatory markers: CSF	Usually, normal	Mild to moderately elevated in up to 50% of cases	Elevated in > 90% of cases
Inflammatory markers: serum	Usually, normal	Sometimes mildly elevated	Sometimes elevated
MR imaging Parenchymal findings	Unilateral ischemic lesions (T2/FLAIR ± DWI)	Unilateral multifocal or bilateral ischemic lesions (T2/FLAIR ± DWI)	• White and/or gray matter T2/FLAIR lesions, not restricted to vascular territories. • Leptomeningeal and/or lesional enhancement (impaired blood-brain barrier)
MR imaging Vessel wall imaging	Vessel wall thickening and enhancement	Vessel wall thickening and enhancement	Normal
Angiography (CTA, MRA, or catheter angiography)	Proximal arterial stenosis	• Proximal and distal arterial stenosis or • isolated proximal disease with evidence of progression > 3 mo	Normal
Biopsy	Not indicated	Not indicated	Indicated (intramural and perivascular lymphocytic infiltrates)

Abbreviations: AN-cPACNS, angiography-negative cPACNS; APNP-cPACNS, angiography-positive nonprogressive cPACNS; APP-cPACNS, angiography-positive progressive cPACNS; cPACNS, childhood primary angiitis of central nervous system; IICP, increased intracranial pressure.
Modified from Smitka M, Bruck N, Engellandt K, Hahn G, Knoefler K, von der Hagen M. Clinical Perspective on Primary Angiitis of the Central Nervous System in Childhood (cPACNS). *Front Pediatr.* 2020;8.

show irregular unilateral stenosis and/or dilatation of the distal ICA and circle of Willis[16] (**Fig. 3**). VWI can reveal vessel wall thickening and contrast wall enhancement due to intramural inflammation.[17,18] During the acute stage (within the first few weeks), vessel wall inflammation can propagate in the affected vascular territory but remains unilateral and does not extend into previously unaffected vascular territory. If this occurs, the condition should be reclassified as APP-cPACNS.

APP-cPACNS often presents with both focal and diffuse neurologic deficits. These diffuse deficits can have an insidious onset and occur days to weeks before diagnosis, including difficulty with concentration, cognitive dysfunction, and mood and personality changes.[13] The vessel wall inflammation and parenchymal lesions in APP-cPACNS are more extensive, commonly affecting more than one vascular territory and occurring bilaterally, typically involving both proximal and distal vessel segments. This is supported by imaging studies that show more widespread involvement of the cerebral vasculature in this subtype.[5]

AN-cPACNS frequently presents with diffuse neurologic deficits, such as severe encephalopathy, extensive focal deficits, and seizures as well as systemic features such as fever and fatigue.[19] The disease course can vary, with some children presenting with a meningitis-like illness and rapidly progressive disease, whereas others may have insidious cognitive deficits over several weeks or months, headaches, or focal seizures.[20]

Imaging studies in AN-cPACNS usually do not show ischemic lesions but rather enhancing white matter abnormalities and leptomeningeal enhancement in about 50% of children.[15] Because inflammation is limited to small vessels, both MRA and VWI are typically normal. Therefore, the diagnosis is often based on indirect signs and markers of inflammation and resultant ischemia, such as parenchymal and leptomeningeal enhancement. Owing to the potential for rapid disease progression and none of the clinical and imaging findings are specific for AN-cPACNS, an extensive evaluation is necessary with a brain biopsy often required to confirm the diagnosis (**Fig. 4**).[19,20]

SECONDARY CENTRAL NERVOUS SYSTEM VASCULITIS
Secondary Central Nervous System Vasculitis Related to Infection

Secondary CCV is often caused by infections, with various microorganisms such as viruses, bacteria, fungi, or parasites being associated with CNS vasculitis. The imaging patterns can vary depending on the complications and causative pathogens, which may include meningitis, subdural empyema, and subarachnoid/parenchymal ring-enhancing lesions.[21]

Viruses
Varicella zoster virus (VZV) is a significant infectious cause of CNS vasculitis in children. Both large and small vessels can be affected, and the spectrum of VZV vasculitis includes ischemic infarction of the brain and spinal cord, aneurysm formation, subarachnoid hemorrhage, cerebral hemorrhage, and arterial dissection (**Fig. 5**).[22,23] When children present with focal cerebral vasculopathy and arterial

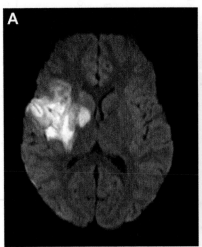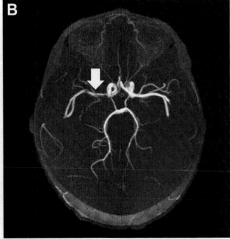

Fig. 3. Angiography-positive nonprogressive childhood primary angiitis of the central nervous system (APNP-cPACNS) in a 5-year-old boy presenting with sudden-onset right side weakness. Diffusion-weighted imaging (*A*) shows acute infarction in the right basal ganglia and right peri-insular region. (*B*) MRA shows focal narrowing in the right middle cerebral artery M1 segment (*arrow*).

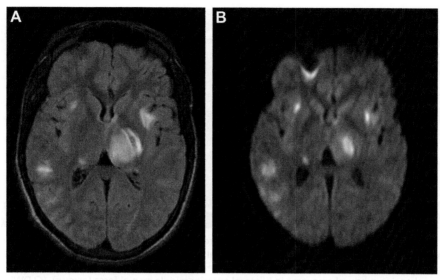

Fig. 4. Biopsy-proven angiography-negative childhood primary angiitis of the central nervous system (AN-cPACNS) in an adolescent presenting with confusion. FLAIR (*A*) and DWI (*B*) depict bilateral multiple hyperintense foci with focally restricted diffusion. No abnormal enhancement is present after gadolinium (not shown).

ischemic infarction, post-varicella angiopathy should be considered in the differential diagnosis.[5] In HIV-infected patients, particularly children and young adults, there is an increased risk of cerebrovascular disease. Aneurysms, vessel occlusion, embolic disease, and venous thrombosis occur in both medium-sized arteries and veins. The aneurysms are usually fusiform and involve the major arteries of the circle of Willis and second- and third-order branches, which distinguishes them from typical berry aneurysms.[10]

The SARS-CoV-2 virus, responsible for COVID-19, can cause acute cerebrovascular inflammation resulting in ischemic and hemorrhagic changes in the brain. However, such complications are less frequently observed in children than in adults.

Imaging studies reveal ischemic changes in the affected region as well as microhemorrhages and alterations in the white matter.[24] VWI scans have demonstrated mostly concentric wall enhancement in the involved vessels, with or without narrowing.[25]

Bacteria

Bacterial meningitis may cause vasculitis and cerebral infarctions in more than one-third of children, with group B *Streptococcus* being most frequently associated with infants under 90 day old and *Streptococcus pneumoniae* is associated in children older than 1 month.[26] Vascular complications tend to manifest early, usually within days to weeks (**Fig. 6**).[23]

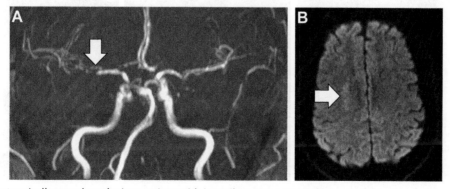

Fig. 5. Post-varicella vasculopathy in a patient with juvenile-onset systemic lupus erythematosus, presenting with acute right-side weakness. (*A*) MRA shows new near total occlusion of right middle cerebral artery distal M1 segment (*arrow*). MRA 6 months earlier was normal (not shown). (*B*) DWI shows acute infarction in the right centrum semiovale (*arrow*).

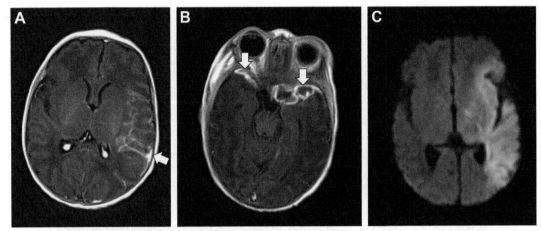

Fig. 6. Bacterial meningitis and subdural empyema of group B *Streptococcus* in a neonate, complicated with vasculitis and acute infarction in the left middle cerebral artery territory. (*A, B*) Post-contrast T1W images at the level of Sylvian fissure show abnormal leptomeningeal enhancement in the left hemisphere (*arrow*) and peripherally enhancing subdural empyema in bilateral anterior middle cranial fossa (*arrows*). (*C*) DWI shows acute infarction in the left middle cerebral artery territory.

Tuberculosis (TB) is the leading cause of chronic meningitis and can result in the accumulation of inflammatory exudates in the basal cisterns of the brain. Children are at a higher risk of developing CNS involvement. In TB-related vasculitis, the base of the brain and Sylvian fissures are the most affected sites, with lenticulostriate and thalamoperforating arteries being the most frequently involved vessels. Ischemic infarctions can be found in up to 41% of patients,[27] and up to 75% of these infarctions are located in the basal ganglia and thalami (Fig. 7).[27,28]

Coccidioides, and *Mucormycosis*, can cause arteritis of the CNS. The spread to the CNS can occur through hematogenous routes or direct extension through the paranasal sinuses and orbits. Vasculitis can manifest as an acute, subacute, or late complication of CNS fungal infection.[10] The imaging characteristics of CNS fungal infections may show ring-enhancing lesions, meningeal enhancement, and ischemic or hemorrhagic stroke.[23]

Fungi

Fungal pathogens play a significant role in patients with leukopenia and immunosuppression. Several fungal agents, most frequently *Aspergillus*, *Candida*,

Secondary Central Nervous System Vasculitis Related to Systemic Vasculitides

Systemic vasculitides sometimes involve the CNS, with a wide range of manifestations, including headaches, vertigo, ataxia, behavioral changes, neuropsychiatric symptoms, consciousness disorders,

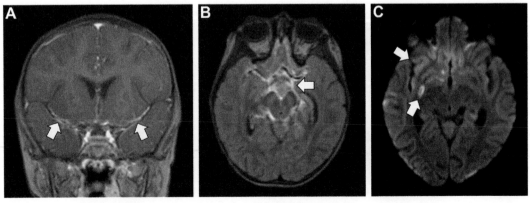

Fig. 7. TB meningitis in a toddler. (*A*) Coronal post-contrast T1W imaging shows leptomeningeal enhancement in the basal cisterns surrounding the bilateral middle cerebral arteries and optic nerves (*arrows*). (*B*) Post-contrast FLAIR shows thick exudate in the basal cisterns (*arrow*). (*C*) DWI shows multifocal acute infarcts (eg, right insula and lentiform nucleus [*arrows*]).

and cerebrovascular events. The incidence of CNS involvement also varies depending on the type of vasculitis.[29]

Childhood-onset Takayasu arteritis

Childhood-onset Takayasu arteritis (c-TA) is the most common pediatric large-vessel vasculitis characterized by granulomatous inflammation involving the aorta and its major branches, leading to stenosis, occlusion, dilatation, and/or aneurysm formation.[30] Up to 71% of patients with c-TA may experience craniocervical arteries involvement.[30–32] Although TA mainly affects the large vessels, intracranial vascular involvement is not uncommon, ranging from 4.9% to 42.9%, presenting mostly with stenosis and/or occlusion and rarely aneurysm formation (Fig. 8).[33–35]

Kawasaki disease

Kawasaki disease (KD) is a common medium vessel vasculitis in children under the age of 5 years.[36] Neurologic symptoms are observed in up to 33% of KD cases, with half of these children presenting with neurologic symptoms as the primary or initial manifestation.[37] Although neurologic symptoms are common, MR imaging and MRA findings are frequently normal. This suggests that cerebral involvement in KD affects small diameter vessels. Abnormal neuroimaging findings in KD include cerebral and cerebellar ischemia and infarcts (Fig. 9), which may be attributed to arterial vasculitis, multiple embolisms, myocarditis, hypokinetic myocardium, or intravenous immunoglobulin(I-VIG)-related thrombosis.[38,39] Other imaging findings in the acute stage may include subdural effusion, subarachnoid hemorrhage from cerebral artery aneurysm rupture,[38,40,41] white matter hyperintensities,[42] microhemorrhages,[43] and regional hypoperfusion[44] (see Fig. 9). It is noteworthy that in a population-based study, KD was associated with a 3.19-fold increase in subsequent cerebrovascular disease, particularly in patients less than 5 year old.[45]

Childhood-onset polyarteritis nodosa

Childhood-onset polyarteritis nodosa (cPAN) is a type of severe systemic necrotizing vasculitis that impacts medium-sized vessels and has an unknown cause. This disease typically affects muscular arteries, particularly the renal and other internal organs' arteries, leading to microaneurysm formation, aneurysm rupture, thrombosis, organ ischemia or infarction, and has a substantial risk of long-term morbidity. Children with cPAN may experience neurologic symptoms, with cranial nerve palsies, headache, visual impairment, seizure, and stroke being the most common presentations, affecting up to 15.4% of them.[46,47] c-PAN patients' most frequent neuroimaging findings include focal or multifocal ischemia and hemorrhage, along with vascular findings on VWI such as wall thickening, small aneurysms, and stenosis[10] (Fig. 10).

Immunoglobulin A vasculitis/henoch-schoenlein purpura

Henoch-schoenlein purpura (HSP) is the most common systemic vasculitis in childhood, characterized by non-granulomatous inflammation of small blood vessels with predominant immunoglobulin A (IgA)1 immune deposits. Although neurologic involvement in HSP is infrequent, it can occur in up to 10% of cases, especially in patients with a severe disease course and multiorgan involvement.[48] These manifestations typically seem in younger children within 2 weeks of onset.[49] The most prevalent CNS symptoms include changes in consciousness, headache, dizziness, and seizures.[29,49] These symptoms may result from sequelae of direct IgA cerebral vasculitis

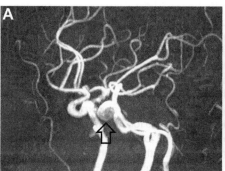
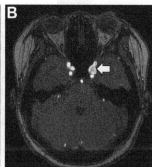
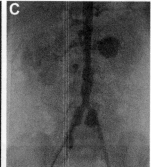

Fig. 8. Childhood-onset Takayasu arteritis in a 7-year-old girl, presenting with severe headaches. Maximal intensity projection (*A*) and axial (*B*) time-of-flight MRA images show fusiform aneurysmal dilatation of left cavernous internal carotid artery (*arrows*). (*C*) Abdominal aortogram shows aneurysmal dilatation of infrarenal abdominal aorta and multiple variable-sized aneurysms in superior mesenteric, bilateral renal, and iliac arteries. (*Courtesy of* H Chen, MD, Taichung, Taiwan).

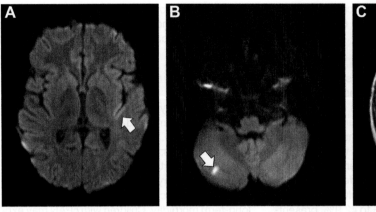
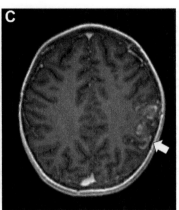

Fig. 9. Kawasaki disease in a 4-year-old boy, complicated with recurrent small acute infarcts at 2 to 3 weeks after onset of fever. (A, B) Axial DWI images show small acute infarcts in the left insula and right cerebellum (arrows). (C) Post-contrast T1W imaging shows increased leptomeningeal enhancement in the left parietal lobe (arrow).

involvement or arterial hypertension in the setting of nephritis. The typical neuroimaging results for HSP include posterior reversible encephalopathy, which occurs in patients with severe hypertension, and multifocal ischemic lesions in two or more vascular territories. Intraparenchymal hemorrhages can also be observed in patients without severe hypertension.[49]

Pediatric-onset Behcet's disease
Behcet's disease (BD) is a chronic inflammatory disease that can affect any artery or vein, regardless

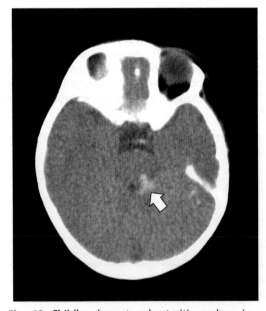

Fig. 10. Childhood-onset polyarteritis nodosa in a toddler, presenting with vomiting. Head CT showed a small intraparenchymal hemorrhage in the left dorsal pons-superior cerebellar peduncle (arrow). Brain MRA and VWI are negative (not shown).

of its type or size. Based on studies from different ethnic and geographic areas, up to 20% of BD cases present early in childhood, and up to 59.6% of cases have neurologic involvement, which may include headache, dizziness, cranial nerve palsy, and stroke.[50,51] Neuro-BD neuroimaging findings can typically be categorized into two forms: parenchymal form and non-parenchymal vascular form. The parenchymal form is characterized by T2-hyperintense lesions that usually affect the brainstem, mesodiencephalic junction, basal ganglia, spinal cord, and cerebral white matter (Fig. 11).[52] The non-parenchymal form comprises cerebral venous thrombosis and pseudotumor cerebri. Compared with adult BD, neuro-Behcet children more commonly present with non-parenchymal form, particularly with cerebral venous thrombosis.[53]

Secondary Central Nervous System Vasculitis Related to Rheumatic and Inflammatory Disease

Juvenile-onset systemic lupus erythematosus
The prevalence of CNS vasculitis in juvenile-onset systemic lupus erythematosus (SLE) remains uncertain. In a post-mortem study, CNS vasculitis was identified in approximately 7% to 10% of patients.[54] In more than half of juvenile-onset neuropsychiatric SLE cases, the MR imaging results are normal. When there are abnormalities, the most frequent findings are focal white matter hyperintensity on T2W (33%) followed by brain atrophy.[55] It is essential to test the antiphospholipid antibody titer in neuropsychiatric SLE patients, as both cerebral vasculitis and antiphospholipid syndrome may present with thrombo-occlusive events but have different underlying pathologies and require distinct treatments (Fig. 12).[54] Small vessel involvement may necessitate brain biopsy for diagnosis.[56]

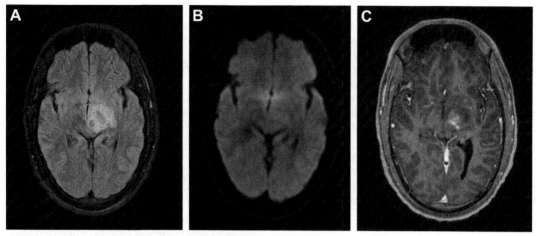

Fig. 11. Parenchymal form neuro-Behcet's disease in a young adult with new ataxia. A focal signal abnormality is present in the left mesodiencephalic junction showing hyperintensity on FLAIR (*A*), no restricted diffusion on DWI (*B*), and increased enhancement after gadolinium administration (*C*).

Pediatric Sjögren's syndrome

Neurologic involvement occurs in 5% to 23% of children with primary Sjogren's syndrome (SS).[57] The most frequent neuroimaging finding in cases of SS with focal CNS disease is the presence of T2-hyperintense lesions in the periventricular or subcortical white matter, which may be enhanced, resembling the lesions seen in multiple sclerosis.[58] The exact mechanism behind these manifestations is not entirely clear, but it is thought to be related to immune-mediated vasculopathy and demyelination.[58]

Inflammatory bowel disease

In children with IBD, there is an elevated risk of arterial and venous strokes due to numerous factors. These may include thromboembolism resulting from large arterial disease, dissection, small

vessel disease, cardioembolism, endocarditis, complications related to anti-tumor necrosis factor (TNF)-α therapy, and vasculitis.[59] However, it is worth noting that vasculitis is a rare occurrence in this population, with only a few reported cases.[60]

Juvenile dermatomyositis

Juvenile dermatomyositis is the most common inflammatory myopathy in children, primarily characterized by systemic capillary vasculopathy. CNS involvement in this condition is a rare occurrence, with only a few case reports including multiple lacunar infarcts, progressive multifocal encephalopathy, and possibly treatment-related PRES.[61–63]

Hemophagocytic lymphohistiocytosis

Hemophagocytic lymphohistiocytosis (HLH) is a hyperinflammatory condition marked by excessive

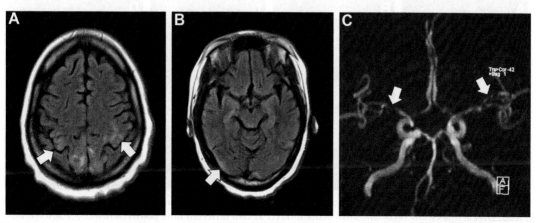

Fig. 12. A young adult with SLE small- and medium-sized vasculitis presenting with seizures. (*A, B*) Axial FLAIR imaging shows multiple cortical-subcortical hyperintense foci (*arrows*). (*C*) MRA shows diffuse irregularity and narrowing of bilateral anterior and middle cerebral arteries and their branches (*arrows*).

immune activation, which can manifest in both primary (familial) and secondary (acquired) forms. In children, CNS involvement has been observed in up to 73% of cases, regardless of the presence of systemic HLH.[64] The patterns of CNS involvement detected by MR imaging can be divided into two distinct groups. The first group (pattern 1) displays significant parenchymal disease with three subtypes: multifocal white matter, brainstem-predominant, and cerebellitis. The second group (pattern 2) exhibits nonspecific imaging findings.[65] It is important to note that CNS-restricted HLH can resemble vasculitis in histopathology, and therefore, genetic testing is crucial to distinguish between these two diagnoses.[66]

Secondary Central Nervous System Vasculitis Related to Rare Genetic Diseases

Deficiency of adenosine deaminase type 2
Deficiency of Adenosine Deaminase type 2 (DADA2) is a rare genetic condition resulting from a mutation of the *ADA2* gene that encodes adenosine deaminase 2 protein. DADA2 is characterized by early-onset PAN-like systemic inflammatory syndrome and frequent CNS involvement. Strokes are the most common manifestation in children with DADA2, followed by CN3 palsy, optic nerve disorders, sensorineural hearing loss, and transverse myelitis (Fig. 13).[67] Compared with PAN, DADA2 tends to present at a younger age (4 years vs 7 years) and is associated with a higher risk of neurologic complications, including ischemic infarcts and hemorrhages as well as increased mortality.[68]

Aicardi–Goutières syndrome
Aicardi–Goutières syndrome (AGS) is a diverse collection of genetic inflammatory encephalopathies caused by various genes. It is characterized by white matter abnormalities, brain atrophy, and intracranial calcifications seen on CT scans.[69] In addition, the SAMHD1 gene mutation may present with medium-sized vessel stenosis/occlusion in the circle of Willis or moyamoya disease.[70]

Secondary Central Nervous System Vasculitis Related to Drug, Radiation, or Malignancy

Drug-induced CCV
A variety of medications, including antibiotics, chemotherapy drugs, and illegal substances, have been found to cause vasculitis. In cases related to drug abuse, particularly involving cocaine and methamphetamine, cerebral vasculitis typically presents with multifocal infarcts or hemorrhages.[71] Chronic cocaine abuse has also been linked to Moyamoya vasculopathy.[72] Another drug, minocycline, commonly used to treat bacterial infections, has been known to induce serious PAN-like necrotizing vasculitis, albeit rarely.[73] Immune checkpoint inhibitors, increasingly used to treat various malignancies, can lead to vasculitis, affecting temporal arteritis, aortitis, and CNS vasculitis.[74] The use of granulocyte-colony stimulating factor to prevent neutropenia has been associated with a rare complication of large-vessel arteritis of carotid arteries.[75]

Radiation-induced CCV
Cranial radiation can cause vascular damage in several ways, such as atherosclerosis, vasculitis, thrombosis, and aneurysm formation. The damage can manifest as ischemic and hemorrhagic strokes, lacunar lesions, vascular stenosis/occlusion, moyamoya syndrome, and vascular malformations. These injuries often occur slowly over many years, even decades after radiation exposure.[76]

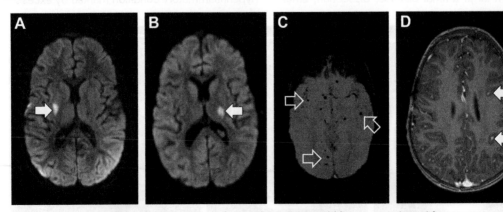

Fig. 13. Deficiency of adenosine deaminase 2 (DADA2) in a 2-year-old boy, presenting with recurrent strokes. (A, B) Axial DWI images show recurrent small acute infarcts at two different time points (*arrows*). (C) Susceptibility-weighted imaging shows multiple microhemorrhages bilaterally, at the gray-white matter junction (some are pointed by open *arrows*). (D) Post-contrast T1W imaging shows scattered foci of leptomeningeal enhancement (*arrows*) without associated restricted diffusion on DWI (not shown).

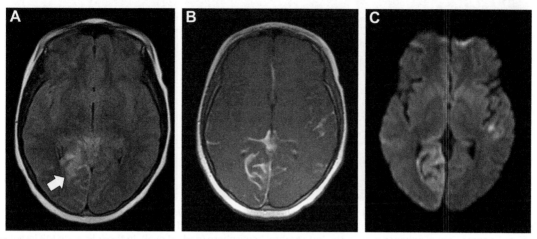

Fig. 14. Acute myeloid leukemia complicated by acute infarction in a teenager. Axial (*A*) FLAIR, (*B*) post-contrast T1-weighted imaging and (*C*) DWI revealed diffuse leptomeningeal sulcal FLAIR hyperintensity, enhancement and associated acute infarction bilaterally, involving the right occipital lobe (*arrow* in *A*).

Malignancy-induced CCV

Hematologic malignancies are the most common type of malignant diseases associated with cerebral vasculitis. In the cases of myelodysplastic syndrome/myeloproliferative neoplasm, temporal arteritis with or without multiorgan PAN-like vasculitis have been reported (Fig. 14). Both Hodgkin and non-Hodgkin lymphomas may be linked to isolated cerebral vasculitis or systemic vasculitis. In addition, "PAN-like" vasculitis is occasionally observed in hairy cell leukemia, a rare lymphoid neoplasm.[77]

Imaging-based differential diagnoses of CCV

The range of potential diagnoses for a child suspected of having cerebral vasculitis is extensive and includes noninflammatory vasculopathies, vasospasm, non-vasculitic inflammatory disease, infection, metabolic disease, and malignancy (Figs. 15 and 16).[5] Table 4 provides a summary of imaging-based differential diagnoses, categorized by the size of vessels involved.

Although brain biopsy is the gold standard for diagnosing AN-cPACNS, some conditions can be difficult to diagnose even with biopsy due to overlapping histopathological findings that resemble small vessel cPACNS which can present with frank vasculitis, intramural lymphocytic infiltration, or perivascular lymphocytic inflammation on histologic examinations.[66] In a study of 21 cases with initial AN-cPACNS diagnoses, even after considering clinical, laboratory, imaging, and biopsy

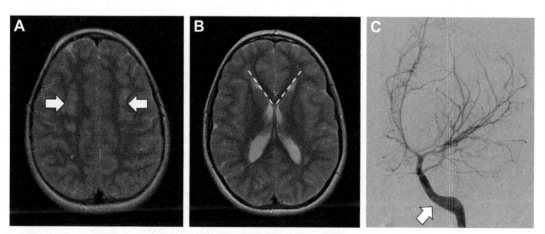

Fig. 15. Mimic of childhood cerebral vasculitis: ACTA2 mutation. Axial T2W imaging shows bilateral confluent hyperintense signal abnormalities (*arrows, A*) and V-shaped anterior corpus callosum (*dashed line, B*). Catheter angiogram of left internal carotid artery (*C*) depicts fusiform dilatation of left proximal internal carotid artery (*arrow*). The left anterior cerebral and middle cerebral arteries and their branches appear attenuated and stretched.

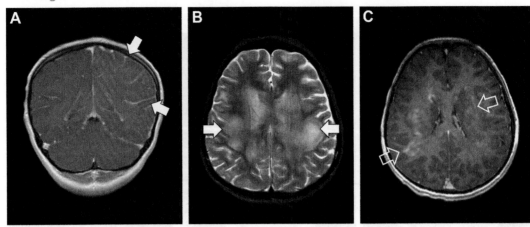

Fig. 16. Mimic of childhood cerebral vasculitis: myelin oligodendrocyte glycoprotein antibody disease (MOGAD) in a 10-year-old girl presenting with seizures. (*A*) Post-contrast T1-weighted imaging of initial MR imaging shows diffuse leptomeningeal enhancement in the left cerebral hemisphere (dashed oval). In the follow-up MR imaging after 2 months, axial T2-weighted imaging (*B*) shows multiple new non-restricting bilateral T2-hyperintense lesions (*arrows*) with ill-defined enhancement on post-contrast T1-weighted imaging (open *arrows*) (*C*).

Table 4
Imaging-based differential diagnoses of children with suspected cerebral vasculitis

Sizes of Affected Vessels	Differential Diagnosis
Medium to large (angiography-positive)	• Noninflammatory vasculopathies: • Dissection, thromboembolic disease, hemoglobin disorders, antiphospholipid syndrome, fibromuscular dysplasia, collagen vascular disorders, focal cerebral angiopathy (Marfan syndrome, Ehlers–Danlos syndrome, among others), and moyamoya disease (idiopathic). • Cerebral vasospasm: channelopathies, including familial hemiplegic migraine, calcium channelopathy, reversible cerebral vasoconstriction syndrome (RCVS) • Genetic syndromes with associated vasculopathy: NF1, Down syndrome, PHACES, CADASIL, Fabry disease, homocystinuria, ACTA2, MYH11 • Other syndromes with associated cerebral vasculopathy: Cogan syndrome (vasculopathy plus inflammatory eye disease and vestibuloauditory dysfunction), Susac syndrome (noninflammatory vasculopathy resulting in retinopathy, hearing loss and encephalopathy)
Small (angiography-negative)	• Nonvasculitic inflammatory disease: demyelinating disease acute disseminated encephalomyelitis (ADEM), multiple sclerosis, myelin oligodendrocyte glycoprotein antibody disease (MOGAD), antibody-mediated inflammatory disease anti-N-methyl D-aspartate receptor (NMDAR) encephalitis, antibody-mediated limbic encephalitis, neuromyelitis optica (NMO), Hashimoto encephalitis, post-mycoplasma encephalitis, celiac disease-associated encephalitis, PANDAS), T-cell-mediated inflammatory brain disease (Rasmussen encephalitis), and granulomatous inflammatory brain diseases (neurosarcoidosis, ANCA-associated vasculitis) • Infection (TB, human polyomavirus 2 [JC virus]) • Metabolic diseases with associated inflammatory and ischemic brain lesions: mitochondrial encephalomyopathy, lactic acidosis and stroke-like episodes (MELAS), Rolandic mitochondrial encephalomyopathy (ROME), polymerase gamma deficiency • Malignancy: angiocentric lymphoma

Modified from Twilt M, Benseler SM. Childhood Central Nervous System Vasculitis. In: Sawhney S, Aggarwal A, eds. *Pediatric Rheumatology: A Clinical Viewpoint.* Springer; 2017:509 to 524.

results, 14 (66.7%) diagnoses were revised an average of 4.5 years after the initial diagnosis. The most common diagnostic revision was AN-cPACNS changed to myelin oligodendrocyte glycoprotein antibody disease (MOGAD) (*n* = 9), followed by CNS-restricted HLH (*n* = 3), anti-GABA$_A$ receptor encephalitis, and AGS.[66] This highlights the possibility of MOGAD being an underrecognized mimic of AN-cPACNS in children and emphasizes the importance of now readily available noninvasive serum antibody or genetic testing, which can help avoid unnecessary invasive biopsy procedures.[78,79]

SUMMARY

CCV is a rare but potentially devastating condition that can cause significant morbidity and mortality. Early and accurate diagnosis is crucial for prompt treatment and better outcomes. Imaging plays a vital role in the diagnosis of CCV, with MR imaging being the most sensitive modality. Radiologists should be familiar with the imaging findings of several types of vasculitis. In addition, clinicians should be aware of the various mimics of cerebral vasculitis and the limitations of imaging as well as the need for biopsy in some cases for definitive diagnosis. A multidisciplinary approach, involving radiologists, neurologists, rheumatologists, and other specialists, is essential for the management of CCV.

CLINICS CARE POINTS

- Magnetic resonance imaging (MRI), including MRA and vessel wall imaging, is pivotal in detecting characteristic cerebral abnormalities, such as parenchymal lesions and vascular abnormalities aiding in the accurate diagnosis and monitoring of childhood cerebral vasculitis.

- Conventional angiography and MRA reveal crucial vascular features, including vessel wall irregularities, stenosis, and aneurysmal dilatation, which are indicative of childhood cerebral vasculitis, assisting in distinguishing it from other neurological conditions, as well as differentiating between angiography-positive and angiography-negative vasculitis.

- A biopsy remains a valuable diagnostic tool to confirm the presence of vasculitis, particularly in angiography-negative cases.4. Early and accurate diagnosis is crucial for prompt treatment and better outcomes of childhood cerebral vasculitis.

DISCLOSURE

The authors have nothing to disclose.

REFERENCES

1. Jennette JC, Falk RJ, Bacon PA, et al. 2012 revised International Chapel Hill Consensus Conference Nomenclature of Vasculitides. Arthritis Rheum 2013; 65(1):1–11.
2. Schnabel A, Hedrich CM. Childhood Vasculitis. Front Pediatr 2018;6:421.
3. Twilt M, Benseler SM. Childhood Central Nervous System Vasculitis. In: Sawhney S, Aggarwal A, editors. Pediatric rheumatology: a clinical Viewpoint. Singapore: Springer; 2017. p. 509–24.
4. Sag E, Batu ED, Ozen S. Childhood systemic vasculitis. Best Pract Res Clin Rheumatol 2017;31(4):558–75.
5. Gupta N, Hiremath SB, Aviv RI, et al. Childhood Cerebral Vasculitis. Clin Neuroradiol 2022. https://doi. org/10.1007/s00062-022-01185-8.
6. Salvarani C, Brown RD Jr, Christianson TJH, et al. Adult Primary Central Nervous System Vasculitis Treatment and Course: Analysis of One Hundred Sixty-Three Patients. Arthritis Rheumatol 2015;67(6):1637–45.
7. de Graeff N, Groot N, Brogan P, et al. European consensus-based recommendations for the diagnosis and treatment of rare paediatric vasculitides - the SHARE initiative. Rheumatol Oxf Engl 2019; 58(4):656–71.
8. Eleftheriou D, Cox T, Saunders D, et al. Investigation of childhood central nervous system vasculitis: magnetic resonance angiography versus catheter cerebral angiography. Dev Med Child Neurol 2010; 52(9):863–7.
9. Soun JE, Song JW, Romero JM, et al. Central Nervous System Vasculopathies. Radiol Clin 2019; 57(6):1117–31.
10. Abdel Razek AAK, Alvarez H, Bagg S, et al. Imaging Spectrum of CNS Vasculitis. Radiographics 2014; 34(4):873–94.
11. Rafay MF, Shapiro KA, Surmava AM, et al. Spectrum of cerebral arteriopathies in children with arterial ischemic stroke. Neurology 2020;94(23):e2479–90.
12. Smitka M, Bruck N, Engellandt K, et al. Clinical Perspective on Primary Angiitis of the Central Nervous System in Childhood (cPACNS). Front Pediatr 2020;8. Available at: https://www.frontiersin.org/articles/10. 3389/fped.2020.00281. Accessed February 3, 2023.
13. Benseler SM, Silverman E, Aviv RI, et al. Primary central nervous system vasculitis in children. Arthritis Rheum 2006;54(4):1291–7.
14. Gowdie P, Twilt M, Benseler SM. Primary and Secondary Central Nervous System Vasculitis. J Child Neurol 2012;27(11):1448–59.
15. Aviv RI, Benseler SM, Silverman ED, et al. MR imaging and angiography of primary CNS vasculitis of

childhood. AJNR Am J Neuroradiol 2006;27(1): 192–9.

16. Aviv RI, Benseler SM, DeVeber G, et al. Angiography of primary central nervous system angiitis of childhood: conventional angiography versus magnetic resonance angiography at presentation. AJNR Am J Neuroradiol 2007;28(1):9–15.

17. Küker W, Gaertner S, Nagele T, et al. Vessel wall contrast enhancement: a diagnostic sign of cerebral vasculitis. Cerebrovasc Dis Basel Switz 2008;26(1): 23–9.

18. Mandell DM, Matouk CC, Farb RI, et al. Vessel wall MRI to differentiate between reversible cerebral vasoconstriction syndrome and central nervous system vasculitis: preliminary results. Stroke 2012; 43(3):860–2.

19. Benseler SM, deVeber G, Hawkins C, et al. Angiography-negative primary central nervous system vasculitis in children: a newly recognized inflammatory central nervous system disease. Arthritis Rheum 2005;52(7):2159–67.

20. Hutchinson C, Elbers J, Halliday W, et al. Treatment of small vessel primary CNS vasculitis in children: an open-label cohort study. Lancet Neurol 2010;9(11): 1078–84.

21. Shen G, Shen X, Pu W, et al. Imaging of cerebrovascular complications of infection. Quant Imaging Med Surg 2018;8(10):1039–51.

22. Gilden D, Cohrs RJ, Mahalingam R, et al. Varicella zoster virus vasculopathies: diverse clinical manifestations, laboratory features, pathogenesis, and treatment. Lancet Neurol 2009;8(8):731–40.

23. Younger DS, Coyle PK. Central Nervous System Vasculitis due to Infection. Neurol Clin 2019;37(2): 441–63.

24. Lee MH, Perl DP, Steiner J, et al. Neurovascular injury with complement activation and inflammation in COVID-19. Brain 2022;awac151. https://doi.org/ 10.1093/brain/awac151.

25. Md Noh MSF, Abdul Rashid AM, Mohd Zain NR. The Spectrum of Vessel Wall Imaging (VWI) Findings in COVID-19-Associated Neurological Syndromes: A Review. Cureus 2023. https://doi.org/10.7759/cureus. 37296.

26. Dunbar M, Shah H, Shinde S, et al. Stroke in Pediatric Bacterial Meningitis: Population-Based Epidemiology. Pediatr Neurol 2018;89:11–8.

27. Patkar D, Narang J, Yanamandala R, et al. Central nervous system tuberculosis: pathophysiology and imaging findings. Neuroimaging Clin N Am 2012; 22(4):677–705.

28. Fugate JE, Lyons JL, Thakur KT, et al. Infectious causes of stroke. Lancet Infect Dis 2014;14(9):869–80.

29. Held M, Sestan M, Kifer N, et al. Cerebrovascular involvement in systemic childhood vasculitides. Clin Rheumatol 2023. https://doi.org/10.1007/s100 67-023-06552-5.

30. Danda D, Goel R, Joseph G, et al. Clinical course of 602 patients with Takayasu's arteritis: comparison between Childhood-onset versus adult onset disease. Rheumatology 2021;60(5):2246–55.

31. Fan L, Zhang H, Cai J, et al. Clinical course and prognostic factors of childhood Takayasu's arteritis: over 15-year comprehensive analysis of 101 patients. Arthritis Res Ther 2019;21(1):31.

32. Aeschlimann FA, Barra L, Alsolaimani R, et al. Presentation and Disease Course of Childhood-Onset Versus Adult-Onset Takayasu Arteritis. Arthritis Rheumatol 2019;71(2):315–23.

33. Johnson A, Emery D, Clifford A. Intracranial Involvement in Takayasu's Arteritis. Diagnostics 2021; 11(11):1997.

34. Guo Y, Du J, Li T, et al. Clinical features and risk factors of intracranial artery disease in patients with Takayasu arteritis. Clin Rheumatol 2022;41(8):2475–81.

35. Hoffmann M, Corr P, Robbs J. Cerebrovascular findings in Takayasu disease. J Neuroimaging Off J Am Soc Neuroimaging 2000;10(2):84–90.

36. McCrindle BW, Rowley AH, Newburger JW, et al. Diagnosis, Treatment, and Long-Term Management of Kawasaki Disease: A Scientific Statement for Health Professionals From the American Heart Association. Circulation 2017;135(17):e927–99.

37. Liu X, Zhou K, Hua Y, et al. Neurological involvement in Kawasaki disease: a retrospective study. Pediatr Rheumatol 2020;18(1):61.

38. Stojanović VD, Radovanović TD, Koprivšek KM, et al. Kawasaki Disease Complicated with Cerebral Vasculitis and Severe Encephalitis. Ann Indian Acad Neurol 2020;23(2):228–32.

39. Wada Y, Kamei A, Fujii Y, et al. Cerebral infarction after high-dose intravenous immunoglobulin therapy for Kawasaki disease. J Pediatr 2006;148(3):399–400.

40. Wang L, Duan H, Zhou K, et al. Kawasaki Disease Complicated by Late-Onset Fatal Cerebral Infarction: A Case Report and Literature Review. Front Pediatr 2021;9:598867.

41. Ahn JH, Phi JH, Kang HS, et al. A ruptured middle cerebral artery aneurysm in a 13-month-old boy with Kawasaki disease. J Neurosurg Pediatr 2010; 6(2):150–3.

42. Laukka D, Parkkola R, Hirvonen J, et al. Brain white matter hyperintensities in Kawasaki disease: A case–control study. Front Neurosci 2022;16. Available at: https://www.frontiersin.org/articles/10.3389/ fnins.2022.995480. Accessed March 24, 2023.

43. Gitiaux C, Kossorotoff M, Bergounioux J, et al. Cerebral vasculitis in severe Kawasaki disease: early detection by magnetic resonance imaging and good outcome after intensive treatment. Dev Med Child Neurol 2012;54(12):1160–3.

44. Hikita T, Kaminaga T, Wakita S, et al. Regional cerebral blood flow abnormalities in patients with kawasaki disease. Clin Nucl Med 2011;36(8):643–9.

45. Lin CH, Lai JN, Lee IC, et al. Kawasaki Disease May Increase the Risk of Subsequent Cerebrovascular Disease. Stroke 2022;53(4):1256–62.

46. Eleftheriou D, Dillon MJ, Tullus K, et al. Systemic Polyarteritis Nodosa in the Young: A Single-Center Experience Over Thirty-Two Years. Arthritis Rheum 2013;65(9):2476–85.

47. Falcini F, La Torre F, Vittadello F, et al. Clinical overview and outcome in a cohort of children with polyarteritis nodosa. Clin Exp Rheumatol 2014;32(3 Suppl 82):S134–7.

48. Du L, Wang P, Liu C, et al. Multisystemic manifestations of IgA vasculitis. Clin Rheumatol 2021;40(1): 43–52.

49. Garzoni L, Vanoni F, Rizzi M, et al. Nervous system dysfunction in Henoch–Schönlein syndrome: systematic review of the literature. Rheumatology 2009;48(12):1524–9.

50. Yıldız M, Köker O, Adrovic A, et al. Pediatric Behçet's disease - clinical aspects and current concepts. Eur J Rheumatol 2020;7(Suppl 1):S38–47.

51. Yildiz M, Haslak F, Adrovic A, et al. Pediatric Behçet's Disease. Front Med 2021;8. Available at: https://www.frontiersin.org/articles/10.3389/fmed.2021.627192. Accessed April 5, 2023.

52. Koçer N, Islak C, Siva A, et al. CNS Involvement in Neuro-Behçet Syndrome: An MR Study. AJNR Am J Neuroradiol 1999;20(6):1015–24.

53. Uluduz D, Kürtüncü M, Yapıcı Z, et al. Clinical characteristics of pediatric-onset neuro-Behçet disease. Neurology 2011;77(21):1900–5.

54. Smith EMD, Lythgoe H, Hedrich CM. Vasculitis in Juvenile-Onset Systemic Lupus Erythematosus. Front Pediatr 2019;7. Available at: https://www.frontiersin.org/articles/10.3389/fped.2019.00149. Accessed April 16, 2023.

55. Al-Obaidi M, Saunders D, Brown S, et al. Evaluation of magnetic resonance imaging abnormalities in juvenile onset neuropsychiatric systemic lupus erythematosus. Clin Rheumatol 2016;35(10): 2449–56.

56. Rowshani AT, Remans P, Rozemuller A, et al. Cerebral vasculitis as a primary manifestation of systemic lupus erythematosus. Ann Rheum Dis 2005;64(5):784–6.

57. Virdee S, Greenan-Barrett J, Ciurtin C. A systematic review of primary Sjögren's syndrome in male and paediatric populations. Clin Rheumatol 2017;36(10): 2225–36.

58. Soliotis FC, Mavragani CP, Moutsopoulos HM. Central nervous system involvement in Sjogren's syndrome. Ann Rheum Dis 2004;63(6):616–20.

59. Ferro JM, Oliveira Santos M. Neurology of inflammatory bowel disease. J Neurol Sci 2021;424:117426.

60. Sy A, Khalidi N, Dehghan N, et al. Vasculitis in patients with inflammatory bowel diseases: A study of 32 patients and systematic review of the literature. Semin Arthritis Rheum 2016;45(4):475–82.

61. Ramanan AV, Sawhney S, Murray KJ. Central nervous system complications in two cases of juvenile onset dermatomyositis. Rheumatology 2001;40(11): 1293–8.

62. Doctor PN, Pophale M, Dazy K. Progressive Multifocal Leukoencephalopathy in a Teenager with Juvenile Dermatomyositis. Pediatrics 2022;149(1 Meeting Abstracts February 2022):834.

63. Besançon A, Brochard K, Dupic L, et al. Presentations and outcomes of juvenile dermatomyositis patients admitted to intensive care units. Rheumatology 2017;56(10):1814–6.

64. Ma W, Li XJ, Li W, et al. MRI findings of central nervous system involvement in children with haemophagocytic lymphohistiocytosis: correlation with clinical biochemical tests. Clin Radiol 2021;76(2):159.e9.

65. Malik P, Antonini L, Mannam P, et al. MRI Patterns in Pediatric CNS Hemophagocytic Lymphohistiocytosis. AJNR Am J Neuroradiol 2021;42(11):2077–85.

66. Stredny CM, Blessing MM, Yi V, et al. Mimics of Pediatric Small Vessel Primary Angiitis of the Central Nervous System. Ann Neurol 2023;93(1):109–19.

67. Barron KS, Aksentijevich I, Deuitch NT, et al. The Spectrum of the Deficiency of Adenosine Deaminase 2: An Observational Analysis of a 60 Patient Cohort. Front Immunol 2022;12. Available at: https://www.frontiersin.org/articles/10.3389/fimmu.2021.811473. Accessed March 26, 2023.

68. Kasap Cuceoglu M, Sener S, Batu ED, et al. Systematic review of childhood-onset polyarteritis nodosa and DADA2. Semin Arthritis Rheum 2021;51(3): 559–64.

69. Abdel-Salam GMH, Abdel-Hamid MS, Mohammad SA, et al. Aicardi-Goutières syndrome: unusual neuroradiological manifestations. Metab Brain Dis 2017; 32(3):679–83.

70. Markovic I, Jocic-Jakubi B, Milenkovic Z. Early arteriopathy in Aicardi–Goutières syndrome 5. Case report and review of literature. NeuroRadiol J 2023. https://doi.org/10.1177/19714009231154677. 19714009231154676.

71. Younger DS. Cerebral vasculitis associated with drug abuse. Curr Opin Rheumatol 2021;33(1):24.

72. Storen EC, Wijdicks EFM, Crum BA, et al. Moyamoya-like Vasculopathy from Cocaine Dependency. Am J Neuroradiol 2000;21(6):1008–10.

73. Martins AM, Marto JM, Johnson JL, et al. A Review of Systemic Minocycline Side Effects and Topical Minocycline as a Safer Alternative for Treating Acne and Rosacea. Antibiotics 2021;10(7):757.

74. Albarrán V, Chamorro J, Rosero DI, et al. Neurologic Toxicity of Immune Checkpoint Inhibitors: A Review of Literature. Front Pharmacol 2022;13. Available at: https://www.frontiersin.org/articles/10.3389/fphar.2022.774170. Accessed April 21, 2023.

75. Yamamoto S, Waki D, Maeda T. Granulocyte-Colony Stimulating Factor-Induced Vasculitis Successfully

Treated With Short-Term Corticosteroid Therapy: A Case Report. Cureus 2021;13(12):e20563.

76. Murphy ES, Xie H, Merchant TE, et al. Review of cranial radiotherapy-induced vasculopathy. J Neuro Oncol 2015;122(3):421–9.

77. Lötscher F, Pop R, Seitz P, et al. Spectrum of Large- and Medium-Vessel Vasculitis in Adults: Neoplastic, Infectious, Drug-Induced, Autoinflammatory, and Primary Immunodeficiency Diseases. Curr Rheumatol Rep 2022;24(10):293–309.

78. Keenan P, Brunner J, Quan AS, et al. Diagnosis and Treatment of Small Vessel Childhood Primary Angiitis of the Central Nervous System (sv-cPACNS): An International Survey. Front Pediatr 2021;9:756612.

79. Gilani A, Kleinschmidt-DeMasters BK. Childhood Small-Vessel Primary Angiitis of the Central Nervous System: Overlap With MOG-Associated Disease. Pediatr Dev Pathol 2022. https://doi.org/10.1177/10935266221121445. 10935266221121444.

Imaging of Amyloid-beta-related Arteritis

Aaron Bangad, BA[a], Mehdi Abbasi, MD[a], Sam Payabvash, MD[b],
Adam de Havenon, MD, MSCI[a,b],*

KEYWORDS

- Cerebral amyloid angiopathy • Aβ-related angiitis • Amyloid-related imaging abnormalities

KEY POINTS

- Cerebral amyloid angiopathy (CAA) is a cerebrovascular disorder that is characterized by the accumulation of amyloid-beta peptide (Aβ) within the brain's leptomeninges and smaller sized blood vessels.
- ABRA is a vasculitis of the central nervous system related to an inflammatory response to Aβ in the vascular walls, which necessitates differentiating ABRA from noninflammatory CAA, as ABRA may require immunosuppressive treatment.
- MR imaging is the most commonly used imaging modality to identify ABRA, where findings may include multiple cortical/subcortical microbleeds, white matter edema, and, on occasion, enhancing lesions, particularly of the leptomeninges, suggestive of inflammation.
- Repeat neuroimaging is crucial in monitoring the response to treatment in ABRA, as changes in imaging findings can reflect alterations in the inflammatory state of the disease.
- Despite advances, imaging findings in ABRA often overlap with other conditions, and the definitive diagnosis often requires a brain biopsy, which presents its own risks. Thus, continued refinement of noninvasive diagnostic techniques is needed.

Cerebral amyloid angiopathy (CAA) is a largely age-dependent cerebrovascular disorder that is characterized by the accumulation or deposition of amyloid-beta (Aβ) peptide within the leptomeninges and the smaller sized blood vessels.[1] In CAA the deposition of Aβ causes the vessels and their walls to become fragile, and this fragility often manifests as lobar intracerebral hemorrhages (ICHs) or asymptomatic accumulation of microhemorrhages or superficial siderosis.[2] The symptoms of this deposition may also include focal neurologic symptoms, cognitive impairment, or transient neurologic symptoms.[3–5] CAA is also recognized as a major contributor of Alzheimer's disease pathogenesis.[6–9] In typical CAA there is no vessel wall inflammation as a result of the Aβ

and patients typically have a slow or stepwise progression.[10] However, this article will focus on Aβ-related angiitis (ABRA) and CAA-related inflammation (CAA-RI), which are rare but serious inflammatory complication of CAA.[11–13]

The presence of Aβ is capable of causing a significant immune response, and there are two specific types of inflammatory responses.[14] On histopathological examination, ABRA is an angiodestructive process characterized by inflammatory infiltration.[15] CAA-RI is characterized by a perivascular inflammatory reaction that surrounds vessels filled with Aβ, but unlike ABRA is not angiodestructive.[11] Both CAA-RI and ABRA share auto-antibodies to Aβ that are central to disease pathogenesis.[16] We will include CAA-RI with

Sources of Funding: Dr A. de Havenon reports NIH/NINDS funding (K23NS105924, R01NS130189, UG3NS130228).
[a] Department of Neurology, Yale University, New Haven, CT, USA; [b] Center for Brain and Mind Health, Yale University, New Haven, CT, USA
* Corresponding author. Department of Neurology, Yale University, 15 York Street, New Haven, CT 06510.
E-mail address: adam.dehavenon@yale.edu

Neuroimag Clin N Am 34 (2024) 167–173
https://doi.org/10.1016/j.nic.2023.09.001
1052-5149/24/© 2023 Elsevier Inc. All rights reserved.

ABRA and collectively call them ABRA because there is significant imaging, treatment, and prognostic overlap.[11] In general, ABRA is rare but treatable with immunosuppression, manifesting mostly in patients above 60 years of age and has several characteristic MR imaging findings (Figs. 1 and 2).[15]

Like other cerebral vasculitides, the clinical manifestation of ABRA involves progressive accumulation of symptoms including headache, focal neurologic symptoms, cognitive dysfunction (encephalopathy), behavioral changes, and seizure.[17,18] In addition, there may be inflammatory changes in cerebrospinal fluid, but that is not specific to ABRA versus other vasculitides.[17] However, the diagnosis of ABRA is important due to implications on the treatment plan. Specifically, ABRA needs to be differentiated from primary central nervous system vasculitis and noninflammatory CAA. Although the most of patients with ABRA will improve with immunosuppression,[19] diagnosis is typically required before starting treatment. Although brain biopsy can provide confirmation of ABRA versus other diagnoses,[8,20] we will discuss neuroimaging findings that are supportive of ABRA.

The most important neuroimaging criterion for ABRA is the presence of MR imaging findings consistent with CAA because ABRA requires underlying CAA. We will discuss additional imaging findings that support the diagnosis of ABRA

subsequently, the notable differences are highlighted in Table 1. CAA is typically defined using the Boston Criteria, which include lobar ICH, cerebral microbleeds (CMBs), and cortical superficial siderosis (cSS); all typically identified on gradient-echo (GRE) sequences on MR imaging.[21] CAA is a common cause of spontaneous lobar ICH, which may first be identified on computed tomography (CT) prompting an MR imaging that subsequently diagnoses CAA.[22] CMBs tend to localize to the areas of the greatest amyloid deposition,[23] are best seen on susceptibility-weighted imaging (SWI) MR imaging sequences, have a diameter of 2 to 10 mm, and in CAA are lobar in location or in the superficial cerebellar regions (cerebellar cortex and vermis).[24–26] cSS is a curvilinear, homogeneous hypointense lesion on GRE or SWI that follows the gyral cortical surface (convexities of the cerebral hemispheres) and may have a "track-like" appearance that results from hemosiderin accumulating at bilateral sides of cortical sulcus.[3]

There are also other MR imaging characteristics that can be seen with CAA, including white matter hyperintensities (WMHs), acute ischemic cortical infarcts, and brain atrophy. For WMHs, the imaging patterns that are indicate CAA include the "multispot" pattern of multiple (ie, >10), bilateral lesions with rounded or oval-like appearance.[3] In more advanced cases, WMHs may be confluent. Such prominent findings may be seen preferentially in

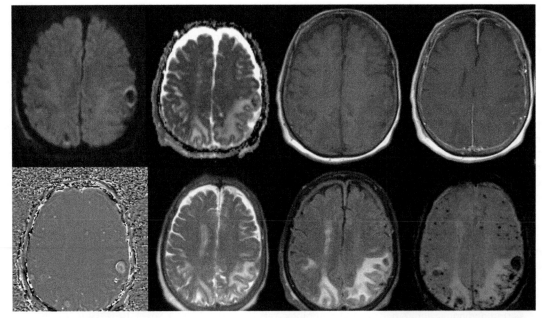

Fig. 1. Suspected ABRA versus CAA-IR in a patient with diffuse juxtracorical microhemorrhage (SWI and phase-map) and associated T2 and FLAIR hyperintensity. There was slight leptomeningeal and dural enhancement on post-contras versus pre-contrast series without any acute diffusion restriction on DWI and ADC series.

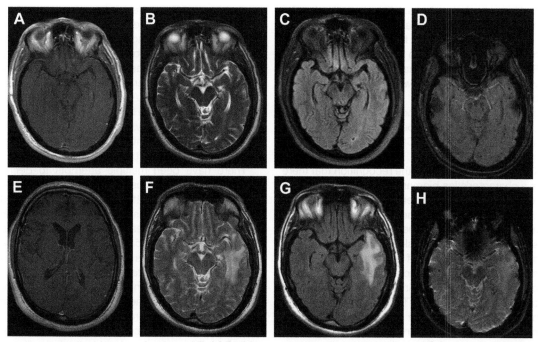

Fig. 2. Treatment response in a patient with ABRA who developed headaches and presented with dysarthria in February 2018 (lower row, *E–H*) which was resolved with immunosuppressive treatment for CAA on December 2021 scan (upper row, *A–D*). There has been interval decrees in subcortical and deep white matter T2 (*B* and *F*) and FLAIR (*C* and *G*) hyper intensity. More foci of microhemorrhage were seen on follow-up 3-T scan (*D*) than baseline 1.5-T (*H*) susceptibility weighted images, but could be due to difference in imaging technique. There was no associated enhancement (on postcontrast series, *A* and *E*) in either time point.

the subcortical parietal and occipital lobes of patients with advanced CAA.[27] Acute ischemic cortical infarcts are punctate hyperintense lesions visible on diffusion-weighted image (DWI) sequencing that are occasionally found in patients with CAA.[28] Histopathological examination of these

lesions has shown that they are related to the Aβ deposition of CAA.[29] Finally, brain atrophy is often present in occipital, temporal, posterior parietal, and medial frontal regions that correspond to areas having higher vascular Aβ burden in CAA.[30] This atrophy is particularly notable in white matter areas,

Table 1
Frequent imaging and symptomatic findings that assist in distinguishing between inflammatory and noninflammatory cerebral amyloid angiopathy

Inflammatory CAA	Noninflammatory CAA
Frequent leptomeningeal enhancement; leptomeningeal disease	Infrequent leptomeningeal processes
Infiltrative white matter abnormalities, asymmetric, occasional edema	The presence of WMHs with a "multispot" pattern of multiple (ie, >10), bilateral lesions with rounded or oval-like appearance
Vascular imaging, including digital subtraction angiography, tends to be unremarkable	The presence of acute ischemic cortical infarcts, which are punctate hyperintense lesions visible on DWI sequencing
Patients often present with progressive symptoms reflecting the inflammation including cognitive decline (encephalopathy), behavioral change, headache, and seizure	Patients are more likely to present with focal neurologic symptoms from lobar ICH

and is suggested to be the primary mechanism for the cognitive dysfunction associated with CAA.[31]

There are also more highly specific imaging methods that are used to diagnose CAA, such as Florbetapir-PET, which has been shown to label vascular Aβ in patients with CAA.[32] It has been conclusively shown that this molecular imaging can directly identify distinct Aβ pathology in living patients,[33,34] but it is expensive and not routinely available. Additionally, CSF biomarkers can be measured to determine the presence of Aβ.[35] This method is based on the recognition that there is a characteristics biomarker profile present as a result of CAA and that there is a global accumulation of Aβ species.[36] There are also other biomarkers of interest for the neuroimaging of CAA, such as peak width of skeletonized mean diffusivity. This is a metric of evaluating whole brain network connectivity, and it has been shown to be altered in CAA, resulting in differences in processing speed.[37] PiB-PET, which is noninvasive, has also been shown to detect cerebrovascular beta-amyloid and may serve as a method for identifying the extent of CAA in living patients.[38,39]

Patients with ABRA typically present with progressive symptoms reflecting the underlying inflammation including cognitive decline (encephalopathy), behavioral change, headache, and seizure, whereas noninflammatory CAA is more likely to present with focal neurologic symptoms from lobar ICH (see Table 1).[5] Multiple publications have reported that ABRA is associated with the apolipoprotein E ε4 allele, which could help distinguish it from noninflammatory CAA or other vasculitides.[15,40,41] Additional MR imaging findings that are consistent with ABRA reflect active inflammation in broad terms and thus the MR imaging study requires gadolinium contrast. In a cohort of 27 biopsy-proven cases of ABRA (including CAA-RI) and 27 cases of noninflammatory CAA, the ABRA cases had a much higher incidence of leptomeningeal enhancement (70.4% vs 7.4%, P<.001). The sensitivity and specificity of leptomeningeal enhancement for ABRA was 70.4% and 92.6%, respectively.[11] However, this comparison did not include patients with other vasculitides. In addition, a minority of ABRA patients (3 of 27) had diffuse WMH and edema, mimicking a low-grade glioma, which was not associated with acute ICH (Fig. 3).[11] A second publication of 2 patients with ABRA found that the white matter edema could become severe enough to lead to cerebral herniation and death when untreated.[38]

Vascular imaging, including digital subtraction angiography, tends to be unremarkable in ABRA, which is in contrast to primary and secondary vasculitis of the central nervous system where luminal irregularities are considered an important component to the diagnosis.[12] Although vessel wall MR imaging (or "black blood" MR imaging) seems appealing to assist in the diagnosis of ABRA,[42-44] there is often vessel wall enhancement in noninflammatory CAA, making it less useful for identifying ABRA.[10,45] However, more studies are needed to understand whether vessel wall MR imaging is capable to identifying a larger spectrum of inflammation that may be seen before ABRA.

There have been multiple attempts to define criteria that would be useful for identifying ABRA, including an original attempt in 2011,[13] followed by a more comprehensive approach in 2016 led by the group which created the influential Boston Criteria for CAA identification.[46] The intent of these classification systems is to prevent brain biopsies if possible. The 2016 criteria, compared 17 individuals with biopsy-proven CAA-RI to 37 with noninflammatory CAA. The neuroimaging criteria included WMHs that are asymmetric and extend to the immediately subcortical white matter (probable CAA-RI) or simply extend to the immediately subcortical white matter (possible CAA-RI).[46] Although such criteria are not definitive diagnoses, they are helpful for delineating the disease. Ultimately, the decision to pursue or not pursue a brain biopsy is performed on a case-by-case basis and incorporates elements of provider and patient preference as well as balancing of the risks and benefits.

Amyloid-related imaging abnormality (ARIA) refers to the iatrogenic manifestation of ABRA/CAA-RI, often in the context of the administration of monoclonal antibodies designed to reduce amyloid burden.[47] Lecanemab, aducanumab, and gantenerumab have all been associated with the development of ARIA.[48] There are 2 specific types of ARIA: ARIA-E, which refers to focal or confluent vasogenic edema on FLAIR imaging, and ARIA-H, which refers to CMBs or cSS on GRE or SWI sequences.[49] There are also spontaneous ARIA-like presentations, which similar to above, include vasogenic edema consistent of WMH focal areas, and hemorrhages consistent with CMBs and cSS. Both spontaneous ARIA-like and therapy-induced ARIA are mediated by the immune system but equally affected by genetic and vascular risk factors.[50] CAA-RI and ABRA can both increase the risk of ARIA, and ARIA and CAA-RI/ABRA can coexist.[20] In addition, ARIA, ABRA, and CAA-RI share similar MR imaging abnormalities and similar clinical features, as well as association with the apolipoprotein E ε4 allele.[51] However, unlike ABRA that involves both perivascular and transmural inflammation, ARIAs are more similar to

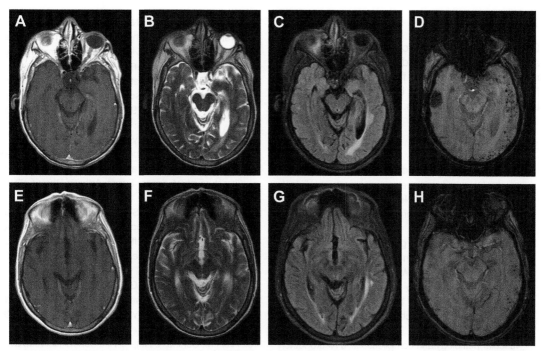

Fig. 3. Interval progression of CAA-IR from April 2020 (lower rows E-H) to March 2022 (upper rows, *A–D*) in a patient whose biopsy showed cerebral and leptomeningeal amyloid angiopathy, with perivascular and leptomeningeal macrophages, and interstitial microglial cells. There was interval progression in the left temporal lobe punctuate foci of microhemorrhage (*D* and *H*—SWI series) and adjacent periventricular white matter hyperintensity (*F* and *D*, T2-weighted images, *G* and *C*, FLAIR series). There was no associated enhancement (on postcontrast series, *A* and *E*) at either time point.

CAA-RI in that they largely involve perivascular inflammation.[52]

SUMMARY

Inflammation of small vessels in the brain due to immunogenicity related to amlyoid-beta vascular deposition can manifest in ABRA, CAA-RI, or ARIA. The variety of abnormal imaging findings that these conditions can lead to are detailed above, but are not entirely pathognomonic. Because the majority of patients with ABRA or CAA-RI will improve with immunosuppression,[19] it is of critical importance that the vast array of potential imaging findings indicate inflammatory CAA are documented, understood, and screened for when appropriate. As such, when clinical suspicion for inflammation caused by amlyoid-beta is present, obtaining an MR imaging to screen for any of the above findings is important toward developing a diagnosis and effective treatment plan. Although final confirmation may require brain biopsy, these findings are a guide toward identifying the inflammation early. In addition, it is important to repeat MR imaging scans at regular intervals to understand evolution of the abnormal findings and their potential improvement or resolution in response to treatment.

CLINICS CARE POINTS

- CAA can be both inflammatory and non-inflammatory and the treatment plan depends on assessing the state of the disease. The latter form includes ABRA and CAA-RI.

- The presumed diagnosis of ABRA or CAA-RI requires an MRI of the brain with contrast and is often supplemented with testing of the cerebrospinal fluid for evidence of inflammation.

- The defintive diagnosis of ABRA or CAA-RI is pathologic and because brain biopsy has non-trivial morbidity, it is only pursued in selected cases with clinical uncertainty.

- Empiric treatment of ABRA or CAA-RI consists of aggressive immunosuppression of variable duration, typically titrated to the severity of disease and response to treatment.

- Many patients have remission of ABRA or CAA-RI, but in others it can be progressive and even lead to fatal complications, typically hemorrhagic stroke.

DISCLOSURE

Dr A. de Havenon has received investigator initiated clinical research funding from the AAN, has received consultant fees from Integra and Novo Nordisk, royalty fees from UpToDate, and has equity in TitinKM and Certus.

REFERENCES

1. Banerjee G, Samra K, Adams ME, et al. Iatrogenic cerebral amyloid angiopathy: an emerging clinical phenomenon. J Neurol Neurosurg Psychiatry 2022. https://doi.org/10.1136/jnnp-2022-328792. jnnp-2022-328792.

2. Viswanathan A, Greenberg SM. Cerebral amyloid angiopathy in the elderly. Ann Neurol 2011;70(6):871–80.

3. Charidimou A, Gang Q, Werring DJ. Sporadic cerebral amyloid angiopathy revisited: recent insights into pathophysiology and clinical spectrum. J Neurol Neurosurg Psychiatry 2012;83(2):124–37.

4. Mandybur TI. Cerebral amyloid angiopathy: the vascular pathology and complications. J Neuropathol Exp Neurol 1986;45(1):79–90.

5. Eng JA, Frosch MP, Choi K, et al. Clinical manifestations of cerebral amyloid angiopathy-related inflammation. Ann Neurol 2004;55(2):250–6.

6. Ghiso J, Tomidokoro Y, Revesz T, et al. Cerebral amyloid angiopathy and alzheimer's disease. Hirosaki Igaku Hirosaki Med J 2010;61(Suppl): S111–24.

7. Ellis RJ, Olichney JM, Thal LJ, et al. Cerebral amyloid angiopathy in the brains of patients with Alzheimer's disease: the CERAD experience, Part XV. Neurology 1996;46(6):1592–6.

8. Theodorou A, Palaiodimou L, Malhotra K, et al. Clinical, Neuroimaging, and Genetic Markers in Cerebral Amyloid Angiopathy-Related Inflammation: A Systematic Review and Meta-Analysis. Stroke 2023;54(1):178–88.

9. Secondary Ischemic Stroke Prevention | SpringerLink Internet. Available at: https://link.springer.com/article/10.1007/s13311-023-01352-w. Accessed March 20, 2023.

10. Hao Q, Tsankova NM, Shoirah H, et al. Vessel Wall MRI Enhancement in Noninflammatory Cerebral Amyloid Angiopathy. Am J Neuroradiol 2020;41(3): 446–8.

11. Salvarani C, Morris JM, Giannini C, et al. Imaging Findings of Cerebral Amyloid Angiopathy, Aβ-Related Angiitis (ABRA), and Cerebral Amyloid Angiopathy–Related Inflammation. Medicine (Baltim) 2016;95(20):e3613.

12. Scolding NJ, Joseph F, Kirby PA, et al. Abeta-related angiitis: primary angiitis of the central nervous system associated with cerebral amyloid angiopathy. Brain J Neurol 2005;128(Pt 3):500–15.

13. Chung KK, Anderson NE, Hutchinson D, et al. Cerebral amyloid angiopathy related inflammation: three case reports and a review. J Neurol Neurosurg Psychiatry 2011;82(1):20–6.

14. Rohm Z. Amyloid Beta-Related Angiitis: A Rare Cause of CNS Vasculitis (P3.422). Neurology Internet. 2018 Apr 10 ;90(15 Supplement). Available at: https://n.neurology.org/content/90/15_Supplement/P3.422. Accessed May 10. 2023.

15. Danve A, Grafe M, Deodhar A. Amyloid beta-related angiitis–a case report and comprehensive review of literature of 94 cases. Semin Arthritis Rheum 2014; 44(1):86–92.

16. Piazza F, Greenberg SM, Savoiardo M, et al. Anti-amyloid β autoantibodies in cerebral amyloid angiopathy-related inflammation: implications for amyloid-modifying therapies. Ann Neurol 2013; 73(4):449–58.

17. Salvarani C, Hunder GG, Morris JM, et al. Aβ-related angiitis: comparison with CAA without inflammation and primary CNS vasculitis. Neurology 2013; 81(18):1596–603.

18. Amin M, Uchino K, Hajj-Ali RA. Central Nervous System Vasculitis: Primary Angiitis of the Central Nervous System and Central Nervous System Manifestations of Systemic Vasculitis. Rheum Dis Clin Internet. 2023 May 2 ;0(0). Available at: https://www.rheumatic.theclinics.com/article/S0889-857X(23)00042-X/fulltext. Accessed June 1, 2023.

19. Kinnecom C, Lev MH, Wendell L, et al. Course of cerebral amyloid angiopathy-related inflammation. Neurology 2007;68(17):1411–6.

20. Werring DJ, Sperling R. Inflammatory cerebral amyloid angiopathy and amyloid-modifying therapies: variations on the same ARIA? Ann Neurol 2013; 73(4):439–41.

21. Greenberg SM, Charidimou A. Diagnosis of Cerebral Amyloid Angiopathy: Evolution of the Boston Criteria. Stroke 2018;49(2):491–7.

22. Chen SJ, Tsai HH, Tsai LK, et al. Advances in cerebral amyloid angiopathy imaging. Ther Adv Neurol Disord 2019;12. 1756286419844113.

23. Dierksen GA, Skehan ME, Khan MA, et al. Spatial relation between microbleeds and amyloid deposits in amyloid angiopathy. Ann Neurol 2010;68(4): 545–8.

24. Wardlaw JM, Smith EE, Biessels GJ, et al. Neuroimaging standards for research into small vessel disease and its contribution to ageing and neurodegeneration. Lancet Neurol 2013;12(8):822–38.

25. Martinez-Ramirez S, Romero JR, Shoamanesh A, et al. Diagnostic value of lobar microbleeds in individuals without intracerebral hemorrhage. Alzheimers Dement J Alzheimers Assoc 2015;11(12):1480–8.

26. Greenberg SM, Vernooij MW, Cordonnier C, et al. Cerebral microbleeds: a guide to detection and interpretation. Lancet Neurol 2009;8(2):165–74.

27. Charidimou A, Boulouis G, Haley K, et al. White matter hyperintensity patterns in cerebral amyloid angiopathy and hypertensive arteriopathy. Neurology 2016;86(6):505–11.

28. van Veluw SJ, Charidimou A, van der Kouwe AJ, et al. Microbleed and microinfarct detection in amyloid angiopathy: a high-resolution MRI-histopathology study. Brain J Neurol 2016;139(Pt 12):3151–62.

29. Ter Telgte A, Scherlek AA, Reijmer YD, et al. Histopathology of diffusion-weighted imaging-positive lesions in cerebral amyloid angiopathy. Acta Neuropathol 2020;139(5):799–812.

30. Cortical atrophy in patients with cerebral amyloid angiopathy: a case-control study - PubMed Internet. Available at: https://pubmed.ncbi.nlm.nih.gov/27180034/. Accessed April 29, 2023.

31. Fotiadis P, Reijmer YD, Van Veluw SJ, et al. White matter atrophy in cerebral amyloid angiopathy. Neurology 2020;95(5):e554–62.

32. Gurol ME, Becker JA, Fotiadis P, et al. Florbetapir-PET to diagnose cerebral amyloid angiopathy: A prospective study. Neurology 2016;87(19):2043–9.

33. Clark CM, Schneider JA, Bedell BJ, et al. Use of Florbetapir-PET for Imaging β-Amyloid Pathology. JAMA 2011;305(3):275–83.

34. Murali Doraiswamy P, Sperling RA, Coleman RE, et al. Amyloid-β assessed by florbetapir F 18 PET and 18-month cognitive decline. Neurology 2012;79(16):1636–44.

35. Renard D, Castelnovo G, Wacongne A, et al. Interest of CSF biomarker analysis in possible cerebral amyloid angiopathy cases defined by the modified Boston criteria. J Neurol 2012;259(11):2429–33.

36. Banerjee G, Ambler G, Keshavan A, et al. Cerebrospinal Fluid Biomarkers in Cerebral Amyloid Angiopathy. J Alzheimers Dis JAD 2020;74(4):1189–201.

37. Raposo N, Zanon Zotin MC, Schoemaker D, et al. Peak Width of Skeletonized Mean Diffusivity as Neuroimaging Biomarker in Cerebral Amyloid Angiopathy. AJNR Am J Neuroradiol 2021;42(5):875–81.

38. Johnson KA, Gregas M, Becker JA, et al. Imaging of amyloid burden and distribution in cerebral amyloid angiopathy. Ann Neurol 2007;62(3):229–34.

39. Yamin G, Teplow DB. Pittsburgh Compound-B (PiB) binds amyloid β-protein protofibrils. J Neurochem 2017;140(2):210–5.

40. Moussaddy A, Levy A, Strbian D, et al. Inflammatory Cerebral Amyloid Angiopathy, Amyloid-β-Related Angiitis, and Primary Angiitis of the Central Nervous System: Similarities and Differences. Stroke 2015;46(9):e210–3.

41. Wu JJ, Yao M, Ni J. Cerebral amyloid angiopathy-related inflammation: current status and future implications. Chin Med J (Engl). 2021;134(6):646–54.

42. Alexander MD, Yuan C, Rutman A, et al. High-resolution intracranial vessel wall imaging: imaging beyond the lumen. J Neurol Neurosurg Psychiatry 2016;87(6):589–97.

43. Lehman VT, Brinjikji W, Kallmes DF, et al. Clinical interpretation of high-resolution vessel wall MRI of intracranial arterial diseases. Br J Radiol 2016;89(1067). 20160496.

44. Bley TA, Wieben O, Vaith P, et al. Magnetic resonance imaging depicts mural inflammation of the temporal artery in giant cell arteritis. Arthritis Care Res 2004;51(6):1062–3.

45. McNally JS, Sakata A, Alexander MD, et al. Vessel Wall Enhancement on Black-Blood MRI Predicts Acute and Future Stroke in Cerebral Amyloid Angiopathy. AJNR Am J Neuroradiol 2021;42(6):1038–45.

46. Auriel E, Charidimou A, Gurol ME, et al. Validation of Clinicoradiological Criteria for the Diagnosis of Cerebral Amyloid Angiopathy-Related Inflammation. JAMA Neurol 2016;73(2):197–202.

47. Zedde M, Pascarella R, Piazza F. CAA-ri and ARIA: Two Faces of the Same Coin? Am J Neuroradiol Internet. 2023 Jan 12. Available from: https://www.ajnr.org/content/early/2023/01/12/ajnr.A7759. Accessed June 1, 2023.

48. de Souza A, Tasker K. Inflammatory Cerebral Amyloid Angiopathy: A Broad Clinical Spectrum. J Clin Neurol 2023;19(3):230–41.

49. Sperling RA, Jack CR, Black SE, et al. Amyloid Related Imaging Abnormalities (ARIA) in Amyloid Modifying Therapeutic Trials: Recommendations from the Alzheimer's Association Research Roundtable Workgroup. Alzheimers Dement J Alzheimers Assoc 2011;7(4):367–85.

50. Antolini L, DiFrancesco JC, Zedde M, et al. Spontaneous ARIA-like Events in Cerebral Amyloid Angiopathy–Related Inflammation. Neurology 2021;97(18):e1809–22.

51. Grasso D, Castorani G, Borreggine C, et al. Cerebral amyloid angiopathy related inflammation: A little known but not to be underestimated disease. Radiol Case Rep 2021;16(9):2514–21.

52. Kozberg MG, Perosa V, Gurol ME, et al. A practical approach to the management of cerebral amyloid angiopathy. Int J Stroke 2021;16(4):356–69.

Printed and bound by CPI Group (UK) Ltd, Croydon, CR0 4YY

03/10/2024

01040365-0017